# MORE 4U!

## This Clinics series is available online.

**Here's what you get:**

- Full text of EVERY issue from 2002 to NOW
- Figures, tables, drawings, references and more
- Searchable: find what you need fast

   Search [ All Clinics ▼ ] for [            ] [GO]

- Linked to MEDLINE and Elsevier journals
- E-alerts

**INDIVIDUAL SUBSCRIBERS**

Click **Register** and follow instructions

You'll need an account number

## LOG ON TODAY. IT'S FAST AND EASY.

Your subscriber account number is on your mailing label →

```
This is your copy of:
THE CLINICS OF NORTH AMERICA
CXXX        2296532-2        2        Mar 05
J.H. DOE, MD
531 MAIN STREET
CENTER CITY, NY  10001-001
```

**BOUGHT A SINGLE ISSUE?** Sorry, you won't be able to access full text online. Please subscribe today to get complete content by contacting customer service at 800 645 2552 (US and Canada) or 407 345 4000 (outside US and Canada) or via email at elsols@elsevier.com.

**NEW!**

## Now also available for INSTITUTIONS

Works/Integrates with MD Consult

Available in a variety of packages: Collections containing 14, 31 or 50 Clinics titles

Or Collection upgrade for existing MD Consult customers

Call today! 877-857-1047 or e-mail: mdc.groupinfo@elsevier.com

ELSEVIER

BRUCE H. THIERS, MD, Consulting Editor

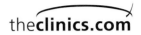

# DERMATOLOGIC CLINICS

Psychocutaneous Disease

MADHULIKA A. GUPTA, MD, FRCPC
Guest Editor

October 2005 • Volume 23 • Number 4

**SAUNDERS**
An Imprint of Elsevier, Inc.
PHILADELPHIA   LONDON   TORONTO   MONTREAL   SYDNEY   TOKYO

**W.B. SAUNDERS COMPANY**
*A Division of Elsevier Inc.*

1600 John F. Kennedy Boulevard • Suite 1800 • Philadelphia, Pennsylvania 19103-2899

http://www.theclinics.com

**DERMATOLOGIC CLINICS**  Volume 23, Number 4
October 2005  ISSN 0733-8635
Editor: Alexandra Gavenda  ISBN 1-4160-2818-8

Copyright © 2005 by Elsevier Inc. All rights reserved. No part of this publication may be reproduced or transmitted in any form or by any means, electronic or mechanical, including photocopy, recording, or any information retrieval system, without written permission from the Publisher.

Single photocopies of single articles may be made for personal use as allowed by national copyright laws. Permission of the publisher and payment of a fee is required for all other photocopying, including multiple or systematic copying, copying for advertising or promotional purposes, resale, and all forms of document delivery. Special rates are available for educational institutions that wish to make photocopies for non-profit educational classroom use. Permissions may be sought directly from Elsevier's Rights Department in Philadelphia, PA, USA at Tel.: (+1) 215-239-3804; Fax: (+1) 215-239-3805; E-mail: healthpermissions@elsevier.com. Requests may also be completed on-line via the Elsevier homepage (http://www.elsevier.com/locate/permissions). In the USA, users may clear permissions and make payments through the Copyright Clearance Center, Inc., 222 Rosewood Drive, Danvers, MA 01923, USA; Tel.: (+1) 978-750-8400; Fax: (+1) 978-750-4744, and in the UK through the Copyright Licensing Agency Rapid Clearance Service (CLARCS), 90 Tottenham Court Road, London W1P 0LP, UK; Tel.: (+44) 171-436-5931; Fax: (+44) 171-436-3986. Other countries may have a local reprographic rights agency for payments.

The ideas and opinions expressed in *Dermatologic Clinics* do not necessarily reflect those of the Publisher. The Publisher does not assume any responsibility for any injury and/or damage to persons or property arising out of or related to any use of the material contained in this periodical. The reader is advised to check the appropriate medical literature and the product information currently provided by the manufacturer of each drug to be administered to verify the dosage, the method and duration of administration, or contraindications. It is the responsibility of the treating physician or other health care professional, relying on independent experience and knowledge of the patient, to determine drug dosages and the best treatment for the patient. Mention of any product in this issue should not be construed as endorsement by the contributors, editors, or the Publisher of the product or manufacturers' claims.

*Dermatologic Clinics* (ISSN 0733-8635) is published quarterly by Elsevier Inc. Corporate and editorial offices: 1600 John F. Kennedy Boulevard, Suite 1800, Philadelphia, PA 19103-2899. Accounting and circulation offices: 6277 Sea Harbor Drive, Orlando, FL 32887-4800. Periodicals postage paid at Orlando, FL 32862, and additional mailing offices. Subscription prices are USD 205 per year for US individuals, USD 314 per year for US institutions, USD 236 per year for Canadian individuals, USD 368 per year for Canadian institutions, USD 260 per year for international individuals, USD 368 per year for international institutions, USD 103 per year for US students, and USD 130 per year for international students. International air speed delivery is included in all *Clinics* subscription prices. All prices are subject to change without notice. POSTMASTER: Send address changes to *Dermatologic Clinics*, W.B. Saunders Company, Periodicals Fulfillment, Orlando, FL 32887-4800. **Customer Service: 1-800-654-2452 (US). From outside of the US, call (+1) 407-345-4000.** E-mail: hhspcs@harcourt.com.

*Reprints.* For copies of 100 or more, of articles in this publication, please contact the Commercial Reprints Department, Elsevier Inc., 360 Park Avenue South, New York, New York 10010-1710. Tel.: (212) 633-3813; Fax: (212) 462-1935; E-mail: reprints@elsevier.com.

The *Dermatologic Clinics* is covered in *Index Medicus, Current Contents/Clinical Medicine, Excerpta Medica, Chemical Abstracts,* and *ISI/BIOMED.*

Printed in the United States of America.

## PSYCHOCUTANEOUS DISEASE

## CONSULTING EDITOR

**BRUCE H. THIERS, MD,** Professor and Chair, Department of Dermatology, Medical University of South Carolina, Charleston, South Carolina

## GUEST EDITOR

**MADHULIKA A. GUPTA, MD, FRCPC,** Professor, Department of Psychiatry, University of Western Ontario; and Mediprobe Research Incorporated, London, Ontario, Canada

## CONTRIBUTORS

**GIONATA BUGGIANI, MD,** Medical Doctor and Resident in Dermatology, University Unit of Physical Therapy and Dermatology, University of Florence, Florence, Italy

**SANTOSH K. CHATURVEDI, MD, MRCPsych,** Professor (Psychiatry), National Institute of Mental Health and Neurosciences, Bangalore, India

**MARY-MARGARET CHREN, MD,** Associate Professor in Residence, University of California at San Francisco; and Director, Health Services Research Enhancement Award Program, San Francisco Veterans Affairs Medical Center, San Francisco, California

**CARL D'ARCY, PhD,** Professor and Director, Applied Research, Department of Psychiatry, College of Medicine, Royal University Hospital, University of Saskatchewan, Saskatoon, Saskatchewan, Canada

**CHARLES N. ELLIS, MD,** Professor, Department of Dermatology, University of Michigan Medical School, Ann Arbor, Michigan

**TIFFANY FIELD, PhD,** Director, Touch Research Institutes, University of Miami School of Medicine, Miami, Florida

**ANDREW Y. FINLAY, MBBS, FRCP,** Professor (Dermatology), Department of Dermatology, Wales College of Medicine, Cardiff University, Cardiff, United Kingdom

**DÓNAL G. FORTUNE, ClinPsyD, PhD,** Senior Clinical Psychologist, Department of Behavioral Medicine, University of Manchester School of Medicine, Hope Hospital, Salford Royal Hospitals NHS Trust, Manchester, United Kingdom

**RICHARD G. FRIED, MD, PhD,** Yardley Dermatology Associates, Yardley, Pennsylvania

**BARBARA A. GILCHREST, MD,** Professor and Chair, Department of Dermatology, Boston University School of Medicine, Boston, Massachusetts

**CHRISTOPHER E.M. GRIFFITHS, MD,** Professor (Dermatology), Hope Hospital, Salford Royal Hospitals NHS Trust, Manchester, United Kingdom

**ADITYA K. GUPTA, MD, PhD,** Professor, Division of Dermatology, Department of Medicine, University of Toronto, Toronto; and Mediprobe Research Incorporated, London, Ontario, Canada

**MADHULIKA A. GUPTA, MD, FRCPC,** Professor, Department of Psychiatry, University of Western Ontario; and Mediprobe Research Incorporated, London, Ontario, Canada

**NITIN GUPTA, MD,** Consultant Psychiatrist, South Staffordshire Healthcare NHS Trust, Margaret Stanhope Centre, Burton upon Trent, Staffordshire, United Kingdom

**PETER R. HULL, MD, PhD(Med), FFDerm(SA), FRCPC,** Professor (Medicine); and Head, Division of Dermatology, Department of Medicine, Royal University Hospital, University of Saskatchewan, Saskatoon, Saskatchewan, Canada

**ANDREW M. JOHNSON, PhD,** Assistant Professor, Faculty of Health Sciences, University of Western Ontario, London, Ontario, Canada

**CAROLINE S. KOBLENZER, MD,** Clinical Professor (Dermatology), University of Pennsylvania; and Faculty, Institute of the Psychoanalytic Center of Philadelphia, Philadelphia, Pennsylvania

**JOHN KOO, MD,** Professor and Vice-Chairman, Department of Dermatology, University of California San Francisco Medical Center, San Francisco, California

**RUTH A. LANIUS, MD, PhD,** Associate Professor and Director, Traumatic Stress Program, Department of Psychiatry, University of Western Ontario, London, Ontario, Canada

**CHAI SUE LEE, MD,** Assistant Professor, Department of Dermatology, University of California Davis Medical Center, Sacramento, California

**VICTORIA J. LEWIS, BMedSci, MBBS, MRCP,** Specialist Registrar in Dermatology, Department of Dermatology, Wales College of Medicine, Cardiff University, Cardiff, United Kingdom

**TORELLO LOTTI, MD,** Director, Centro Interuniversitario di Dermatologia Biologica e Psicosomatica, University of Florence; Full Professor, Chairman, and Director, University Unit of Physical Therapy and Dermatology; and Professor (Dermatology and Venereology), University of Florence, Florence, Italy

**STEFANO PALLANTI, MD,** Professor (Psychiatry); Associate Professor; Director, Institute of Neuroscience, University of Florence, Florence, Italy; and Adjunct Professor, Mount Sinai School of Medicine, New York, New York

**EMILIANO PANCONESI, MD,** Professor Emeritus, Department of Dermatology, University of Florence, Florence, Italy

**HELEN L. RICHARDS, ClinPsyD, PhD,** Consultant Clinical Psychologist, Dermatology Center, University of Manchester School of Medicine, Hope Hospital, Salford Royal Hospitals NHS Trust; and Senior Clinical Lecturer, Academic Department of Clinical Psychology, Wythenshawe Hospital, University of Manchester, Manchester, United Kingdom

**CHRYS DELLING SCHMULTS, MD,** Assistant Professor, Department of Dermatology, University of Pennsylvania Medical Center, Philadelphia, Pennsylvania

**GURCHARAN SINGH, MD,** Professor and Department Head, Department of Dermatology and Sexually Transmitted Disease, Sri Devaraj Urs Medical College, Tamaka, Kolar, India

**PHILIP D. SHENEFELT, MD, MS,** Associate Professor (Medicine), Division of Dermatology and Cutaneous Surgery, Department of Medicine, College of Medicine, University of South Florida, Tampa, Florida

**DAN J. STEIN, MD, PhD,** Director, MRC Research Unit on Anxiety and Stress Disorders, Department of Psychiatry, University of Stellenbosch, Tygerberg; Professor, University of Cape Town, Cape Town, South Africa; and Chairman, Department of Psychiatry, University of Florida, Gainesville, Florida

**MAURO URPE, PhD,** Psychologist, Centro Interuniversitario di Dermatologia Biologica e Psicosomatica; and University Unit of Physical Therapy and Dermatology, University of Florence, Florence, Italy

**BESSEL A. VAN DER KOLK, MD,** Professor (Psychiatry), Boston University School of Medicine, Brookline, Massachusetts

**BAVANISHA VYTHILINGUM, FCPsych,** Research Psychiatrist, MRC Research Unit on Anxiety and Stress Disorders, Department of Psychiatry, University of Stellenbosch, Tygerberg, South Africa

## FORTHCOMING ISSUES

January 2006
> **Sunscreens**
> Zoe D. Draelos, MD, *Guest Editor*

April 2006
> **Nail Disorders and Their Management**
> Aditya K. Gupta, MD, PhD, *Guest Editor*

July 2006
> **Women's Dermatology**
> Kathryn Schwarzenberger, MD, *Guest Editor*

## RECENT ISSUES

July 2005
> **Advanced Cosmetic Surgery**
> Neil S. Sadick, MD, *Guest Editor*

April 2005
> **Dermatologic Therapy**
> David I. McLean, MD, and
> W. Stuart Maddin, MD, *Guest Editors*

January 2005
> **Advanced Surgical Reconstructive Techniques**
> Marc D. Brown, MD, *Guest Editor*

---

**THE CLINICS ARE NOW AVAILABLE ONLINE!**

Access your subscription at:
http://www.theclinics.com

# CONTENTS

**Preface** xiii
Madhulika A. Gupta

**Psychiatric Evaluation of the Dermatology Patient** 591
Madhulika A. Gupta, Aditya K. Gupta, Charles N. Ellis, and Caroline S. Koblenzer

> Over one third of dermatologic disorders have significant psychiatric comorbidity. The impact of the skin disorder on quality of life, the role of psychosocial stressors, and use of substances should be assessed. Major depressive disorder is the most frequently encountered psychiatric disorder in dermatology and is often associated with suicide risk. Other psychiatric syndromes comorbid with dermatologic disorders include obsessive-compulsive disorder, social phobia, posttraumatic stress disorder associated with dissociation and conversion symptoms, body image pathologies, delusional disorder, and a wide range of personality disorders. This article reviews psychiatric guidelines that may be used to assess psychopathology in the dermatology patient.

**Psychosomatic Factors in Dermatology** 601
Mauro Urpe, Stefano Pallanti, and Torello Lotti

> Psychosomatics describes any aspect of dermatology with psychologic or psychiatric elements. Dermatologists know that a significant proportion of their practice involves patients for whom psychologic elements either partially or sometimes entirely dominate their presenting chief complaints. This article explores the role of psychosomatic factors in dermatologic disorders. The authors discuss the clinical interface between psychiatry, psychology and dermatology and the interpretation of possible relationships between cutaneous diseases, the role of the mind, and psychotherapeutic interventions.

**Stress and Psychoneuroimmunologic Factors in Dermatology** 609
Mauro Urpe, Gionata Buggiani, and Torello Lotti

> There is clinical and experimental evidence that the brain can start, influence, and stop biologic skin events. Studies suggest that the skin, as a relevant part of the "diffuse brain," can modify the quality of perceptions and feelings. The immune and the endocrine systems seem to represent the protagonists of the modulation of those events and, in this context, psychosocial stressors and interventions can lead to global health changes of great interest for dermatologists.

### The Emotional Impact of Chronic and Disabling Skin Disease: A Psychoanalytic Perspective
Caroline S. Koblenzer

619

> This article discusses some major early factors that influence the evolving psychologic development, which in turn helps determine the emotional impact that chronic or disabling skin disease may have on patients' lives. If the emotional environment, encompassed by the infant-caretaker relationship, is less than optimal, the stability of the body image may be compromised, self-esteem diminished, and affect less well handled and the somatic expression of emotional content may ensue. Each of these is important in dermatology, as is the nature of the disease and the capacity of families and of society to adapt. Psoriasis, atopic dermatitis, and acne are used as examples.

### Psychosomatic Factors in Dermatology: Special Perspectives for Application in Clinical Practice
Emiliano Panconesi

629

> The identification of psychosomatic factors in dermatology has always been one of the principal themes in the history of this field and in the personal experience and research of the author. After a brief review of some of the milestones in the area of psychosomatic factors in dermatology, the author presents the criteria dictated by clinical experience, in the absence to date of more precise scientific data, for the individuation of such psychosomatic factors in clinical practice.

### Stigma Experience in Skin Disorders: An Indian Perspective
Santosh K. Chaturvedi, Gurcharan Singh, and Nitin Gupta

635

> Dermatologic disorders generally have a major impact on patients' daily activities, psychologic and emotional state, and social relationships. The intensity of impact of skin disease on an individual person is extremely variable, however, and depends on natural history of the disorder; the patient's demographic characteristics, personality, character, and value; the patient's life situation; and the attitudes of society. Social stigma toward dermatologic disorders in the Indian society is quite widespread, especially toward leprosy. Dermatologists are expected to consider quality of life issues along with social aspects, nature of disorder, efficacy, and tolerability of various therapeutic options to optimize relief and comfort to their patients.

### Psychosocial Aspects Of Aging Skin
Madhulika A. Gupta and Barbara A. Gilchrest

643

> Many older individuals use products and procedures to conceal or delay the signs of aging. For most, this provides a helpful ego boost, but some individuals seeking such procedures suffer from pathologies such as eating disorders and body dysmorphic disorder. The impact of aging skin may include social anxiety and social isolation. Poor self-image is associated with chronic illness and fewer preventive health behaviors, such as exercise. Aged appearance, especially in women, is also associated with workplace discrimination. Patients should therefore be offered treatments for aging skin while maintaining realistic treatment expectations; and the dermatologist should ensure that society's negative views about aging are not necessarily reinforced.

### Psychologic Trauma, Posttraumatic Stress Disorder, and Dermatology 649
Madhulika A. Gupta, Ruth A. Lanius, and Bessel A. Van der Kolk

Psychologic trauma refers to events (such as sexual assault, major earthquake, or plane crashes) that overwhelm an individual's capacity to cope. Psychologic trauma can result in chronic and recurring dermatologic symptoms that persist after the trauma subsides. Examples are cutaneous sensory flashbacks (which may be fragments of the sensory component of the traumatic experience), autonomic hyperarousal (with symptoms such as profuse sweating or flare-up of an underlying stress-reactive dermatosis), conversion symptoms (such as numbness, pain, or other medically unexplained cutaneous symptoms), and cutaneous self-injury (manifesting in many forms, including trichotillomania, dermatitis artefacta, and neurotic excoriations—tension-reducing behaviors in patients who have posttraumatic stress disorder).

### Depression and Skin Disease 657
Richard G. Fried, Madhulika A. Gupta, and Aditya K. Gupta

The occurrence of depression in association with dermatologic disease is common. Psychiatric disturbance is reported in approximately 30% of dermatology patients. Depression can have varied presentations and is more relevant clinically in dermatology patients during critical psychosocial periods of development. Early recognition and treatment of depression associated with skin disorders can lead to improved therapeutic outcomes and may avert disastrous outcomes, including suicide.

### Acne, Depression, and Suicide 665
Peter R. Hull and Carl D'Arcy

Acne is a common disorder that may have a considerable psychologic impact including anxiety and depression. Depression and suicide occur frequently in adolescents and young adults. Although case reports suggest an association between isotretinoin and depression and suicide, more rigorous observational studies and epidemiologic studies, using different designs, have not shown any effect of isotretinoin use in increasing the occurrence of depression and suicide. It is prudent for the practitioner to continue to use isotretinoin to treat severe acne, while at the same time informing patients and their relatives that depressive symptoms should be actively assessed at each visit and, if necessary, referral to a psychiatrist and a discontinuation of isotretinoin should be considered.

### Obsessive-Compulsive Disorders and Dermatologic Disease 675
Bavanisha Vythilingum and Dan J. Stein

Obsessive-compulsive disorder and obsessive-compulsive spectrum disorders are often associated with dermatologic manifestations. The phenomenology is discussed and possible animal models explored. Treatment involves both pharmacotherapy and cognitive behavior therapy. Many of these patients experience considerable shame over their behavior and may be reluctant to acknowledge the existence of a psychiatric disorder. The dermatologist's approach to this patient is discussed.

### Psychologic Factors in Psoriasis: Consequences, Mechanisms, and Interventions 681
Dónal G. Fortune, Helen L. Richards, and Christopher E.M. Griffiths

This article examines the English-language research literature concerning psychologic aspects of psoriasis published since 1995. The literature is concerned with (1) the consequences of psoriasis in terms of quality of life, disability, depression, anxiety, and stigmatization and factors that may predict such outcomes; (2) potential mechanisms of the interaction between psychologic factors, stress, and the pathophysiology of psoriasis; and (3) examination of the clinical utility of psychologic interventions on extent of psoriasis and psychologic distress. The implications of the findings are discussed with reference to future directions for research and practice.

## Psychoneuroimmunodermatology of Atopic Dermatitis: From Empiric Data to the Evolutionary Hypothesis 695
Stefano Pallanti, Torello Lotti, and Mauro Urpe

Atopic dermatitis is a pruritic skin disease affecting predominantly young people. There is evidence that psychologic stress constitutes an increased risk for atopy and influences the disease's clinical course. This risk is believed mediated by the effects of stress on neuroimmunoregulation, which in turn modulates the hypersensitivity response and involves immunoglobulin E–mediated inflammation, helper T-cell 2 predominance, and eosinophilia. This article examines theoretic perspectives and other behavioral dimensions, such as maternal caring behavior, infant response to stress, temperament, and the so-called "hygiene hypothesis." The Darwinian framework and the mental scenario are examined. These processes may be akin to the generation of antibodies by the immune system.

## Evaluating Clinical Rating Scales for Evidence-Based Dermatology: Some Basic Concepts 703
Madhulika A. Gupta, Andrew M. Johnson, and Mary-Margaret Chren

Evidence-based dermatology has necessitated the development of rating scales that measure multidimensional and abstract constructs, such as quality of life. This article discusses some basic psychometric concepts, such as reliability, validity, standardization, and measurement precision, which need to be considered when choosing a clinical rating instrument. Also discussed is the impact of these parameters on increasing the statistical power of a clinical trial.

## A Critical Review of Quality-of-Life Scales for Psoriasis 707
Victoria J. Lewis and Andrew Y. Finlay

Psoriasis can have a major impact on the lives of patients who have psoriasis and many different methods are described to measure this effect. This article describes four general health measures, six dermatology-specific measures, four psoriasis-specific measures, and four utility measure concepts that are used in psoriasis. For each of these, the extent of validation, including reliability of each measure and correlation with other measures, is described. The experience of use of each measure is summarized and key references listed. Advice is given concerning strategy for choosing which measures to use.

## Massage Therapy for Skin Conditions in Young Children 717
Tiffany Field

Two studies are reviewed that highlight the positive effects of massage therapy on skin conditions in young children. In the first study, children being treated on a burn trauma unit received 30-minute massages before debridement or dressing change. The children who received massage therapy were more relaxed during the procedure. In the study on children with eczema, those who were massaged during the application of their skin medication showed less anxiety after the massage sessions. Across the massage period the children also showed an improved clinical condition including less redness, lichenification, scaling, excoriation, and pruritus.

### Complementary Psychocutaneous Therapies in Dermatology 723
Philip D. Shenefelt

> The skin and the nervous system develop side by side in the fetus and remain intimately interconnected and interactive throughout life. Because of the skin-nervous system interactions, there is a significant psychosomatic or behavioral component to many dermatologic conditions. This permits complementary nonpharmacologic psychotherapeutic interventions, such as acupuncture, aromatherapy, biofeedback, cognitive-behavioral therapy, hypnosis, placebo, and suggestion, to have positive impacts on many dermatologic diseases. Complementary pharmacologic psychotherapeutic interventions, such as herbs and supplements, also may help improve some dermatologic disorders.

### Psychopharmacologic Therapies in Dermatology: An Update 735
Chai Sue Lee and John Koo

> Many patients who have skin disorders have associated psychosocial issues. Psychotropic agents with improved side-effect profiles are available to allow physicians who are not psychiatrists to manage patients who have psychiatric conditions with agents that are effective, simple to administer, and generally well tolerated. Dermatologists who wish to help their patients who have psychodermatologic conditions can enhance their armamentarium by becoming familiar with the use of a few selected psychotropic agents. This article reviews the current status and future directions of psychopharmacology for the major types of psychopathologies encountered in dermatology practice.

*Current Therapy*

### Laser Treatment of Vascular Lesions 745
Chrys Delling Schmults

> Lasers and other light sources have been developed that remove or improve many vascular lesions that were previously untreatable. Port-wine stains are the most notable example. Vascular lasers and light sources represent a major advance in dermatology for cosmetic and noncosmetic applications. This article reviews the common vascular conditions amenable to laser therapy and the approaches and devices used.

### Cumulative Index 2005 757

# Preface
# Psychocutaneous Disease

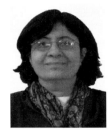

Madhulika A. Gupta, MD, FRCPC
*Guest Editor*

The importance of psychosocial factors in skin disorders is being increasingly recognized because they can have a significant impact upon the overall morbidity associated with these disorders and therefore constitute an important component of treatment outcome. Furthermore, psychosocial morbidity, when untreated, may also have an adverse impact upon the overall response of the skin condition to dermatologic therapies as a result of a wide range of factors including the psychoneuroimmunologic and neuroendocrine changes secondary to stress and the problems with adherence to prescribed dermatologic therapies as a result of a coexisting mental disorder.

There is an overall increase in interest in psychosomatic factors in medical disorders, in part because of a greater demand for evidence-based medicine when comparing various therapies. This has resulted in the consideration of quality of life measures and a more holistic approach to the patient. Practical considerations aside, the increasing availability of psychotropic medications with fewer unacceptable side effects, and recent advances in functional neuroimaging, have further fueled interest in examining the impact of psychosomatic factors in medical conditions. Unlike other organ systems, the integumentary system plays a very special role in psychosomatic medicine because the skin plays an integral role as an organ of communication right from birth and is the primary organ of attachment. The newborn infant's initial physical experience is largely tactile, and the child requires secure holding and hugging to develop physically, neurologically, and psychosocially. Adequate tactile nurturance in early life is necessary for the development of a healthy body image and the capacity for regulation of internal emotional states such as anxiety, anger, and depression. Physical therapies that focus upon touch, such as massage therapy, can have a very beneficial effect upon the course of certain skin conditions in addition to helping the patient's overall emotional well-being. When there is a disruption in this early nurturance due to maternal neglect or abuse, such as sexual abuse of the patient, the impact of the trauma is often focused on the integumentary system, in the form of a wide range of self-injurious behaviors that are observed, for example, in posttraumatic stress disorder, dissociative states, depressive disease, and obsessive-compulsive disorder.

Because the skin remains a vital organ of communication throughout the life cycle, a cosmetically disfiguring skin disorder can have a significant psychosocial impact, especially when it develops during a developmentally critical stage such as adolescence, when the patient is also dealing with emerging body image issues. Therefore, in certain skin disorders, such as acne, the psychosocial impact of the condition can be out of proportion to the clinical severity of the disorder. A cosmetically disfiguring disorder such as psoriasis in a young adult can have a significant impact upon the patient's social and vocational functioning in later life. In the later stages of life, the cutaneous changes associated with photo damage and chronologic aging have important psychosocial implications, especially for women, both socially and in the workplace.

The skin plays an important role as an organ of communication in all cultures because of its primary role in attachment during infancy; however, other sociocultural, climatic, and economic factors possibly determine the specific factors associated with stigma experienced by patients in different cultures who have skin disorders or aging skin. This issue of the *Dermatologic Clinics* features articles that address some of these issues and provide some practical clinical guidelines for the psychosocial assessment and management of the dermatologic patient.

Madhulika A. Gupta, MD, FRCPC
*Department of Psychiatry*
*University of Western Ontario*
*London, ON, Canada*

*Mediprobe Research Inc.*
*645 Windermere Road*
*London, ON N5X 2P1, Canada*
*E-mail address:* magupta@uwo.ca

# Psychiatric Evaluation of the Dermatology Patient

Madhulika A. Gupta, MD, FRCPC[a,b,*], Aditya K. Gupta, MD, PhD[b,c], Charles N. Ellis, MD[d], Caroline S. Koblenzer, MD[e,f]

[a]*Department of Psychiatry, University of Western Ontario, London, ON, Canada*
[b]*Mediprobe Research Inc, London, ON, Canada*
[c]*Division of Dermatology, Department of Medicine, University of Toronto, Toronto, ON, Canada*
[d]*Department of Dermatology, University of Michigan Medical School, Ann Arbor, MI, USA*
[e]*Department of Dermatology, University of Pennsylvania, Philadelphia, PA, USA*
[f]*Institute of the Psychoanalytic Center of Philadelphia, Philadelpia, PA, USA*

The psychiatric comorbidity in some dermatologic disorders is often one of the most important indices of the overall disability associated with the condition [1–6]. Significant psychiatric and psychosocial comorbidity is present in at least 30% of dermatologic patients. As a general guideline, psychiatric pathology is important in the cutaneous associations of primary psychiatric disorders, such as delusional states, and some of the self-inflicted dermatoses, such as dermatitis artefacta; and a wide range of primary dermatologic disorders that have psychiatric comorbidity. When assessing the dermatologic patient, it is best to adopt a multidimensional biopsychosocial approach, which allows for the relative contributions of biologic, psychiatric, and psychosocial factors, because it may not be possible clearly to determine whether a psychiatric syndrome is primary or entirely secondary to the dermatologic condition.

## General psychiatric evaluation

### History

It is important to maintain the well-defined boundaries of a doctor-patient relationship. The boundary issues become even more important if the clinician is doing both a physical and psychiatric assessment. If the patient seems uneasy or unwilling to discuss their psychiatric history, they should be referred to a mental health professional with whom they are willing to consult. Patients often think that if the dermatologist is enquiring about psychiatric factors he or she must think that "they are crazy" or that "the problem is not real" or "in their mind." It is important to acknowledge to the patient ahead of time with a comment like: "Emotional factors, such as stress and depression, can affect physical health; for example, stress can bring on a heart attack or ulcers. I know that what you describe is exactly what you experience. I would like to know if stress or your emotions may be affecting your skin problem."

It is important to evaluate the patient within the context of his or her developmental stage and social setting. A cosmetically disfiguring condition during adolescence or early adult life has been shown to have a much greater impact on socialization and occupational functioning than a similar condition in a middle-aged patient. Evaluation of the social support network of the patient is essential because it can affect the degree of stigma that the patient experiences.

In doing a history of the present illness (Box 1) [7] make a general enquiry about the impact of the disorder on the quality of life, which assesses the psychosocial burden of the disorder by addressing the impact of the skin condition on the social, emotional, physical, and vocational-occupational functioning of the patient. A question that is helpful in assessing the impact of the skin disorder on the quality of life is

* Corresponding author. 645 Windermere Road, London, ON N5X 2P1, Canada.
  E-mail address: magupta@uwo.ca (M.A. Gupta).

**Box 1. Some guidelines for the psychiatric evaluation of the dermatologic patient**

*History of present illness*

1. Impact of the skin disorder on the quality of life
   - What does your condition stop you from doing?
   - Is your skin disorder affecting your social life?
   - Is your skin disorder affecting your sexual functioning?
   - Are you frequently worried about the reaction of others to your skin disorder?
   - Are you regularly anticipating negative comments about your skin condition from strangers?
   - Does your skin disorder affect how you feel about yourself?
   - Do you feel anxious or depressed as a result of your skin disorder?
   - Is your skin condition affecting your functioning at school or work?
   - Do people at school or work treat you differently because of your skin condition?
   - Has your skin condition had an adverse effect on your financial state?
   - Does your skin condition interfere with your sleep on a regular basis?
   - Is the pain or itching caused by your skin condition very distressing for you?
2. Role of psychosocial stressors
   - Does psychologic stress cause your skin disorder to flare up? If yes, have you been experiencing a lot of stress lately?
   - Do you feel that you have to deal with a lot of daily hassles that others do not have to cope with because of your skin condition?
   - Do you have a past history of trauma or abuse that is a recurring source of stress for you?
3. History of substance abuse
   - How much alcohol do you drink (if at all) during an average week?
   - Do you think there is a relation between your use of alcohol and your skin condition?

*Mental status examination*

1. Appearance
   A depressed patient may appear disheveled and withdrawn; a highly obsessive-compulsive individual may appear immaculately groomed and controlled.
   Discrepancy between patient's perception of their appearance and the clinician's perception may indicate an underlying body image disorder.
2. Speech (eg, slow or hesitant speech may be present in a depressed patient; a manic patient typically presents with fast, pressured speech)
3. Sensorium: orientation to time, place, and person
   Concentration, memory, capacity for abstract thinking
   Insight (eg, does the patient deny his or her illness)
   Dissociation: involves a disruption in the usually integrated functions of consciousness, memory, identity, or perception, and is often underrecognized in dermatology. Patients with dissociation often have no memory of actions or events (eg, patients with dermatitis artefacta) and may be misdiagnosed as malingerers.
4. Mood and affect
   Mood defines the pervasive emotion that colors the patient's perception of the world (eg, is the patient depressed, anxious, irritable, anhedonic; have loss of interest in most things that were previously enjoyable)? It is important to recognize that in

major depression anhedonia may be the only mood-related symptom (ie, the patient may not acknowledge that he or she is feeling depressed or tearful).

Affect defines the outward expression of the patient's inner experiences (eg, is the affect restricted, in a depressive or severely obsessive-compulsive patient).

5. Thought

Thought form refers to the productivity of thought (eg, does the patient have an overabundance or paucity of ideas, is there continuity of thought or is there a lack of a cause and effect relationship in the patient's thinking process. Most dermatologic patients are not likely to have problems with thought form, because they are encountered in severe psychotic disorders, such as schizophrenia or acute mania.

Thought content disorder typically encountered in dermatology may present as obsessions and compulsions, phobias, hypochondriacal, or suicidal preoccupations.

Thought disturbance can manifest as a delusion, which is defined as a false belief, based on incorrect inference about external reality, which is firmly held by the patient despite objective contradictory proof.

6. Perception

Perceptual abnormalities present as hallucinations involving any of the senses. In dermatology haptic hallucinations or hallucinations related to touch are encountered in delusional states and organic brain disorders secondary to brain disease and drug withdrawal. Hallucinations of smell may be present with delusions of bromhidrosis.

Flashbacks are transient disturbances in perception, including perceptions of touch or pain, which are reminiscent of earlier experiences. Flashbacks, when not associated with hallucinogen abuse, may be the feature of posttraumatic stress disorder secondary to a traumatic life experiences including abuse. This is often underrecognized in dermatology.

*Data from* Manley MRS. Psychiatric interview, history, and mental status examination. In: Sadock BI, Sadock VA, editors. Kaplan & Sadock's comprehensive textbook of psychiatry, Vol. 1. Philadelphia: Lippincott Williams & Wilkins; 2000. p. 652–65.

asking the patient what their skin condition prevents them from doing. When addressing the physical impact of the skin disorder, in addition to enquiring about symptoms that are specific to the disorder, enquiries about general and nonspecific symptoms, such as pervasive sleep difficulties, pain, and itching, should be made, because they may have a major impact on the overall physical well-being of the patient. The role of psychosocial stressors in the onset or exacerbation of the skin condition is very important. It is important to enquire about the role of daily hassles associated with having to cope with the skin disorder, because this in turn may cause a flare-up of a stress-reactive dermatosis. Unresolved traumatic experiences, resulting from both abuse or neglect during early life, can be an ongoing source of stress and result in heightened autonomic reactivity or a posttraumatic stress disorder, which may in turn lead to exacerbations of a stress-reactive skin disorder. Some situations that can culminate in neglect include physical absence of the mother or caretaker, emotional absence of the mother or caretaker caused by depression, or inconsistent parenting. Another component is a history of substance abuse, such as alcohol, and its impact on the skin disorder.

*Mental status examination*

It is helpful to have a logical and systematic approach that facilitates diagnosis (see Box 1) [7]. At a practical level, the busy dermatologist is likely to focus on the area where there may be a problem.

## Major depressive disorder

Major depressive disorder [8] is one of the most commonly encountered psychiatric disorders in dermatology [1,4]. Major depressive disorder is characterized by one or more major depressive episodes. Depression is a recurrent disorder and over half of patients who have experienced one major depressive episode are expected to have a second episode. About two thirds of patients suffering from a major depressive episode experience complete remission of symptoms (ie, they stay symptom free between episodes). Among the remaining one third the symptoms remit only partially or not at all and this group of patients typically requires long-term therapy. Chronic medical conditions (eg, chronic recurrent skin disorders) are a known risk factor for more persistent episodes of depression.

A major depressive episode [8] is associated with at least 2 weeks of depressed mood or loss of interest or pleasure in activities that the patient previously found pleasurable or interesting. The anhedonia in depression can also manifest as social withdrawal, which may be mistakenly attributed to the cosmetic impact of the dermatologic disorder. Secondly, anhedonia may be the only mood-related symptom in major depression, because patients may not acknowledge that they are feeling sad or tearful. Sometimes the most prominent affect may be one of anxiety and agitation rather than sadness and depression. It is important not to misdiagnose these symptoms as being representative of a primary anxiety disorder. The mood changes in depression are accompanied by four or more symptoms that represent a change from the previous functioning of the patient including psychomotor agitation or retardation; difficulties with initiating and maintaining sleep or conversely, hypersomnia nearly every day; decrease or increase in appetite; fatigue or loss of energy; feelings of worthlessness or excessive or inappropriate guilt; indecisiveness; decreased concentrating ability; and recurrent thoughts of death with or without suicidal ideation.

Some depressed patients may complain of cutaneous dysesthesia, such as pain and burning sensations, for which no physical basis can be identified. These symptoms may represent masked depression or depressive equivalents, because some patients lack psychologic insight and may deny an underlying depressive disorder [1]. Some other patients with primary depressive disease may become preoccupied with relatively minor dermatologic problems, such as minimal hair loss. More severe depressive disease can present with mood-congruent delusions (eg, of having an incurable skin disease or delusions that their skin is rotting or emitting a foul odor).

Suicidal ideation has been reported in a wide range of dermatologic disorders including psoriasis and acne [9,10]. The peak incidence of acne is during midadolescence, a life stage that is also associated with a high incidence of depressive disease and body image disorders. This may be one reason why the prevalence of psychiatric morbidity, including depressive disease in even mild to moderate acne, is relatively high in some instances. It is important to recognize that the severity of depression and suicidal ideation do not necessarily correlate with the clinical severity of symptoms (ie, patients with mild dermatologic disease can have severe psychiatric morbidity). The psychomotor agitation experienced by some patients can be associated with hair-pulling, rubbing, scratching, or picking of the skin. Some symptoms, such as sleep difficulties, can complicate other dermatologic symptoms, such as pruritus.

The suicide rate in the United States is 12 per 100,000 [11]. Suicide is a central feature of depressive disease and 50% of all persons who commit suicide are depressed [11]. Fifteen percent of individuals with major depression eventually kill themselves. Among men the suicide rate peaks after age 45 years and among women after age 65 years [11]. After age 75 years, the suicide rate rises in both sexes. Women attempt suicide four times more frequently than men; however, men commit suicide three times more often than women.

Currently, there is a rapid rise in suicide rates among males between 15 and 24 years [11]. Suicidal behavior in the adolescent patient may not be solely caused by the psychosocial impact of the skin disorder. The social impact of a cosmetically disfiguring skin disorder may be the last straw, however, that precipitates suicidal behavior in the adolescent.

## Assessment of suicide risk

No combination of risk factors has adequate specificity or sensitivity to select those patients with suicidal thinking who go on to attempt suicide [12]. Asking patients about suicide does not put the idea into their heads; indeed, a truly suicidal patient is often relieved to be asked about suicide [12]. The clinician should not avoid bringing up the subject of suicide, because of the concern that the potentially suicidal patient will become more suicidal. It is important to offer the patient a private setting when enquiring about suicide. It is appropriate to ask a question like: "Have things been so bad that you

> **Box 2. Personal and demographic risk factors for suicide**
>
> 1. *Psychiatric disorder:* Over 90% of patients who commit suicide have a psychiatric disorder, such as major depressive disorder (50% of cases of suicide), and substance abuse and dependence, such as alcohol abuse (25% of cases of suicide). Other psychiatric disorders include psychotic states, such as schizophrenia and postpartum psychosis.
> 2. *Chronic illness and chronic pain:* Fifty percent of patients who attempt suicide have a physical illness, especially chronic disease and chronic pain. Severe pruritus and cosmetically disfiguring skin conditions have also been associated with a higher frequency of suicidal thoughts [9,10,13]. In some patient groups, such as the adolescent patient, even clinically mild skin disease has been associated with suicide [9].
> 3. *History of suicide threats and attempts:* Patients with a prior history of attempting suicide have a five to six times increased risk of trying again; between 25% and 50% of completed suicide victims have a history of having made a prior attempt. Even the apparently manipulative and chronic patients who make repeated threats often eventually succeed in killing themselves. All suicide threats should be taken seriously and managed as a psychiatric emergency.
> 4. *Age and gender:* The suicide rate among adolescents and young adults has increased markedly over the recent years. Generally, risk increases with age (peak incidence among men at age 75 years, among women from 55–65 years). Women attempt suicide three to four times more frequently than men; however, men are two to three times more successful in committing suicide than women.
> 5. *Marital status:* Risk greatest in those that never married, followed by those who are widowed, separated, or divorced.
> 6. *Employment status:* Unemployed and unskilled individuals are at greater risk.
> 7. *Access to lethal means:* Such as firearms, is a risk factor.
>
> *Data from* Refs. [11,12].

have thought of hurting yourself or ending your life?" and "Have you had thoughts about killing yourself?". It is important not to try to talk the patient out of their suicidality, because premature or inappropriate reassurances may be misconstrued by the patient as a lack of empathy or as a lack of permission to speak about their suicidal thoughts.

In addition to the personal and demographic factors for suicide (Box 2) [12], the patient should be asked about suicidal thoughts; the degree to which the patient intends to act on his or her suicidal thoughts and suicidal plans (eg, has the patient made a plan); and are the planned means available to the patient. Suicidality has legal implications. The clinician's assessment should be well documented. If the clinician is unsure, it is safest to obtain an emergency psychiatric consultation. Patients who are suicidal may require involuntary hospitalization. Patients who are not imminently suicidal but have suicidal thoughts can be sent home, with a definite follow-up plan. Such patients should not be sent home alone and the clinician should ensure that the patient has adequate support at home, for example by talking to the patient's family members.

*Obsessive-compulsive disorder*

Obsessive-compulsive disorder is characterized by recurrent obsessions or compulsions severe enough to be time-consuming or cause marked distress or significant impairment [8]. Obsessions are persistent ideas, thoughts, impulses, or images that are experienced as intrusive and inappropriate and that cause marked anxiety and distress to the patient. Compulsions are repetitive behaviors or mental acts, such as counting, the goal of which is to prevent or reduce anxiety or distress, which results from the obsessive thoughts. To evaluate obsessive-compulsive disorder a patient may be asked: "Do you ever have repetitive thoughts (about washing your hands or picking your skin or plucking hair from your body, and so forth; enquire about whatever behavior is relevant, depending on the presenting problem) that you wish you could stop but you are not able to stop?" Because patients are often embarrassed about their compulsive behaviors, they may not volunteer information about the problem unless specifically asked. Some of the obsessive-compulsive behaviors encountered in dermatology include fears of contamination and excessive hand washing, excessive grooming, hair plucking, trichotillomania, onychophagia, picking of a minor irregularity in the skin or lesions on the skin, and repetitive bathing or scratching [14,15].

The patient with obsessive-compulsive disorder feels driven to perform the compulsive act, such as hand washing, in response to an obsession that, if resisted, produces anxiety. The compulsive scratching of obsessive-compulsive disorder is often the underlying psychopathology in prurigo nodularis, and may exacerbate a primary skin disorder, such as psoriasis, eczema, and other pruritic conditions, or cause flare-ups of acne. A concern with dermatologic symptoms that are not consistent with objective dermatologic evaluation may represent underlying obsessive-compulsive disorder, rather than a primary disorder of body image, in the patient who has difficulty tolerating even a minor imperfection in their complexion.

*Social phobia (social anxiety disorder)*

Social phobia is characterized by a marked or persistent fear of one or more social or performance situations in which embarrassment may occur [8]. Patients may fear that they will act in a way or show anxiety symptoms that are humiliating or embarrassing. For example, some patients with hyperhidrosis and rosacea often perspire or blush more prominently in embarrassing situations and may develop a social phobia as a result. Exposure to the feared social situation almost always provokes anxiety, which may take the form of a situationally bound panic attack, which in turn also results in an exaggerated autonomic reactivity of the skin. In social phobia the individual recognizes that the fear is excessive or unreasonable; however, intense anxiety results if the feared situation is not avoided. The anxious anticipation or distress in the feared social or performance situation interferes significantly with the individual's overall functioning. Social phobia is also encountered in patients with cosmetically disfiguring skin disorders [16], such as psoriasis and acne [1,4], especially those who have been teased or ridiculed about their skin disorder at some time earlier in their lives. Patients with social phobia are typically underdiagnosed because the very nature of their disorder prevents them from attending clinics and doctors offices where they have to face large numbers of relatively unfamiliar people.

*Posttraumatic stress disorder (dissociation and conversion symptoms)*

Symptoms related to posttraumatic stress disorder tend to be underrecognized in dermatology [4]. Psychologic trauma refers to events that are outside the range of human experience, such as sexual assault, terrorists' attack, or a plane crash. For children, traumatic experiences also include emotional neglect, without the threat of actual violence or injury. The central clinical features of posttraumatic stress disorder [8] include the persistent re-experience of extremely traumatic or stressful life experiences or life events, which can manifest as recurrent and intrusive thoughts, dreams, flashbacks, or physical symptoms. In posttraumatic stress disorder there is a persistent avoidance of stimuli associated with the trauma and this can manifest as dissociative symptoms. Posttraumatic stress disorder secondary to childhood neglect and abuse, especially sexual abuse, is often the underlying psychiatric pathology in dermatologic patients who self-induce their lesions. Posttraumatic stress disorder is often complicated by substance abuse disorders and this often becomes the main focus in treatment, and the underlying trauma tends to get overlooked. When dissociative symptoms are a prominent feature of the posttraumatic stress disorder, the patient may not have recollection of the fact that they self-induced their lesions [17–19] and may be misdiagnosed as malingerers or attentions seekers.

Posttraumatic stress disorder, dissociation, and self-injury can be the underlying psychiatric disturbance in some cases of trichotillomania, prurigo nodularis, and dermatitis artefacta or may complicate the course of other dermatologic conditions, such as acne excoriée or the exacerbation of psoriatic lesions secondary to the Koebner phenomenon. If the clinician suspects that dissociative symptoms are the basis for the dermatologic problem, emphasis by the clinician that the lesions are self-induced, when the patient reports that they do not recall self-inducing the lesions, may make the patient more anxious and mistrustful. Because dissociation is likely also to affect other major areas of functioning, however, a more productive line of enquiry is to ask about general symptoms of dissociation. To screen for typical dissociative symptoms, the clinician may ask the following: "Have there been instances when you are not able to account for what you did or where you had been, for hours at a time?"; "Have there been instances where you found yourself in a place, such as a shopping mall, and did not know how you got there?"; "Have there been times when others have remarked that they had seen you in some place, but you have no recollection of being there?".

Another symptom that is underrecognized in dermatology, and that is typically associated with psychologic trauma, is conversion. Conversion symptoms were referred to as hysterical symptoms in the earlier literature, and have been referred to as somatoform dissociation in the more recent literature. In conversion, psychologic conflicts are manifested through somatic symptoms. The essential feature of conversion disorder is the presence of symptoms or deficits affecting sensory function or voluntary motor control that suggest a general medical or neurologic condition. Classically, most conversion symptoms present as pseudoneurologic symptoms, such as hysterical paralysis and seizures; however, symptoms and deficits can also affect the sensory system [8], and manifest as anesthesia with loss of sensations of touch and pain, and other cutaneous sensory syndromes including bouts of unexplained pruritus.

Some conversion symptoms may also represent flashbacks and body memories [20] of abuse, such as the development of a wheal where the patient had been hit as a child or pruritus vulvae in reaction to past sexual abuse. Patients who are experiencing acute conversion symptoms related to earlier trauma may also be vulnerable to misconstruing the intentions of the dermatologist who is physically examining them, because they are in a state where they are reliving their traumatic experiences. For example, in the dissociated state the patient may misinterpret the clinician's touch as sexual assault.

*Body dysmorphic disorder and other body image pathologies*

Body dysmorphic disorder presents as a preoccupation with an imagined defect in appearance; or if a slight anomaly is present, the individual's concern is excessive [8]. Body dysmorphic disorder is also referred to as "dysmorphophobia" and "dermatologic nondisease" [21] in the dermatologic literature. Body dysmorphic disorder should be suspected when there is a significant discrepancy between the patient's perception of their appearance and the clinician's evaluation of the patient. The complaints in body dysmorphic disorder commonly involve imagined or slight flaws of the face or head, such as thinning hair, acne, wrinkles, scars, vascular markings, paleness or redness of the complexion, swelling, facial disproportion or asymmetry, or excessive facial hair.

Some associated features of body dysmorphic disorder include repetitive behaviors, such as excessive grooming behavior. This may manifest as excessive hair combing, hair removal, hair picking or picking of the skin, or ritualized make-up application. The main purpose of the repetitive behavior is to improve or hide the perceived defect in the appearance. Many individuals may camouflage their perceived defect or deformity with make-up, clothing, or hair.

Most individuals with body dysmorphic disorder experience marked distress over their supposed deformity that often leads to vocational and social impairment. In some instances body dysmorphic disorder can be life-threatening because patients may resort to extreme behaviors to deal with a perceived defect in their appearance (eg, they may use razor blades or knives to remove these "defects"). In some patients the preoccupation with a minimal or imagined defect in appearance can reach delusional proportions.

Patients with eating disorders, such as anorexia nervosa and bulimia nervosa, which have a peak incidence during adolescence, often present with excessive concerns about various aspects of their skin in addition to concerns about their weight and shape [22]. Maintenance of an abnormally low body weight in association with secondary amenorrhea, frequent fluctuations in body weight, and history of compulsive exercising are some clues that there may be an underlying eating disorder. Typically, patients do not disclose that they have an eating disorder and the wide range of dermatologic [23,24] complications related to starvation, bingeing and purging, abuse of laxatives, and other related symptoms [8] may be the first sign that an eating disorder is present.

Acne has a peak incidence during midadolescence, a life stage that is associated with a high incidence of eating disorders. The hormonal changes associated with frequent bingeing and purging can cause flare-ups of acne, whereas dietary restriction is often associated with an improvement in the acne. Recurrent flare-ups of acne in an adolescent patient may be an indication of an underlying bulimic disorder [25].

*Delusional disorder and other psychotic symptoms*

The essential feature of delusional disorder [8] is the presence of one or more nonbizarre delusions that persist for at least 1 month. A delusion is defined as a false belief, based on faulty or incorrect interpretation of external reality that is not consistent with the patients' cultural background or intelligence that cannot be corrected by reasoning. A delusion that is frequently referenced in the dermatologic literature is delusion of parasitosis. The delusion may be associated with tactile or olfactory hallucinations that are related to the theme of the delusion (eg, a crawling sensation under the skin in association with delusions of parasitosis, or a delusion that one is emitting a foul odor from an orifice of the body). This can occur in conjunction with delusions of reference where the patient believes that everyone around them is talking about the odor that they are emitting. Certain hallucinations related to touch may in part be related to an organic brain syndrome or peripheral degenerative changes that may cause some cutaneous dysesthesia.

A delusional state may coexist with a major depressive episode in which the patient experiences delusions that are congruent with his or her depressed mood, and typically represents a more severe form of depressive disease. Delusions of disfigurement may be a feature of body dysmorphic disorder. If the delusion or hallucination becomes more bizarre and is clearly implausible and not derived from normal life experience (eg, a complaint that aliens are putting electricity though the body and causing the patient to feel a stinging sensation in the skin), the diagnosis of schizophrenia should be considered.

*Personality disorders*

Personality disorder [8] is defined as an enduring pattern of inner experience and behavior that is pervasive across a wide range of personal and social situations and deviates markedly from the expectations of the individual's culture and is pervasive and inflexible. This enduring pattern is manifested in two or more of the following areas [8]: cognition (ie, ways of perceiving and interpreting self, others, and events); affectivity (ie, the range, intensity, lability, and appropriateness of emotional response); interpersonal functioning; and impulse control. The personality disorders that are most frequently encountered in dermatology include borderline, narcissistic, histrionic, and obsessive-compulsive personality disorders [8].

Borderline personality disorder is associated with a pattern of instability in interpersonal relationships, affects, and self-image, and impulsive behaviors, such as self-induced injury, for which they may present to the dermatologist. Such patients are often difficult because their instability in interpersonal relationships and self-image are also manifested in their relationship with their dermatologist and other health care providers. Such patients often try to split or play one professional against the other, and at times may be very unreasonable, manipulative, and demanding.

Narcissistic personality disorder presents with a pattern of grandiosity, need for admiration, and often a lack of empathy for others. Some such patients may place an inordinate importance on their appearance and the approval of others, and face a psychiatric crisis including suicidal ideation when faced with a cosmetically disfiguring skin disorder or the normal changes of aging. The patient with a histrionic personality disorder presents with excessive emotionality and is attention seeking and may self-induce skin lesions to gain attention.

In obsessive-compulsive personality disorder there is a pattern of preoccupation with orderliness, perfectionism, and control. Unlike OCD (described previously), the patient with obsessive-compulsive personality disorder presents with an enduring pattern that is pervasive. An obsessive-compulsive personality disorder may be a feature in patients with compulsive behaviors, such as compulsive washing and picking of the skin, or patients with excessive body image concerns where the patient is bothered by a minor or nonexistent imperfection in their skin. Some patient with body dysmorphic disorder have underlying obsessive-compulsive symptoms, rather than primarily body image-related problems.

**Summary**

Because psychiatric comorbidity is present in about a third of dermatology patients it is often essential for the dermatologist to be able to assess the mental state of the patient. It is important to maintain clear boundaries in the doctor-patient relationship, especially when the dermatologist is dealing with both the physical and psychiatric aspects of the disorder. A biopsychosocial approach is helpful, where the relative contributions of both dermatologic and psychosocial factors are considered. An enquiry about the impact of the skin disorder on the quality of life, role of psychosocial stressors including early traumatic life experiences, and substance abuse should be part of the assessment. Depressive disease is one of the most frequently encountered psychiatric disorders in dermatology and is associated with a high incidence of suicide. Some of the other psychiatric disorders that are comorbid with dermatologic disorders include obsessive-compulsive disorder; social phobia; posttraumatic stress disorder; body image pathologies, such as body dysmorphic disorder and eating disorders; delusional disorder; and a range of personality disorders. This article outlines some guidelines for assessing these psychiatric disorders in the dermatologic patient.

# References

[1] Gupta MA, Gupta AK. Psychodermatology: an update. J Am Acad Dermatol 1996;34:1030–46.

[2] Gupta MA, Gupta AK. Psychiatric and psychological comorbidity in patients with dermatologic disorders. Am J Clin Dermatol 2003;4:833–42.

[3] Picardi A, Abeni D, Renzi C, et al. Treatment outcome an incidence of psychiatric disorders in dermatologic out-patients. J Eur Acad Dermatol Venereol 2003;17: 155–9.

[4] Woodruff PWR, Higgins EM, Du Vivier AWP, et al. Psychiatric illness in patients referred to a dermatology-psychiatry clinic. Gen Hosp Psychiatry 1997;19:29–35.

[5] Sampogna F, Picardi A, Chren MM, et al. Association between poorer quality of life and psychiatric morbidity in patients with different dermatological conditions. Psychosom Med 2004;66:620–40.

[6] Picardi A, Abeni D, Melchi CF. Psychiatric morbidity in dermatological outpatients: an issue to be recognized. Br J Dermatol 2000;143:983–91.

[7] Manley MRS. Psychiatric interview, history, and mental status examination. In: Sadock BI, Sadock VA, editors. Kaplan & Sadock's comprehensive textbook of psychiatry, vol. 1. Philadelphia: Lippincott Williams & Wilkins; 2000. p. 652–65.

[8] American Psychiatric Association. Diagnostic and statistical manual of mental disorders (DSM IV-TR), 4th edition. Text revision. Washington: American Psychiatric Association; 2000.

[9] Gupta MA, Gupta AK. Depression and suicidal ideation in dermatology patients with acne, alopecia areata, atopic dermatitis and psoriasis. Br J Dermatol 1998;139:846–50.

[10] Cotterill JA, Cunliffe WJ. Suicide in dermatological patients. Br J Dermatol 1997;137:246–50.

[11] Sadock BJ, Sadock VA. Kaplan and Sadock's pocket book of clinical psychiatry. 3rd edition. Philadelphia: Lippincott Williams and Wilkins; 2001. p. 261–74.

[12] Hyman SE. The suicidal patient. In: Hyman SE, Tesar GE, editors. Manual of psychiatric emergencies. 3rd edition. Boston: Little, Brown and Company; 1994. p. 21–7.

[13] Gupta MA, Schork NJ, Gupta AK, et al. Suicidal ideation in psoriasis. J Dermatol 1993;32:188–90.

[14] Stein DJ, Hollander SE. Dermatology and conditions related to obsessive-compulsive Disorder. J Am Acad Dermatol 1992;26:237–42.

[15] Hatch ML, Paradis C, Friedman S, et al. Obsessive-compulsive disorder in patients with chronic pruritic conditions: case studies and discussion. J Am Acad Dermatol 1992;26:549–51.

[16] Kent G, Keohane S. Social anxiety and disfigurement: the moderating effects of fear of negative evaluation and past experiences. Br J Clin Psychol 2001; 40:23–34.

[17] Gupta MA, Gupta AK, Chandarana PC, et al. Dissociative symptoms and the self-induced dermatoses: a preliminary empirical study [abstract]. Psychosom Med 2000;62:116.

[18] Shelley WB. Dermatitis artefacta induced in a patient by one of her multiple personalities. Br J Dermatol 1981;105:587–9.

[19] Gupta MA, Gupta AK, Haberman HF. The self-inflicted dermatoses: a critical review. Gen Hosp Psychiatry 1987;9:45–52.

[20] Van der Kolk BA. The body keeps the score: memory and the evolving psychobiology of posttraumatic stress. Harv Rev Psychiatry 1994;1:253–65.

[21] Cotterill JA. Dermatologic non-disease: a common and potentially fatal disturbance of cutaneous body image. Br J Dermatol 1981;104:611–9.

[22] Gupta MA, Gupta AK. Dissatisfaction with skin appearance among patients with eating disorders and non-clinical controls. Br J Dermatol 2001;145:110–3.

[23] Gupta MA, Gupta AK. Dermatological complications. Eur Eat Disord Rev 2000;8:134–43.

[24] Gupta MA, Gupta AK, Haberman HF. Dermatologic signs in anorexia nervosa and bulimia nervosa. Arch Dermatol 1987;123:1386–90.

[25] Gupta MA, Gupta AK. The psychological comorbidity in acne. Clin Dermatol 2001;19:360–3.

# Psychosomatic Factors in Dermatology

Mauro Urpe, PhD[a,b], Stefano Pallanti, MD[c,d], Torello Lotti, MD[a,b],*

[a]Centro Interuniversitario di Dermatologia Biologica e Psicosomatica, University of Florence, Florence, Italy
[b]University Unit of Physical Therapy and Dermatology, University of Florence, Florence, Italy
[c]Institute of Neuroscience, University of Florence, Florence, Italy
[d]Mount Sinai School of Medicine, New York, New York, USA

The skin is the largest organ and determines to a great extent appearance and plays a major function in social and sexual communication. The skin constitutes what René Thom calls an interface, serving as an envelope that simultaneously limits or contains the body, conditions exchanges between inside and outside, and, most important for dermatologists and psychologists, presents a "visible" self, even perhaps an "aesthetic" self [1]. A healthy normal skin is essential for a person's physical and mental well-being and a sense of self-confidence. Most skin diseases alter the body surface that constitutes the self-image in interpersonal relationships. Perception of surface alteration as a handicap and its evaluation and somatopsychic repercussions in terms of quality and quantity of damage vary from individual to individual and from dermatosis to dermatosis. With advances in generic and specific instruments measuring quality of life, there is now a greater appreciation of how skin diseases affect children and adults [2,3]. The field of psychodermatology has developed as a result of increased interest and understanding of the relationship between skin disease and various psychologic factors [4]. Patients with real and perceived imperfections in important body image areas (eg, the face, scalp, hands, and genital area) are prone to psychologic distress [5,6]. Blemishes on other parts of the body also can cause distress and require treatment [7]. Patients with body dysmorphic disorder, acne, psoriasis, and vitiligo and particularly men and women with facial conditions are more likely to have reactive depression and be at risk of suicide [8,9].

Several studies have indicated that people with cutaneous disease experience a heightened level of distress, as measured by the General Health Questionnaire and structured diagnostic interviews [10,11]. These patients benefit from clinical interventions because their level of distress typically declines with successful treatment [12]. Because psychosomatic factors in dermatologic disorders have been estimated to be present in at least one third of dermatology patients, effective management of the skin condition involves consideration of the associated emotional factors [13,14]. The placebo response in certain dermatologic conditions is more than 30%, which further emphasizes the importance of psychosomatic factors [15,16]. This article summarizes some cutaneous diseases in which psychosomatic factors and psychiatric and psychologic conditions seem to play an important role.

* Corresponding author. Department of Dermatology, University of Florence, Via della Pergola 58/60, Florence, 50121 Italy.
E-mail address: tlotti@unifi.it (T. Lotti).

## More recent developments in psychosomatic dermatology

*Acne*

Acne's effect on psychosocial and emotional problems is comparable to the effects of arthritis, back pain, diabetes, epilepsy, and disabling asthma [17]. Acne has a demonstrable association with depression, anxiety, and feelings of social isolation; it affects personality, emotions, self-image, self-esteem, and the ability to form relationships [17–19]. Acne in adolescents affects self-image and assertiveness, factors that are important in forming friendship and personality traits. It seems that adolescents are more influenced by the psychosocial effects of acne than older patients [20].

The literature pertaining to the somatopsychic aspect of acne varies in that not all reports support a causal link with emotional dysfunction. Some studies report no relationship between acne and anxiety [21], whereas other studies report that the level of anxiety was increased in patients with acne [22,23] and that the level of anxiety correlated positively with the severity of acne [22]. Yazici and colleagues [24] reported that anxiety and depression levels were higher in patients who thought that acne was affecting their life adversely. Regardless of the degree of severity, patients with acne are at increased risk for anxiety and depression compared with the normal population. Acne negatively affects quality of life, and the greater the impairment secondary to the disease, the greater the level of anxiety and depression. The study of psychosomatic and psychologic effects of acne is significant because acne is one of one of most common diseases in dermatologic practice. Gupta and Gupta [25] showed that acne is associated with higher depression scores than other dermatologic conditions. The relatively high depression scores among mildly to moderately affected patients with noncystic acne further underline the profound impact of even mild-to-moderate acne on body image.

*Atopic dermatitis*

Results of several studies on atopic dermatitis indicate that psychologic factors, such as perceptions of stigma, depression, self-esteem, anxiety, and fear of negative evaluation, and disease severity were independently associated with quality of life. Wittkowski and colleagues [26] found that perception of stigma, disease severity, and depression seem to play an important role in predicting atopic dermatitis–related quality of life in these patients. Further dermatologic studies are needed to evaluate exactly what is the role of psychosomatic factors in predicting severity of disease and its course.

*Psoriasis*

The degree of pruritus in patients with psoriasis and atopic dermatitis is strongly correlated to depressive psychopathology [13,25,27]. Patients have feelings of physical and sexual unattractiveness and helplessness, anger, and frustration. The disease is associated with increased alcohol consumption and smoking [28]. Women seem to report greater impairment of quality of life, whereas men report greater work-related stress. Psoriasis is rarely a life-threatening disease. The course of the disease varies greatly, however. Psoriasis may induce different kinds of stressful experiences with which patients must cope [29]. Patients with psoriasis report that their disease leads to various psychologic and psychosomatic consequences, such as feelings of anger, depression, shame, anxiety, and social isolation [30].

*Alopecia areata*

Alopecia areata has long been associated with multiple etiopathogenic factors; its cause is still unclear. Psychologic and psychopathologic factors have been analyzed as modulators of neuroendocrinologic, vascular, and immunologic variables [31]. Adjustment disorders, generalized anxiety disorders, and depressive episode were the most prevalent psychiatric diagnoses in patients with alopecia areata. These findings are in accordance with the results of the few studies performed on adults with alopecia areata [32,33], general dermatologic patients [34], and children with alopecia areata. Concerning personality, the highest scores were obtained for obsessive, anxious, and dependent traits. The characteristic of alexithymia is closely related to psychosomatic disease [35] and manifests itself through the patients' operative way of thinking. Patients are oriented toward action, are pragmatic, have new fantasies, and have difficulty expressing emotions; this can result in a greater interiorization of stress, which may alter immune responses related to cytokines and neuropeptides [36].

*Vitiligo*

Vitiligo is one of the diseases whose manifestations most often cause alarm and psychologic problems in patients. Although the somatopsychic aspect (ie, the influence of the cutaneous alteration on the mind) is preponderant in this condition, one cannot exclude the influence of emotions, stress, and deep psychic conflicts in triggering the onset and affecting its course in predisposed subjects. Because vitiligo is a long-lasting disease, it is at increased risk of becoming a major aspect of conflict in the daily life of patients and their families. The skin lesions on the face and hands (these localizations are frequent in vitiligo) can be seen by any casual observer, and this may make it impossible for the patient to work, especially if the occupation requires direct interactions with the public, such as salesperson, physician, or childcare worker. Lesions on the genitals are fraught with meaning and anguish for affected patients. Many young patients with vitiligo localized on the genitals (or with particularly evident genital lesions) think they will be repugnant to a sexual partner and consider themselves obliged to meet only in the dark. In consideration of the psychologic impact of a skin disease such as vitiligo, according to Ginsburg [37], the patient's life situation is confirmed to be poor, including social support network, attitudes of intimates, work experiences, and actual experiences of rejection. Patients with vitiligo can be extremely sensitive to the way others perceive them, and they often withdraw because they anticipate being rejected. The impact is profound. Patients can experience subjective emotional distress; some seek professional help and experience interference with various aspects of employment ("I am simply existing") or use tension-lessening, oblivion-producing substances such as alcohol. Feelings of embarrassment and self-consciousness and perception of discrimination are predominant in patients younger than 40 and members of working class.

A significant discrepancy between the patient's and dermatologist's assessment of disease severity is usually a sign that psychosocial factors contribute to the overall morbidity associated with the disease [38,39]. Papadopoulos and colleagues [40] found that vitiligo patients encounter a significantly higher number of stressful life events than matched patients affected with skin disease not thought to associated with stress. These results suggest that psychologic distress may have contributed to the onset of their vitiligo. Another study suggests that personality characteristics, such as alexithymia and insecure attachment, and poor social support increase the susceptibility to vitiligo, possibly through deficits in emotional regulation or reduced ability to cope with stress [41]. Nearly all vitiligo patients feel distressed and stigmatized by their condition. The self-image of the vitiligo patient decreases considerably and may lead to significant depression, low self-esteem, and social isolation [42].

**Psychodynamic perspective: the hole in the ego**

Referring to dynamics and structure of the psychosomatic process of some skin disease, the authors agree with Ammon, a pioneer in this field, on the existence of a hole in the ego, which can be filled by the symptom to prevent disintegration of personality [43,44]. In this way, skin diseases can be understood as a hole in the skin-ego—a visible demonstration on the skin of ego defects. Patients gain attention from others and contact to themselves through their skin and their illness. From this perspective, some skin diseases can indicate profound psychic problems concerning the entire human being. The unity of body-mind is inseparably connected with the environment [45]. The ego structure of a person is developed and differentiated by social energetic experiences in human relationships. Ammon [43,44,46] introduced the concept of social energy functions as a transmitter among society, groups, and the individual. The ego structure of a human being consists of manifested social energy. The deficit in the ego structure could be interpreted in this context as the root of the illness. Skin disease could be an expression of afflicted central ego functions. In healthy development, skin expresses and receives continuously caressing and erotic contact and can be used aggressively in a constructive way. Similar to other patients reacting through their body, the personality structure of patients with skin diseases finds its expression in feelings of emptiness, nonexistence, and incapacity to admit emotions. These patients could be far away from their emotions, unable to admit arguing and aggression, leading to the well-known psychic phenomenon that Sifneos [47] called "alexithymia."

**Sexuality and skin conditions**

The dermatologist may not recognize that behind the young acne patient's insistence on therapeutic intervention are hidden problems of timidity and inhibition or other more relevant problems. Pasini [48] discussed situations in which behind episodes of psoriatic exacerbation, one can find a personality in a state of abandon, and behind hyperhidrosis and erythrophobia, a true phobic–anxious personality.

When diseases need repeated topical treatments that impede direct skin contact, modifications in the real and affective distances of contact with the patient may result and trigger the process of desocialization [48]. In applying Hall's scheme [49] to dermatologic disturbances, it can be said with Pasini's thought that these disturbances lead to a modification of the interpersonal distances and the passage from an intimate distance to a greater distance of the patient from his or her social environment. Modifications in the emotional and affective distance may have particularly negative repercussions on a couple's sexual relationship [48]. Such events are sometimes explicit, but more often they are masked by nearly pure somatic symptoms. Panconesi [50] affirmed that many requests on the part of adolescents for treatment of acne serve to express a desire for and at the same time fear of contact with the other sex. Many consultations for venereal disease and, even more, the phobia of contagion can be expressions of a negative moral judgment regarding sexuality. Pasini [48] also illustrated cases in which consultation by men for loss of hair could mask a decline in virility; requests for checkups are an evident expression of sexual anxiety. Many situations require a sexual anamnesis that departs from the specific symptom taking into consideration of the sexual deficit in its current and remote meanings. Dermatologists must consider an attentive assessment of the request and conduct an accurate sexual anamnesis that permits establishment of a pathogenetic diagnosis that takes into account the somatic, intrapsychic, and relational factors underlying the symptom presented [48].

## Psychosomatic interventions

### Psychoanalytic treatment

Psychoanalytic treatment is not usual for psychosomatic dermatologic diseases. Its application is restricted to persons motivated to comprehend themselves in a profound way through treatment that is extremely costly in terms of time and money. It is based on the assumption that psychosomatic patients are in general incapable of accepting intrapsychic conflicts and their unconscious dimension and tend to submit to the physician only somatic disturbances according to classic defensive dynamics [51–55].

### Biofeedback

The most commonly used biofeedback techniques measure and provide simultaneously auditory or visual feedback of galvanic skin resistance, skin temperature, electromyography, or electroencephalography [56]. As reported by Shenefelt [57] in his systematic review, cutaneous problems with an autonomic nervous system component can be improved by biofeedback with or without associated hypnosis. With training, individuals can learn consciously how to alter the autonomic response, and with enough repetition they may establish new habit patterns. Hypnosis or autogenic training may enhance the effects obtained by biofeedback. A large study of Raynaud's patients compared hand-warming results using different biofeedback methods and found that attention to emotional and cognitive aspects of biofeedback training was important [57,58] for the final result. Biofeedback of muscle tension via electromyography can be used to enhance the teaching of relaxation. Relaxation can have a positive effect on inflammatory and emotionally triggered skin conditions, such as acne, atopic dermatitis, lichen planus, neurodermatitis, psoriasis, and urticaria, with a complex mechanism that is operating also through influencing immunoreactivity [59]. Patients who have low hypnotic ability may be especially suitable for this type of relaxation training. Biofeedback also was used along with multiagent antihistamines in a multimodal approach to reduce the urticaria [57]. For patients with medium to high hypnotic ability, hypnosis may be employed in cognitive-behavioral therapy to produce desensitization, facilitate relaxation, or produce imagined aversive experiences [60]. Especially with aversion therapy, it is much easier and safer to have the patient experience the aversive stimulus in the imagination than in real life. For patients with low hypnotic ability, biofeedback may be more appropriate [57].

### Supportive counseling

Supportive counseling encompasses a wide range of types of psychologic intervention that can be applied by any physician who pays attention to the disturbances reported by a patient. Approaches range from reassurance to clarification regarding the exact nature of the disease, to the point of triggering what Balint [61] calls the "flash." In such a case, the physician transmits a flash of comprehension to the patient. Early rational clarification of the symptoms can prevent the development of an obsessive vicious circle regarding illness and the consequent chronicity of the clinical pattern [62]. Sarti and Cossidente [62] advise the necessity to remember patients who refuse an approach with psychiatric or psychologic consultation and limit their recognition of disease to the somatic sphere because they have chosen the dermatologist as the sole referee. Sarti and Cossidente [62] further suggest keeping in mind the suggestions made by the Balint groups to nonpsychiatrists interested in following the psychologic problems of their patients through a possibility for verification with global psychotherapeutic scope. Balint groups nowadays are used in some medical disciplines, especially in oncology, but are desirable also in dermatology [61]. Sarti and Cossidente [62] suggest that these moments of support and clarification are available and help the physician to face sometimes complex problems with more self-assurance and favor progressive enrichment of his or her therapeutic repertoire.

*Cognitive-behavioral therapy*

In behavioral therapy [63], in contrast to psychoanalysis, one starts out with theoretical formulations and their experimental verification and only subsequently proceeds with practical application. This method historically came about through an attempt to apply the laws of experimental psychology to clinical practice [64]. According to this theory [65], behavioral disturbances depend on the patient's individual learning processes. The aim of behavioral therapy techniques is modification of behavior that is considered nonadaptive to the individual. Nonadaptive habits are weakened and eliminated, whereas adaptive habits are reinforced. From behaviorism is derived cognitivism. Cognitive theory is based on the assumption that the human being is an active builder of reality and not a passive agent of external information [66,67]. Individual expectations and assumptions about the world can have significant implications for one's emotional reactions to that world and for individual behavior [68,69].

In dermatology, cognitive–behavioral techniques have given good results in atopic dermatitis, psoriasis, acne vulgaris, alopecia areata, and pruritus sine materia and in certain psychiatric disorders that often first present to the dermatologist, such as Ekbom's syndrome and body dysmorphophobia [70,71]. This method draws in part on the cognitive therapies of identifying dysfunctional negative self-talk and substituting positive self-talk or reframing the thought picture by offering a new perspective. A more detailed description of systematic desensitization, aversion therapy, operant techniques, and assertiveness training as applied to dermatology is provided by Bär and Kuypers [72]. Scratching in atopic dermatitis can become a conditioned response [73,74], often associated with and exacerbated by feelings of anxiety or hostility. Ratliffe and Stein [75] reported improvement of neurodermatitis in a 22-year-old man using aversion therapy techniques.

Rosenbaum and Ayllon [76] successfully used habit reversal treatment for neurodermatitis. They taught awareness of the scratching behavior; reviewed the inconveniences produced by the habit; developed a competing response practice of isometric exercise using fist clenching, which was incompatible with scratching; and did symbolic rehearsal. Psychosomatic triggering or exacerbation of urticaria was ameliorated in a young professional woman using cognitive–behavioral therapy with specific self-talk and relaxation techniques.

Systematic desensitization [77] is perhaps one of the most commonly used cognitive–behavioral therapy techniques. Perfected by Wolpe [78] and Lazarus [79], it represents one possible choice for a therapist in the treatment for phobic behavior in dermatologic contexts. It consists fundamentally of getting the patient used to exposure to the phobic stimulus and inhibiting the anxiety evoked through induction of an antagonistic state. The procedure, based on so-called "counter-conditioning," is not different from the procedure normally used in classic conditioning. Even in the case of counter-conditioning, it is essential to substitute one response (relaxation) for another (fear) in the event of the same situation-stimulus [80–82]. Galassi [69] and others have illustrated cognitive-behavioral methods that can be used successfully with dermatologic patients. Other techniques comprise systematic rational restructuring, which can be divided into four phases: (1) presentation of the rationale of the procedure, (2) overview of irrational assumptions, (3) analysis of the patient's problems in rational terms, and (4) teaching the patient to modify the opinion of himself or herself. This method seems appropriate in the treatment of the anxiety component present in almost all skin conditions. Galassi [69] suggests the use of the systematic rational restructuring technique also in group situations to treat behavioral problems in social settings, particularly in cases involving anxiety resulting from social judgments, such as subjects with dysmorphophobia, which is an important issue in psychosomatic dermatology.

**Summary**

Patients need not only dermatologic problem-solving skills to manage the physical care demands and the changes in lifestyle caused by skin diseases, but also emotion-regulating skills to handle numerous psychosocial tasks related to illness, such as uncertainty, fear, and lack of control. Skin diseases should be measured not only by symptoms, but also by other physical, psychologic, and social parameters. Knowledge of mind–body–environment interactions and interventions can help to improve patients' skin conditions and ultimately their quality of life.

**References**

[1] Panconesi E, Cossidente A, Giorgini S, et al. A psychosomatic approach to dermatologic cosmetology. Int J Dermatol 1983;22:449–54.
[2] Hautmann G, Panconesi E. Vitiligo: a psychologically influenced and influencing disease. Clin Dermatol 1997;15(6):879–90.
[3] Finlay AY, Khan GK. Dermatology Life Quality Index (DLQI). Clin Exp Dermatol 1994;19:210–6.
[4] Koo J, Do JH, Lee CS. Psychodermatology. J Am Acad Dermatol 2000;43:848–53.
[5] Cotterill JA, Cunliffe WJ. Suicide in dermatologic patients. Br J Dermatol 1997;137:246–50.
[6] Cotterill JA. Dermatologic nondisease. Dermatol Clin 1996;14:439–45.
[7] Stewart TW, Savage D. Cosmetic camouflage in dermatology. Br J Dermatol 1972;86:530–2.
[8] Cotterill JA. Body dysmorphic disorder. Dermatol Clin 1996;14:457–63.
[9] Gupta MA, Schork NJ, Gupta AK, et al. Suicidal ideation in psoriasis. Int J Dermatol 1993;32:188–90.
[10] Hughes J, Barraclough B, Hamblin L, et al. Psychiatric symptoms in dermatology patients. Br J Psychiatry 1983;143:51–4.
[11] Root S, Kent G, Al-Abadie M. The relationship between disease severity, disability, and psychological distress in patients undergoing PUVA treatment for psoriasis. Dermatology 1994;189:234–7.
[12] Rubinow D, Peck G, Squillace K, et al. Reduced anxiety and depression in cystic acne patients after successful treatment with oral isotretinoin. J Am Acad Dermatol 1987;17:25–32.
[13] Gupta MA, Gupta AK. Psychodermatology: an update. J Am Acad Dermatol 1996;34:1030–46.
[14] Savin JA, Cotterill JA. Psychocutaneous disorders. In: Champion RH, Burton JL, Ebling FJG, editors. Textbook of dermatology. Oxford: Blackwell Scientific Publications; 1992. p. 2479–96.
[15] Gupta MA, Gupta AK, Haberman HF. Psychotropic drugs in dermatology. J Am Acad Dermatol 1986;14:633–45.
[16] Rudzki E, Borkowski W, Czubalski K. The suggestive effect of placebo on the intensity of chronic urticaria. Acta Allergol 1970;25:70–3.
[17] Mallon E, Newton JN, Klassen AF, et al. The quality of life in acne: a comparison with general medical conditions using generic questionnaires. Br J Dermatol 1999;140:672–6.
[18] Lasek RJ, Chren MM. Acne vulgaris and the quality of life of adult dermatology patients. Arch Dermatol 1998;134:454–8.

[19] Shuster S, Fisher GH, Harris E, et al. The effect of skin disease on self image. Br J Dermatol 1978;99(Suppl 16):18–9.
[20] Lewis-Jones MS, Finlay AY. The Children's Dermatology Life Quality Index (CDLQI): initial validation and practical use. Br J Dermat 1995;132:942–9.
[21] Medanski RS, Handler RM, Medanski DL. Self evaluation of acne and emotion: a pilot study. Psychosomatics 1981;22:379–83.
[22] Wu SF, Kinder BN, Trunnel TN, et al. Role of anxiety and anger in acne patients: a relationship with the severity of the disorder. J Am Acad Dermatol 1988;18:325–32.
[23] Van Der Meeren HLM, Van Der Schaar WW, Van Den Hurk CMAM. The psychological impact of severe acne. Cutis 1985;7:84–6.
[24] Yazici K, Baz K, Yazici AE, Tot S, Demirseren D, Buturak V. Disease-specific quality of life associated with anxiety and depression in patients with acne. J Eur Acad Dermatol Veneorol 2004;18:435–9.
[25] Gupta MA, Gupta AK. Depression and suicidal ideation in dermatology patients with acne, alopecia areata, atopic dermatitis and psoriasis. Br J Dermatol 1998;139:846–50.
[26] Wittkowski A, Richards HL, Griffiths CEM, et al. The impact of psychological and clinical factors on quality of life in individuals with atopic dermatitis. J Psychosom Res 2004;57:195–200.
[27] Gupta MA, Gupta AK, Schork NJ, Ellis CN. Depression modulates pruritus perception: a study of pruritus in psoriasis, atopic dermatitis, and chronic idiopathic urticaria. Psychosom Med 1994;56:36–40.
[28] Finlay AY, Coles EC. The effect of severe psoriasis on the quality of life of 369 patients. Br J Dermatol 1995;132:236–44.
[29] Fortune DG, Main CJ, O'Sullivan TM, et al. Quality of life in patients with psoriasis: the contribution of clinical variables and psoriasis-specific stress. Br J Dermatol 1997;137:755–60.
[30] Gupta MA, Gupta AK, Haberman HF. Psoriasis and psychiatry: an update. Gen Hosp Psychiatry 1987;9(3):157–66.
[31] Ruiz-Doblado S, Carrizosa A, Garcia-Hernandez MJ. Alopecia areata: psychiatric comorbidity and adjustment to illness. Int J Dermatol 2003;42:434–7.
[32] Colon EA, Popkin MK, Callies AL, et al. Lifetime prevalence of psychiatric disorders in patients with alopecia areata. Compr Psychiatry 1991;32:245–51.
[33] Gupta MA, Gupta AK, Watteel GN. Stress and alopecia areata: a psychodermatologic study. Acta Dermatol Veneor 1997;77:296–8.
[34] Woodruff PW, Higgins EM, Du-Vivier J, et al. Psychiatry illness in patients referred to a dermatology-psychiatry clinic. Gen Hosp Psychiatry 1997;19:29–35.
[35] Sifneos PE. The prevalence of alexithymic characteristics in psychosomatics patients. Psychoter Psychosom 1973;22:255–62.
[36] Lotti T, Hautmann G, Panconesi E. Neuropeptides and skin. J Am Acad Dermatol 1995;33:482–96.

[37] Ginsburg JH. The psychological impact of skin disease: an overview. Dermatol Clin 1996;14:473–84.
[38] Porter JR, Beuf AH, Nordlund JJ, et al. Psychological reaction to chronic skin disorders: a study of patients with vitiligo. Gen Hosp Psychiatry 1979;1:73–7.
[39] Gupta MA, Gupta AK. Psychiatric and psychological co-morbidity in patients with dermatological disorders: epidemiology and management. Am J Clin Dermatol 2003;4:833–42.
[40] Papadopoulos L, Bor L, Legg C, et al. Impact of life events on the onset of vitiligo in adults: a preliminary evidence for a psychological dimension in aetiology. Clin Exp Dermatol 1998;23:243–8.
[41] Picardi A, Pasquini P, Cattaruzza MS, et al. Stressful life events, social support, attachment security and alexithymia in vitiligo: a case-control study. Psychother Psychosom 2003;72:150–8.
[42] Mattoo SK, Handa S, Kaur L, et al. Psychiatric morbidity in vitiligo: prevalence and correlates in India. J Eur Acad Dermatol Veneorol 2002;16:573–8.
[43] Ammon GU. Zur genese and struktur psychosomatischer syndrome unter berücksichtigung psychoanalytisch technik [Genesis and structure of psychosomatic syndrome through psychoanalytic technique]. Dyn Psychiat 1972;5:223–51 [in German].
[44] Ammon GU. Das ich-strukturelle und gruppendynamische prinzip bei depression und psychosomatischer erkrankung [The principles of ego structure and dynamic groups in depression and psychomatics]. Dyn Psych 1978;12:445–71.
[45] Ammon GU. Theoretical aspects of milieutherapy. Topeka (KS): Menninger School of Psychiatry; 1959. p. 1–42 [German edition: Berlin: Pinel Publikationen; 1977].
[46] Ammon GU, Ammon GI, Griepenstroh D. Das prinzip von sozialenergie: gleitendes spectrum und regulation [The principles of social energy: spectrum and regulation]. Dyn Psychiat 1981;14:1–15 [in German].
[47] Sifneos PE. Problems of psychotherapy of patients with alexithymic characteristics and physical disease. Psychoter Psychosom 1975;26:65–70.
[48] Pasini W. Sexologic problems in dermatology. Clin Dermatol 1984;2:59–65.
[49] Hall E. The hidden dimension. New York: Doubleday; 1966.
[50] Panconesi E. In tema di infezioni sessuali e dermatosis inestetiche nell'adolescente [On the theme of sexual infections and nonesthetic dermatosis in adolescents]. Proceedings of the Conference at the Sixth National Congress of Sexology, Florence, Italy, September 30–October 2, 1983. Milan: Franco Angeli; 1984 [in Italian].
[51] Thomas K. Autoipnosi e training autogeno [Self-hypnosis and autogenous training]. Roma: Edizioni Mediterranee; 1976. p. 44–9.
[52] Dotti A. Le terapie psicoanalitiche [Psychoanalytic therapies]. In: Pancheri P, editor. Trattato di medicina psicosomatica [Theory of psychosomatic medicine]. Firenze: USES; 1984. p. 1063–79 [in Italian].
[53] Fenichel O. Trattato di psicoanalisi delle nevrosi e delle psicosi [The psychoanalytical theory of neuroses]. Roma: Astrolabio; 1951. p. 33–43 [in Italian].
[54] Haynal A, Pasini W. Medicina psicosomatica [Psychosomatic medicine]. Milano: Masson; 1979. p. 47–9.
[55] Kaplan HI, Sadock BJ. Modern synopsis of comprehensive textbook of psychiatry/ill. Baltimore: Williams & Wilkins; 1981.
[56] Sarti MG. Biofeedback in dermatology. Clin Dermatol 1998;16:711–4.
[57] Shenefelt PD. Biofeedback, cognitive-behavioral methods, and hypnosis in dermatology: is it all in your mind? Dermatol Ther 2003;16:114–22.
[58] Middaugh SJ, Haythornthwaite JA, Thompson B, et al. The Raynaud's Treatment Study: biofeedback protocols and acquisition of temperature biofeedback skills. Appl Psychophysiol Biofeedback 2001;26:251–78.
[59] Tausk FA. Alternative medicine: is it all in your mind? Arch Dermatol 1998;134:1422–5.
[60] Dengrove E. Hypnosis. In: Dengrove E, editor. Hypnosis and behavior therapy. Springfield (IL): Charles C. Thomas; 1976. p. 26–35.
[61] Balint M. The doctor, his patient, and the illness. London: Pitman; 1957.
[62] Sarti MG, Cossidente A. Therapy in psychosomatic dermatology. Clin Dermatol 1984;2:59–65.
[63] Skinner BF. Science and human behavior. New York: McMillan; 1953.
[64] Mosticoni R. Terapia del comportamento [Behavioral therapy]. Roma: Bulzoni; 1979. p. 151–4 [in Italian].
[65] Wolpe J, Lazarus AA. Behavior therapy techniques. New York: Pergamon Press; 1966.
[66] Mahoney MJ. Behavior therapy: some critical comments. Boston: American Psychopathological Association; 1974.
[67] Mahoney MJ. Cognitive and non cognitive views in behaviour modifications. In: Sjoden S, Bates B, Dockens M, editors. Trends in behavior therapy. New York: Plenum Press; 1979.
[68] Beck A. Cognitive therapy: nature and relation to behaviour therapy. Behav Ther 1970;1:184–200.
[69] Galassi F. Cognitive-behavioral techniques. Clin Dermatol 1998;16:715–23.
[70] Ehelers A, Stangier U, Gieler U. Treatment of atopic dermatitis: a comparison of psychological and dermatological approaches to relapse prevention. J Consult Clin Psychol 1995;63:624–35.
[71] Phillips KA. Body dysmorphic disorder: diagnosis and treatment of imagined ugliness. J Clin Psychiatry 1996;57(Suppl 8):61–5.
[72] Bär LHJ, Kuypers BRM. Behaviour therapy in dermatological practice. Br J Dermatol 1973;88:591–8.
[73] Jordan JM, Whitlock FA. Emotions and the skin: the conditioning of the scratch response in cases of atopic dermatitis. Br J Dermatol 1972;86:574–85.
[74] Jordan JM, Whitlock FA. Atopic dermatitis, anxiety and conditioned scratch responses. J Psychosom Res 1974;18:297–9.
[75] Ratliffe R, Stein N. Treatment of neurodermatitis by

behavior therapy: a case study. Behav Res Ther 1968;6:397–9.
[76] Rosenbaum MS, Ayllon T. The behavioral treatment of neurodermatitis through habit reversal. Behav Res Ther 1981;19:313–8.
[77] Wolpe J. Psychotherapy by reciprocal inhibition. Palo Alto (CA): Stanford University Press; 1958.
[78] Wolpe J. Tecniche di terapia del comportamento [Behavioral therapy techniques]. Milano: Franco Angeli; 1972. p. 100–43 [in Italian].
[79] Lazarus AA. Behavior therapy and beyond. New York: McGraw-Hill; 1971.
[80] Panconesi E. Psychosomatic dermatology. Clin Dermatol 1984;2:8–14.
[81] Meazzini P, Galeazzi A. Paure e fobie [Fear and phobias]. Firenze: Giunti-Barbera; 1979. p. 73–4.
[82] Sandier J, Davidson RS. Psychopathology: learning theory, research and applications. New York: Harper & Row; 1973.

# Stress and Psychoneuroimmunologic Factors in Dermatology

Mauro Urpe, PhD[a,b], Gionata Buggiani, MD[c], Torello Lotti, MD[b,]*

[a]Centro Interuniversitario di Dermatologia Biologica e Psicosomatica, University of Florence, Florence, Italy
[b]University Unit of Physical Therapy and Dermatology, University of Florence, Florence, Italy
[c]Department of Dermatology, University of Florence, Florence, Italy

Psychologic and social factors are believed to influence disease processes via two main mechanisms: psychosocial processes and health-oriented behaviors. Psychosocial processes include factors that affect interpretation of and response to life events and stressors, such as mental health and mood factors, personality characteristics, and resources, such as social relationships. Health-oriented behaviors (exercise, nutrition, and smoking) serve as indirect pathways by which psychosocial processes can influence health, as they may be influenced strongly by factors such as mood [1]. Within the domains of psychosocial processes and behavioral health, there are factors believed to serve as resources to enhance health (eg, social support and exercise) and vulnerability (eg, depression and cigarette smoking). These factors can be acute (eg, temporary lack of sleep before writing a grant) or chronic (eg, caregiving for a chronically-ill spouse). According to the biopsychosocial model, these psychosocial factors interact with a person's biologic characteristics (eg, genetic or constitutional) creating a vulnerability to disease processes [2]. Moreover, according to this model, a genetic predisposition to disease development (also known as "diathesis") may remain latent until stress events, which can be represented bypsychosocial factors interacting with a person's biologic characteristics, make the disease unfold.

Psychoneuroimmunology (PNI) was comprehensively described for the first time about 30 years ago. The influence of mental status on the course and outcome of a large number of diseases, however, was suspected long before then. The links between mental and affective disorders and immune status repeatedly were also suggested. PNI is commonly associated with the work of Ader and colleagues [3]. There also is clinical and experimental evidence that the body and mind communicate closely in health and illness. The association between illness and behavioral and psychologic states has been closely investigated recently showing that anxiety, sleep loss, bereavement, and certain external stress factors (eg, family illness, academic stress, unemployment) seem to affect immune function in some way. Not all the measured immune parameters were significantly altered in all these observations, however [4–9]. More available data also seem to link mental affective disorders, such as major depression and mania, with impaired immune function [10–12].

The link between personal relationships and immune function is one of the most significant findings in PNI [13]. When close relationships are discordant, they can be associated with immune disregulation. For example, pervasive differences in endocrine and immune function are associated reliably with hostile behaviors during marital conflict among diverse samples, including newlyweds selected on the basis of stringent mental and physical health criteria and couples married for an average of 42 years [14–18].

* Corresponding author. Department of Dermatology, University of Florence, Via della Pergola, 58/60, 50121 Florence, Italy.
E-mail address: torello.lotti@unifi.it (T. Lotti).

On the basis of findings for negative affect and social support, aspects of personality and coping styles associated with negative moods or social relationships might well demonstrate, under certain circumstances, immunologic disorders. For example, personality and coping styles (repression, rejection sensitivity, attributional style, sociability) are associated with altered levels of leukocytes in peripheral blood counts and with a dysregulation in cellular immune function [19]. Indeed, optimism has been associated with more positive moods, coping, and differences in response to stress among law students in their first year of study, and these differences seemed to mediate optimists' better immune function [20]. In another study, highly hostile individuals exhibited an increase in natural killer (NK)–cell cytotoxity after self-disclosure, greater than that observed in individuals who had lower levels of hostility [21]. This supports the authors' hypothesis that persons high in cynical hostility find disclosure more threatening; no differences between highly hostile and less hostile participants were observed in the nondisclosure condition. The study of individual differences in PNI is in its infancy, but the data are promising. As the data on personality and coping suggest, differences in perceptions and reactions to the same events can provoke different endocrine and immune responses. In fact, neuroendocrine mechanisms may mediate the associations between personality and coping styles and immune function [19].

## Interventions

PNI intervention studies involve different strategies, including hypnosis, relaxation, exercise, classical conditioning, self-disclosure, exposure to a phobic stressor to enhance perceived coping self-efficacy, and cognitive-behavioral therapies with a range of populations [22]. One excellent series of studies demonstrates that 10-week cognitive-behavioral stress management and aerobic-exercise training programs buffer distress responses and immune alterations [23–25].

## How do psychologic factors influence immune function?

The endocrine system serves as a central gateway for psychologic influences on health. Stress and depression can cause the release of pituitary and adrenal hormones that have multiple effects on immune function [26]. For example, negative emotions may also indirectly contribute to immune dysregulation evidenced by proinflammatory cytokine overproduction and repeated chronic or slow-resolving infections or wounds that enhance the secretion of proinflammatory cytokines—a process leading to further inhibition of certain branches of immune responses (eg, decreased levels of interleukin [IL]-2, an important defense against infection)—thus perhaps contributing to the immunodepression of aging [27]. Negative emotions, such as those evoked by depression or anxiety, can affect the immune system effectors directly and either up- or down-regulate proinflammatory cytokine secretion. In addition, negative emotions may also contribute to the self-maintenance mechanisms of chronic infections and pathologic delay in wound healing; two processes that indirectly boost proinflammatory cytokine production.

The relationship between psychiatric syndromes or symptoms and the immune system has been a consistent theme for decades. Early studies of psychotic subjects report various immune alterations, including abnormal levels of lymphocytes [28,29] and weaker-than-normal antibody response to whooping cough (*Bordetella pertussis*) vaccination [30] compared with nonpsychiatric controls. Subsequently, immunologic alterations are reported across a range of psychiatric disorders [31,32]. The majority of psychopathologically focused studies, however, have dealt with immunologic alterations associated with affective and anxiety symptoms and disorders [33–36]. There is consistent evidence that depression and anxiety can enhance the production of proinflammatory cytokines, including IL-6 [33–38]—an significant finding related to the broad literature on the morbidity and mortality associated with depressive and anxiety disorders (discussed later) [33–39]. In addition to syndromal depressive disorders, depressive symptoms can also provoke immune system alterations leading to dysregulation with serious health consequences. Elevated depressive symptoms, for example, are associated with lower $CD8^+$ T-lymphocyte counts and a higher rate of genital herpes simplex virus 2 recurrence over 6 months [34]. Depressive symptoms in HIV-positive homosexual men parallel decreased $CD4^+$ T-cell count, increased B-cell count, and increased immune activation marker HLA-DR, even when standardized for disease stage and health behaviors [36].

The evidence supporting a relationship between psychopathologic symptoms and disorders and immunologic alterations seems convincing. Furthermore, negative affect, a characteristic of most psychopathologic diseases, is conceptualized as a key pathway for other psychologic modifiers of immune function (described later), in particular interpersonal relationships and personality.

## Personality and coping

Personality and coping styles reflect individual differences in appraisal and response to stressors that may influence immune function. Reflecting the broader field of psychosomatic medicine at the time, much of the work before 1970 attempted to link personality traits to various diseases. For example, some researchers attempted to identify personality variables that predisposed individuals to allergic disorders [40–42]; skin reactivity to injected allergens (ie, wheal and flare size) was weaker in individuals who had personality styles described as passive, negative, withdrawn, unhappy, anxious, dissatisfied, and impulsive [4,41–43]. In another arena, relatives of patients who had rheumatoid arthritis and who lacked rheumatoid factor in their serum were more anxious and dysphoric than those who had the factor [44]. Specific personality characteristics, such as academic achievement, motivation, and aggression, are associated with immunologic alterations.

Among cadets at a military academy, high motivation to perform well interacted with poor actual academic performance and predicted greater susceptibility to Epstein-Barr virus (EBV) infection [45]. Aggression, operationalized using *Diagnostic and Statistical Manual of Mental Disorders, Revised Third Edition* antisocial personality disorder symptoms [46], was positively associated with T- and B-cell levels in male military personnel; this effect was independent from testosterone level, age, health status, or behavior [47]. Coping styles associated with altered immunity include repression, denial, escape-avoidance, and concealment. Greater reliance on repressive coping is associated with lower monocyte counts, higher eosinophil counts, higher serum glucose, more self-reported medication-reactions in a retrospective chart review of medical outpatients [48], and higher EBV antibody titres in students (the latter finding suggesting a decrease in memory T-cell response to the latent virus [49]). Among family members of bone marrow transplant patients, escape-avoidance coping coupled with anxiety traits was associated with fewer total T cells and fewer $CD4^+$ T cells; escape-avoidance coping by itself was associated with increased B-cell counts during the period preceding the transplant [50]. Denial coping seemed to have protective effects in homosexual men anticipating HIV-status notification. Among HIV-negative men, denial coping was associated with reduced intrusive thoughts, lower cortisol, and greater lymphocyte proliferation to phytohemagglutinin [51]. Although the majority of these studies were cross-sectional and involved students or young-to-middle–aged adults, one prospective study provided provocative evidence of notable health consequences. Concealment of homosexual identity predicted an accelerated course of HIV over 9 years of disease (assessed by $CD4^+$ T-cell counts), AIDS diagnosis, and AIDS mortality, even when controlling for demographic, health, and psychopathology factors [52]. Personality or coping style associated with emotional or affection regulation is likely to have immunologic correlates and styles that influence interpersonal relationships. In this context, it is not surprising that self-disclosure interventions may have immunologic consequences. For example, high-hostility subjects exhibited greater increases in NK-cell cytotoxicity after self-disclosure than low-hostility subjects (discussed previously). Greater emotional disclosure by students on a written task was associated with lower EBV virus capsid antigen IgG antibody titers than students who expressed less emotion when describing a personal stressful event [49]. Thus, self-disclosure is believed to be a factor associated with the health benefits of psychotherapy. These data are consistent with recent evidence of improvements in disease activity after self-disclosure in patients who had asthma and arthritis [53].

The support provided by social relationships can serve as a buffer during acute and chronic stressors, protecting against immune dysregulation. For example, early studies suggest that lonelier medical students and psychiatric inpatients had poorer cell immune function than their counterparts who reported less loneliness [30–45,47–57]. Subsequent investigators report that lower levels of social support in the context of naturalistic stressors, such as job strain [58], dementia caregiving [59,60], and surgery [61], are associated with poorer immune function. Social support also may be important for immunity during the exposure to short-term stressors, such as examination tasks. Moreover, greater social support is linked with better immune responses to the hepatitis B vaccine in medical students [55]. The link between personal relationships and immune function is one of the strongest findings in PNI spanning diverse populations and stressors [13]. In a sample of men who were HIV-positive, low-perceived emotional support was associated with a more rapid decline in $CD4^+$ T cells, an important marker of HIV-infection progression [62]. Higher NK-cell activity in female patients who had breast cancer was related to high-quality emotional support from husbands or mates, perceived social support from the patients' physicians, and the patients' actively seeking social support as a coping strategy [63]. Disruption of close relationships has well-documented consequences for immune function, whether or not the disruption is the result of bereavement [36–45,47–55] or divorce [58,64,65]. In addition, the maintenance of abrasive close relationships also exerts a toll; among newlywed couples engaged in a 30-minute conflict-resolution task, individuals who exhibited more hostile or negative behaviors during conflict showed greater decrements in functional immune measures 24 hours later [66] and concurrent alterations in stress hormones [63]. Similar patterns emerged in older couples married an average of 42 years [64]. These results were striking, particularly given that the majority of young and old couples had happy marriages; thus, these findings actually may underestimate the physiologic impact of troubled relationships [67].

Furthermore, a well-recognized model of chronic stress (eg, stress of caring for a spouse who has Alzheimer's disease) is linked to a host of immune impairments, including decreased NK response to interferon (IFN)-$\gamma$ and IL-2, poorer lymphoproliferative response to mitogens, impaired antibody response to influenza vaccine, poorer responses to delayed hypersensitivity skin testing, higher levels of the sympathetic neurotransmitter neuropeptide Y, slower wound healing [68], and higher levels of IL-6 F [69]. Moreover, compared with noncaregivers, dementia caregivers exhibited higher percentages and increased numbers of $CD4^+$ and $CD8^+$ cells expressing T-helper cell–2 (Th-2) cytokine and IL-10; but no changes in expression of Th-1 cytokines, IFN-$\gamma$, or IL-2 in these cells were noted, suggesting a stress-related Th-1 to -2 shift. Dementia caregivers also reported more days of infectious illness than noncaregivers [1]. These findings indicate the importance of considering interactions between stress and aging in the context of the additional vulnerability that may be conferred by individual medical history. Repetitive patterns of short-term negative emotions also are believed to constitute chronic stressors [1].

PNI research has thus contributed to the larger literature on social relationships and health by delineating another pathway through which relationships can be beneficial or detrimental to health outcomes.

There now are sufficient data to conclude that immune modulation by psychosocial stressors or interventions can lead to actual health changes. Although changes related to infectious disease and wound healing provide the strongest evidence to date, the clinical importance of immunologic dysregulation is highlighted by increased risks across diverse conditions and diseases related to proinflammatory cytokines [62,63,67–75]. The PNI field has grown tremendously over the past two decades, and the future looks even more promising.

## Psychoneuroimmunology in dermatology

Mental and psychic issues are also important in the genesis or development of many diseases. The psychologic or psychiatric genesis of a skin disease, however, still remains one of the most debated and controversial arguments present in contemporary medicine and academia. This controversy is in part due to the ease with which a poorly understand and hard to treat disease can be labeled as having "psychosomatic pathogenesis". Labeling occurs often in dermatology because it is a field in which "elementary psychosomatic signs" are common (ie, pallor, sweat, horripilation, itch, and redness). Psychologic influence should be considered in dermatologic affections [76] and many common dermatologic diseases have some form of psychomediated pathogenesis that partly accounts for the development of lesions. Clinical observations show a well-defined link between acute or chronic emotional stressors, psychiatric diseases, conflict, hostility, personality, mood, and dermatoses (whether increased, developing, or in remission) and also report positive effects of psychopharmacology and psychotherapy on the same diseases. "Mental" events, such as hypnosis and psychologic stress, can influence delayed-type hypersensitivity responses, ultraviolet B ray–induced erythema, and the genesis of wheals after histamine prick test [77]. Hyperhydrosis, telogen effluvium, idiopathic itch, lichen simplex, rosacea, alopecia areata, vitiligo, seborrhoic dermatitis, psoriasis, acnes, atopic dermatitis, viral warts, herpes simplex, and urticaria all can be associated with some psychomediated mechanism.

The psycho-immune-endocrine-cutaneous system functions as a primary route of communication between mind and body. The skin can be seen as the juncture of the simultaneous and connected activity of brain, immune system, and the skin itself. Neuropeptides, interleukines, and immune-system messengers are the means through which communication among the three entities takes place. $\alpha$–Melanocyte-stimulating hormone ($\alpha$-MSH) is one of the most investigated mediators in this system. $\alpha$-MSH is a neuropeptide whose immune-modulating activity seems to inhibit inflammation generated in the skin [78,79]. It is a 13-amino-acid–polipeptide derived from pro-opiomelanocortin and primarily synthesized by the hypophisis. α-MSH can also be released by the skin when a series of structures not belonging to the nervous system synthesize and release pro-opiomelanocortin, its derivatives, and a series of other substances after the "diffuse-brain" demonstration (substance P, calcitonin gene-related peptide, vasoactive intestinal peptide, neuropeptide Y, etc), which are capable of influencing human sensations, feelings, and behavior [80].

Neuropeptides are released by skin cells and Aδ and C nerve fibers that link the nervous system and the skin itself. α-MSH, in particular, seems to decrease tumor necrosis factor α (TNF-α) and IL-1 release from macrophages and neutrophils and stimulates anti-inflammatory cytokine production (eg, IL-10). Furthermore, α-MSH may regulate the expression of cell mediators on the surface of immune cells. In animal models, the injection of α-MSH into the central nervous system of mice can inhibit cutaneous inflammation caused by topical irritatives and intradermal inoculation proinflammatory cytokines, such as IL-1β, IL-8, leukotriene $B_4$, and platelet activating factor [81]. This may possibly occur through the local release of other neuropeptides, such as vasoactive intestinal peptide and calcitonin gene-related peptide. The mechanism of action, however, still remains partially unknown, but it would seem that these neuropeptides may also act directly by inhibiting proinflammatory cytokine production (TNF- α, IL-6, IL-1, and IL-2) and nuclear factor κB (NF-κB) expression (a proinflammatory transcription factor) by monocytes, macrophages, and neutrophils. Furthermore, α-MSH reportedly decreases IFN-γ release from activated lymphocytes and increase IL-10 production in peripheral blood monocytes [82–84].

α-MSH also seems to interfere with leukocyte migration from blood to sites of inflammation, modifying the expression of leukocyte and endothelial adhesion molecules and endothelial leukocyte and vascular cell adhesion molecules−1. These data suggest that α-MSH and other neuropeptides may function as novel powerful therapeutic antinflammatory agents in dermatology [84].

Only a few clinical and experimental studies, however, have investigated the association of these data and well-defined clinical entities (psoriasis, itch, etc.). A majority of the observations are limited to parallel clinical entities and macroscopic psychologic states. In other words, it is common knowledge that psoriasis is worsened by stress, but no clinical study convincingly reports which defined molecular mechanisms are involved in this phenomenon.

For other dermatoses, more investigation is required. Various speculative etiology and epidemiologic studies of atopic dermatitis are discussed repeatedly [85]. The basic consensus is that this disease consists of complex immunologic reactions that partially are inherited, although a few reports suggest that "allergy" is not always central to the development of atopic dermatitis [86]. Because atopic dermatitis is also a chronic skin disease, psychologic aspects of the disease must also be taken into account. Kasamatsu and colleagues stated that IL-4 serum levels in patients who have atopic dermatitis were significantly higher than those of normal controls [87]. Other investigators report that IFN-γ production by Th-1 and -0 cells predominates IL-4 production by Th-2 and -0 cells in the late and chronic phases of atopic patch tests in patients who have atopic dermatitis. Hashiro and Okumura [88] investigated the relationship between the psychologic and immunologic states in patients who had atopic dermatitis by measuring IL-4 and IFN-γ levels in serum. Although no significant correlation was detected between any pair of psychologic and immunologic results in patients or normal controls, psychologic variables seemed to affect serum IFN-γ significantly and, to a lesser degree, IL-4, in patients who had atopic dermatitis. Trait and state anxiety seem to affect NK-cell activity, although psychosomatic symptoms do not affect NK activity in patients who have atopic dermatitis. In sum, patients who have moderate or severe atopic dermatitis score significantly higher in depressive or anxiety states and, alternatively, show significantly lower NK-cell activity and IL-4 levels in serum than normal controls. Thus, in patients who have atopic dermatitis, psychologic factors seem to affect serum IFN-γ and IL-4, whereas NK activity is affected not by psychosomatic complaints but mainly by anxiety. Patients who have atopic dermatitis may differ from nonaffected ones by low NK-cell activity and slightly higher serum IFN-γ.

Regarding urticaria, in a high percentage of cases of chronic recalcitrant disease, the authors were not able to isolate the antigen or substances provoking the symptoms. This may be because an incomplete number of antigens were tested. Alternatively, it seems that "emotional allergy" [89] is more common than currently acknowledged. Psychologic factors also may contribute to urticaria in which the antigen is well known. Psychosocial and psychiatric factors may act in the pathogenesis of urticaria, increasing the release of neuro- and immunemediators, mainly from mast cells (eg, IL-4, IL-5, IFN-γ, and TNF-α) and release of vasoactive peptides (including histamine) paralleling the pathogenetic pathways of other systemic diseases discussed previously (viral and chronic infections, delayed wound healing, poorer antibody-mediated responses, etc.). There is no evidence, however, of these pathways in urticaria.

There is conclusive evidence of psychoneuroimmune mechanisms in the pathogenesis of vitiligo—a hypomelanotic skin disorder usually aesthetically compromising, so that a somatopsychic rebound seems logical. Vitiligo changes one's personal body image so that maintaining or forming relationships becomes more difficult [90]. Many patients who have vitiligo feel depressed, experience a reduced self-esteem, and perceive a reduction in quality of life [91,92]. Some investigators have examined the role of life stress events as factors provoking the development of vitiligo [93]. Newly diagnosed patients and matched controls were asked to complete the 12-month version of the Schedule of Recent Experience, a questionnaire measuring the frequency and number of stressful life events occurring over a specified period. The results suggest that these patients endure a significantly higher number of stressful life events than do controls, suggesting that psychologic distress may have contributed to the onset of their condition.

The same investigators tested the effect of cognitive-behavioral support therapy on coping with vitiligo and adaptation to the negative effects on body image, self-esteem, and quality of life in adult patients who had vitiligo and in control patients receiving a classic treatment. The study also examined if any psychologic gains acquired from psychologic therapy influenced the progression of the condition itself. Results suggested that patients could benefit from cognitive behavioral therapy in terms of coping with vitiligo. Preliminary evidence also suggests that psychologic therapy may have a positive effect on the progression of the condition itself [94].

The above observations are partly consistent with two of the numerous pathogenetic pathways of vitiligo: the neural and autoimmune hypotheses. Patients who have vitiligo show abnormal secretion of neuromediators (eg, $\beta$-endorphin and metenkephalin) and a higher immunoreactivity to neuropeptide Y and vasoactive intestinal peptide [95]. Not all effects of neuropeptides on melanocytes are known, though the nervous system seems to play a role in activating melanocytes; psychologic and psychiatric issues and chronic stress are demonstrated to be linked to and increase expression of neuropeptide Y and other mediators.

Alternatively, much clinical and experimental evidence suggests a role of humoral and cellular autoimmunity in vitiligo pathogenesis. Alteration in the levels and ratio of $CD4^+$ and $CD8^+$ T-lymphocytes reported in vitiligo are somewhat consistent with the same alterations seen in particular mental states, such as depression, anxiety, chronic stressors, and mood disturbances. These alterations may be strictly linked and altered mental and psychologic states may produce, at least in this context, a portion of the alterations reported in vitiligo pathogenesis [96].

# Summary

Clinical and experimental data supports the brain's ability to start, influence, and stop biologic events in the skin. The skin, as a relevant part of the diffuse brain, can modify the quality of perceptions and feelings, as suggested by relevant studies. The immune and the endocrine systems may act as protagonists of the modulation of these events and, in this context, psychosocial stressors and interventions can lead to global health changes of great interest to dermatologists.

# References

[1] Kiecolt-Glaser JK, Mcguire L, Robles TF, et al. Emotions, morbidity, and mortality. New perspectives from psychoneuroimmunology. Annu Rev Psychol 2002;53:83–107.
[2] Engel GF. The need for a new medical model: a challenge for biomedicine. Science 1977;196:129–36.
[3] Ader R, Cohen N, Felten D. Psychoneuroimmunology: interactions between the nervous system and the immune system. Lancet 1995;345(8942):99–103.
[4] Bartrop RW, Luckhurst C, Lazarus L, et al. Depressed lymphocyte function after bereavement. Lancet 1977; 1:834–6.
[5] Jemmot JB, Borysenko JZ, Borysenko M, et al. Academic stress power motivation and decrease in secretion rate of salivary secretory immunoglobin A. Lancet 1983;1:1400–2.
[6] Kiecolt-Glaser JK, Glaser R, Shuttleworth EC, et al. Chronic stress and immunity in family caregivers of alzheimer's disease victims. Psychosom Med 1987;49: 523–35.
[7] Graham NMH, Chiron R, Bartholomeusz A, et al. Does anxiety reduce the secretion rate of secretory iga in saliva? Med J Aust 1988;148:131–3.
[8] Fell LR, Shut DA. Behavioural and hormonal response to acute surgical stress in sheep. Appl Anim Behav Sci 1989;22:283–94.
[9] Moldofsky H, Lue FA, Davidson JR, et al. Effect of sleep deprivation on human immune function. FASEB J 1989;3:1972–7.

[10] Irwin M, Daniels M, Bloom ET, et al. Life events, depressive symptoms and immune function. Am J Psychiatry 1987;144:437–41.

[11] Irwin M. Depression and immune function. Stress 1988;4:95–103.

[12] Maes M, Bosmans E, Calabrese J, et al. Interleukin-2 and interleukin-6 in schizophrenia and mania: effect of neuroleptics and mood stabilizers. J Psychiatry Res 1995;29:141–52.

[13] Uchino BN, Cacioppo JT, Kiecolt-Glaser JK. The relationship between social support and physiological processes: a review with emphasis on underlying mechanisms. Psychol Bull 1996;119:488–531.

[14] Kiecolt-Glaser JK, Glaser R, Cacioppo JT, et al. Marital conflict in older adults: endocrinological and immunological correlates. Psychosom Med 1997;59:339–49.

[15] Kiecolt-Glaser JK, Malarkey WB, Chee M, et al. Negative behaviour during marital conflict is associated with immunological down-regulation. Psychosom Med 1993;55:395–409.

[16] Kiecolt-Glaser JK, Newton T, Cacioppo JT, et al. Marital conflict and endocrine function: are men really more physiologically affected than women? J Consult Clin Psychol 1996;64:324–32.

[17] Malarkey WB, Kiecolt-Glaser JK, Pearl D, et al. Hostile behavior during marital conflict alters pituitary and adrenal hormones. Psychosom Med 1994;56:41–51.

[18] Mayne TJ, O'leary A, McGrady B, et al. The differential effects of acute marital distress on emotional, physiological and immune functions in martially distressed men and women. Psychol Health 1997;122:77–88.

[19] Segerstrom SC. Personality and the immune system: models methods, and mechanisms. Annu Rev Behav Med 2000;22:180–90.

[20] Segerstrom SC, Taylor SE, Kemeny ME, et al. Optimism is associated with mood, coping and immune change in response to stress. J Pers Soc Psychol 1998;74:1646–55.

[21] Christensen AJ, Edwards DL, Wiebe JS, et al. Effect of verbal selfdisclosure on natural killer cell activity: moderating influence of cynical hostility. Psychosom Med 1996;58:150–5.

[22] Kiecolt-Glaser JK, Glaser R. Psychoneuroimmunology: can psychological interventions modulate Immunity? J Consult Clin Psychol 1992;60:569–75.

[23] Antoni MH. Cognitive behavioural intervention for person with HIV. In: Spira JL, editor. Group therapy for medically ill patients. New York: Guilford Press; 1997. p. 55–91.

[24] Schneiderman N, Antoni M, Ironson G, et al. HIV-1, immunity and behaviour. In: Glaser R, Kiecolt-Glaser JK, editors. Handbook of humane stress and immunity. San Diego: Academic Press; 1994. p. 267–300.

[25] Schneiderman N, Antoni M, Saab PG, et al. Health psychology: psychosocial and biobehavioral aspects of chronic disease management. Annu Rev Psychol 2001;52:555–80.

[26] Rabin BS. Stress immune function and health: the connection. New York: Wiley-Liss & Sons; 1999.

[27] Catania A, Airaghi L, Motta P, et al. Cytokine antagonists in aged subjects and their relation with cellular immunity. J Gerontol Biol Sci Med Sci 1997;52A:B93–7.

[28] Freeman H, Elmadjian F. The relationship between blood sugar and lymphocyte levels in normal and psychotic subjects. Psychosom Med 1947;9:226–33.

[29] Phillips L, Elmadjian F. A Rorschach Tension Score and the Diurnal Lymphocyte Curve in psychotic subjects. Psychosom Med 1947;9:364–71.

[30] Vaughan WTJ, Sullivan JC, Elmadjian F. Immunity and schizophrenia. Psychosom Med 1949;11:327–33.

[31] Kiecolt-Glaser JK, Ricker D, George J, et al. Urinary cortisol levels, cellular immunocompetency, and loneliness in psychiatric inpatients. Psychosom Med 1984;46:15–24.

[32] Appelberg B, Katila H, Rimon R. Plasma interleukin-1 beta and sleep architecture in schizophrenia and other nonaffective psychoses. Psychosom Med 1997;59:529–32.

[33] Appels A, Bar FW, Bar J, et al. Inflammation, depressive symptomatology, and coronary artery disease. Psychosom Med 2000;62:601–5.

[34] Kemeny M, Cohen F, Zegens L. Psychological and immunological predictors of genital herpes recurrence. Psychosom Med 1989;51:195–208.

[35] Koh KB, Lee BK. Reduced lymphocyte proliferation and interleukin-2 production in anxiety Disorders. Psychosom Med 1998;60:479–83.

[36] Kemeny ME, Weiner H, Duran R, et al. Immune system changes after the death of a partner in hiv-positive gay men. Psychosom Med 1995;57:547–54.

[37] Dentino AN, Pieper CF, Rao KMK, et al. Association of interleukin-6 and other biologic variables with depression in older people living in the community. J Am Geriatr Soc 1999;47:6–11.

[38] Maes M, Lin A, Delmeire L, et al. Elevated serum interleukin-6 (IL-6) and IL-6 receptor concentrations in posttraumatic stress disorder following accidental man-made traumatic events. Biol Psychiatry 1999;45:833–9.

[39] Kiecolt-Glaser JK, McGuire L, Robles TF, et al. Emotions, morbidity, and mortality: new perspectives from psychoneuroimmunology. Annu Rev Psychol 2002;53:83–107 [review].

[40] Cassell WA, Fisher S. Body image boundaries and histamine flare reaction. Psychosom Med 1963;25:344–50.

[41] Jacobs MA, Friedman MA, Franklin MJ, et al. Incidence of psychosomatic predisposing factors in allergic disorders. Psychosom Med 1966;28:679–95.

[42] Ely NE, Verhey JW, Holmes TH. Experimental studies of skin inflammation. Psychosom Med 1963;25:264–84.

[43] Solomon GF, Moos RH. The relationship of personality to the presence of rheumatoid factor in asymptomatic relatives of patients with rheumatoid arthritis. Psychosom Med 1965;27:350–60.

[44] Kasl SV, Evans AS, Niederman JC. Psychosocial risk factors in the development of infectious mononucleosis. Psychosom Med 1979;41:445–66.
[45] Granger DA, Booth A, Johnson DR. Human aggression and enumerative measures of immunity. Psychosom Med 2000;62:583–90.
[46] American Psychiatric Association. Diagnostic and statistical manual of mental disorders. 3rd edition. Washington, DC: American Psychiatric Association; 1980.
[47] Jamner LD, Schwartz GE, Leigh H. The relationship between repressive and defensive coping styles and monocyte, eosinophil, and serum glucose levels: support for the opioid peptide hypothesis of repression. Psychosom Med 1988;50:567–75.
[48] Esterling B, Antoni M, Kumar M, et al. Emotional repression, stress disclosure responses, and Epstein-Barr viral capsid antigen titers. Psychosom Med 1990;52:397–410.
[49] Futterman AD, Wellisch DK, Zighelboim J, et al. Psychological and immunological reactions of family members to patients undergoing bone marrow transplantation. Psychosom Med 1996;58:472–80.
[50] Antoni MH, August BA, Laperriere A, et al. Psychological and neuroendocrine measures related to functional immune changes in anticipation Of HIV-1 serostatus notification. Psychosom Med 1990;52:496–510.
[51] Cole SW, Kemeny M, Taylor SE, et al. Accelerated course of human immunodeficiency virus infection in gay men who conceal their homosexual identity. Psychosom Med 1996;58:219–31.
[52] Smyth JM, Stone AA, Hurewitz A, et al. Effects of writing about stressful experiences on symptom reduction in patients with asthma or rheumatoid arthritis: a randomized trial. JAMA 1999;17:1304–9.
[53] Bartrop R, Luckhurst E, Lazarus L, et al. Depressed lymphocyte function after bereavement. Lancet 1977;1:374–7.
[54] Glaser R, Kiecolt-Glaser JK, Bonneau RH, et al. Stress-induced modulation of the immune response to recombinant hepatitis b vaccine. Psychosom Med 1992;54:22–9.
[55] Mitchell JH, Curran CA, Myers RN. Some psychosomatic aspects of allergic diseases. Psychosom Med 1947;9:184–91.
[56] Kiecolt-Glaser JK, Garner W, Speicher C, et al. Psychosocial modifiers of immunocompetence in medical students. Psychosom Med 1984;46:7–14.
[57] Linn BS, Linn MW, Klimas NG. Effects of psychophysical stress on surgical outcome. Psychosom Med 1988;50:230–44.
[58] Kiecolt-Glaser JK, Fisher LD, Ogrocki P, et al. Marital quality, marital disruption, and immune function. Psychosom Med 1987;49:31–4.
[59] Esterling BA, Kiecolt-Glaser JK, Glaser R. Psychosocial modulation of cytokine-induced natural killer cell activity in older adults. Psychosom Med 1996;58:264–72.
[60] Theorell T, Orth-Gomer K, Eneroth P. Slow-reacting immunoglobulin in relation to social support and changes in job strain: a preliminary note. Psychosom Med 1990;52:511–6.
[61] Kiecolt-Glaser JK, Dura JR, Speicher CE, et al. Spousal caregivers of dementia victims: longitudinal changes in immunity and health. Psychosom Med 1991;53:345–62.
[62] Levy SM, Herberman RB, Whiteside T, et al. Perceived social support and tumor estrogen/progesterone receptor status as predictors of natural killer cell activity in breast cancer patients. Psychosom Med 1990;52:73–85.
[63] Malarkey W, Kiecolt-Glaser JK, Pearl D, et al. Hostile behavior during marital conflict alters pituitary and adrenal hormones. Psychosom Med 1994;56:41–51.
[64] Kiecolt-Glaser JK, Glaser R, Cacioppo JT, et al. Marital conflict in older adults: endocrinological and immunological correlates. Psychosom Med 1997;59:339–49.
[65] Kiecolt-Glaser JK, Kennedy S, Malkoff S, et al. Marital discord and immunity in males. Psychosom Med 1988;50:213–29.
[66] Kiecolt-Glaser JK, Malarkey WB, Chee M, et al. Negative behavior during marital conflict is associated with immunological down-regulation. Psychosom Med 1993;55:395–409.
[67] Kiecolt-Glaser JK, Newton T. Marriage and health: his and hers. Psychol Bull 2001;127(4):472–503 [review].
[68] Glaser R, Maccallum R, Laskowski B, et al. Evidence for a shift in the th-1 to th-2 cytokine response associated with chronic stress and aging. J Gerontol A Biol Sci Med Sci 2001;56:M477–82.
[69] Lutgendorf S, Garand L, Buckwalter K, et al. Life stress, mood disturbance, and elevated IL-6 in healthy older women. J Gerontol A Biol Sci Med Sci 1999;54:M434–9.
[70] Papanicolaou DA, Wilder RL, Manolagas SC, et al. The pathophysiologic roles of interleukin-6 in human disease. Ann Intern Med 1998;128:127–37.
[71] Theorell T, Blomkvist V, Jonsson H, et al. Social support and the development of immune function in human immunodeficiency virus infection. Psychosom Med 1995;57:32–6.
[72] Hamerman D. Toward an understanding of frailty. Ann Intern Med 1999;130:945–50.
[73] Ershler W, Keller E. Age-associated increased interleukin-6 gene expression, late-life diseases, and frailty. Annu Rev Med 2000;51:245–70.
[74] Harris T, Ferrucci L, Tracy R, et al. Associations of elevated interleukin-6 And C-reactive protein levels with mortality in the elderly. Am J Med 1999;106:506–12.
[75] Cohen H, Pieper C, Harris T, Rao K, Currie M. The association of plasma IL-6 levels with functional disability in communitydwelling elderly. J Gerontol A Biol Sci Med Sci 1997;52:M201–8.
[76] Panconesi E. Psychosomatic dermatology in stress and skin disease. Clin Dermatol 1984;4:1–272.
[77] Locke SE, Ransil BJ, Zacharie R, et al. Effect of

hypnotic suggestion on the delayed type hypersensitivity response. JAMA 1994;272:47–52.
[78] Luger TA, Scholzen T, Brzoska T, et al. Cutaneous immunomodulation and coordination of skin stress responses by α-MSH. Ann N Y Acad Sci 1998;840: 381–94 [review].
[79] Lotti T, Bianchi B, Ghersetich I, et al. Can the brain inhibit inflammation generated in the skin? The lesson of gamma-melanocyte-stimulating hormone. Int J Dermatol 2002;41(6):311–8 [review].
[80] Lotti T, Hautmann G, Panconesi E. Neuropeptides and skin. J Am Acad Dermatol 1995;33:482–96.
[81] Lipton JM, Macaluso A, Hiltz ME, et al. Central administration of the peptide α-MSH inhibits inflammation in the skin. Peptides 1991;12:795–8.
[82] Lipton JM, Catania A. Antinflammatory actions of the neuroimmunomodulator α-MSH. Immunol Today 1997;18:140–5.
[83] Bhardwaj RS, Schwarz A, Becher E, et al. Proopiomelanocortin-derived peptides induce IL-10 production in human monocytes. J Immunol 1996;156:2517–21.
[84] Luger TA, Lotti T. Neuropeptides: role in inflammatory skin diseases. J Eur Acad Dermatol Venereol 1998;10:207–11.
[85] Rothe MJ, Grant-Kel JM. Atopic dermatitis: an update. J Am Acad Dermatol 1996;35:1–13.
[86] Halbert AR, Weston WL, Morelli JG. Atopic dermatitis: is it an allergic disease? J Am Acad Dermatol 1995;33:1008–18.
[87] Kasamatsu M, Tsuji T, Miura M. A method for quantification of interleukin-4 in serum (sandwich elisa) and IL4 levels in patients with atopic dermatitis. Jpn Allergol 1993;42:878–82.
[88] Hashiro M, Okumura M. The relationship between the psychological and immunological state in patients with atopic dermatitis. J Dermatol Sci 1998;16: 231–5.
[89] Panconesi E, Cossidente A. Dermatologia psicosomatica. In: Panconesi E, editor. Manuale di dermatologia. II edition. Torino (Italy): UTET; 1992.
[90] Hautmann G, Panconesi E. Vitiligo: a psychologically influenced and influencing disease. Psychosom Dermatol 1984;3:78–93.
[91] Porter JR, Beuf AH, Lerner A, et al. Psychosocial effect of vitiligo: a comparison of vitiligo patients with "normal" control subjects, with psoriasis patients, and with patients with other pigmentary disorders. J Am Acad Dermatol 1986;15(2 Pt 1):220–4.
[92] Dent G, Al'Abadie M. Factors affecting responses on Dermatology Life Quality Index items among vitiligo sufferers. Clin Exp Dermatol 1996;214:330–3.
[93] Papadopoulos L, Bor R, Legg C, et al. Impact of life events on the onset of vitiligo in adults: preliminary evidence for a psychological dimension in aetiology. Clin Exp Dermatol 1998;23:243–8.
[94] Papadopoulos L, Bor R, Legg C. Coping with the disfiguring effects of vitiligo: a preliminary investigation into the effects of cognitive-behavioural therapy. Br J Med Psychol 1999;72(Pt3):385–96.
[95] Mozzanica N, Villa ML, Foppa S. Plasma a-melanocyte stimulating hormone, β endorphin, met-enkephalin, and natural killer cell activity in vitiligo. J Am Acad Dermatol 1992;26:693–700.
[96] Lotti T, Hercogova J, editors. Vitiligo: problems and solutions. New York: Marcel Dekker; 2004.

# The Emotional Impact of Chronic and Disabling Skin Disease: A Psychoanalytic Perspective

Caroline S. Koblenzer, MD[a,b],*

[a]Department of Dermatology, University of Pennsylvania, Philadelphia, PA, USA
[b]Institute of the Psychoanalytic Center of Philadelphia, Philadelphia, PA, USA

In Biblical times, and until the Middle Ages, when disease was believed to be an expression of the wrath of God, visited on those who had sinned [1], all diseases of the skin were believed contagious. Even today, some hold this archaic belief. Now it is believed that much of what was considered leprosy in those early times may have been psoriasis [2,3], but skin disease sufferers were excommunicated and condemned to live separately in huts; their garments, sometimes even their houses, were burned; and they were declared dead by the church, their approach announced by horn or bell [3]. In our own times, by contrast, the significance of skin disease, in the context of the general health of patients, tends to be depreciated by the medical community. "It's only a rash" or "it isn't life-threatening" often has been the attitude of colleagues in other fields of medicine; only recently has attention been paid to the significant impact of chronic disfiguring or disabling skin disease on the quality of life of patients and their families. Although sometimes patients express alarm about a transient and eminently treatable skin disease, the focus of this article is on the disorders about which there is most research, that have significant impact, and that tend to be chronic. Psoriasis, atopic dermatitis, and acne are examples, although the principles pertain to the spectrum of dermatologic disorders.

Tables have been constructed within recent years that quantify, in a reproducible manner, the negative impact of skin disease on quality of life for pediatric and adult sufferers [4–7]. This aspect of dermatology, largely neglected until now, is of great relevance in the current political climate where little time per patient is afforded dermatologists; the information generated by these studies serves to justify the appropriate expenditure by the government and other third-party payers for treatments that often are expensive and that may be misunderstood by those outside of the field.

Whereas these tables provide much information about experiencing skin disease at a conscious level, they tell little about the developmental roots or the internal meanings of experiences to patients. It is the goal of this article to explore some of those developmental roots and understand their deeper meanings. Although occasional patients are able to take in stride disease that is disfiguring or disabling, for many patients, the experience of being "different" is frightening, leading to feelings of embarrassment and shame; to feeling stigmatized; or to feeling marked as standing out, as the body of Christ was said to have been marked by the crucifixion (the origin of the word *stigma*).

Disease in any organ inevitably affects the sense of personal integrity, seeming to say, in physical terms, something negative about the totality of the self. Elderly people who are deaf, for example, not infrequently refuse to wear a hearing aid, because such appliances make manifest the aging process, causing individuals to feel less whole. Many women, in like fashion, feel less feminine after surgery for

---

* 1812 Delancey Place, Philadelphia, PA 19103.
  E-mail address: cskpjk@comcast.net

hysterectomy or mastectomy, which result in physical changes that, although not readily evident, affect the totality of the way in which individuals experience self.

How much greater an issue, then, is disease of the skin, that part of the whole that presents to the world, that is the barrier between the self and the outside world, and that is seen first and judged first in any social interaction. The impact of skin conditions on patients and families is complex and depends on several variables. Perhaps most important are the early life experiences of patients and the quality of interaction that takes place between patients and primary caretakers in infancy. It is the nature of this interaction that determines the integrity of the body image, the level of self-esteem that evolves, and the capacity of individuals to adapt [8–11]. Also important are the age at which the condition develops, the nature of the disease itself, the capacity of families to cope, and the capacity of society to accept. Each of these is considered in this article [12], much of which is culled from clinical experience gleaned from working with patients.

## Developmental issues

### Body image

The emotional environment for infants is encompassed by the relationship with the mother or primary caretaker. With an empathic touch, mothers define for infants the physical boundaries of the self and enable infants to discriminate their bodies from the surroundings, the "me" from the "not me" [8,9]. The greater the extent of the empathic touching at this early stage, the closer to reality is the body image that develops [10]. An empathic reciprocity between caretakers and infants, with a mirroring of emotional responses, helps to reinforce the sense of boundaries and at the same time integrate and organize the developing psychic functioning [9,11,13,14]. "Body image" means a cohesive mental representation of the self, with physical and psychic components. This is a dynamic concept, with ongoing changes that must be integrated as the individual matures. The stability and integrity of the body image have great significance in dermatology, because when they are not optimal, the interpretation of symptoms may be faulty, as in body dysmorphic disorder [15], or the skin may be used to provide emotional stimulation or define boundaries, as in dermatitis artifacta [16] or severe atopic dermatitis. The emotional impact of the disease on these patients is profound.

### Self-esteem

It is through this emotional dialog between infants and caretakers that self-esteem is born. Infants who are completely accepted, loved, and admired incorporate these positive feelings into their own personality [17] along with a healthy positive self-esteem and a capacity to accept and cope better with whatever adversities life may bring. Less fortunate infants are likely to have less effective self-esteem regulation, be less flexible, and be less able to adapt. These patients are subject to depression and feelings of embarrassment and humiliation that disrupt every aspect of their lives [18,19].

### Tension regulation

The infantile response to all stimuli is physical. Pain, hunger, anxiety, and discomfort all lead to crying and physical movement, which become progressively more frantic if soothing does not take place. It is the empathic holding, touching, and soothing by caretakers that enable infants gradually to master, and internalize, the capacity to regulate tension [19,20]. When tension regulation is not mastered, then discharge through physical pathways persist into adult life, with the possibility that psychophysiologic symptoms may ensue [21].

It is the success with which each of these infantile tasks, the development of body image and self-esteem and the regulation of tension, is accomplished, that determines to a great extent the degree to which skin disease has an impact on patients emotionally and the characteristics of that impact.

### Age of onset

When children have a congenital abnormality, or one that develops in early infancy, it is the emotional response of the parents that helps to determine the emotional impact. Common examples are vascular or pigmented birthmarks [22], epidermolysis bullosa, and atopic dermatitis. If parents can come to terms with the situation and accept, admire, and love the child, as they would a child without an abnormality, these positive attitudes are incorporated into the child's personality, and the abnormality is accepted as just a part of the self [23]. Such parents are able to focus on and foster the positive aspects of their developing child, permitting healthy self-esteem, firm boundaries, and adaptive capabilities to evolve. As an example, a child who has congenital ichthyosis, who was born to a supportive and united family, was never made to feel different. Her skin was stimulated constantly in a variety of ways by topical treatments, and her strengths were supported by loving parents and grandparents, so that despite her abnormal skin, she had firm boundaries and healthy positive self-esteem and has been able to have a successful professional life, with many meaningful and long term relationships [24], one of which led to the birth of a child.

In conditions where the epidermis is altered grossly, and where the tactile experience and the quality of the infant-caretaker dialog may be impaired, the possibility of body-image issues is real and may result in a personality with borderline features. These patients have painful feelings of emptiness, heightened anxiety, and poor impulse control, and for them, skin disease has a severe emotional impact. This was the case for another patient [24], whose severe atopic dermatitis demanded that his limbs be wrapped constantly by his anxious and emotionally distant mother through much of his early childhood. Wrapping and immobilization was accepted treatment at that time. Because of this, he was denied the needed empathic touching [10,11,14,25], and in his adult life he developed borderline features with feelings of boredom and emptiness. At time he scratched frenetically to affirm his boundaries, comfort himself, and assure himself that he really was there. Because of his early experiences and the persistence of his eczema, this patient had great difficulties with relationships.

When onset of a problem is in later childhood, once the basis of the body image is established, the emotional impact likely is much greater. The altered skin feels alien, not a part of the self and, therefore, alarming. Children feel self-conscious and often ashamed; they also may feel guilty that the rash is something they caused through some real or perceived transgression [26]. Frequently, anxieties focus on issues of body integrity and boundaries—even life itself—and, lacking adequate information or understanding, fantasies about what may happen—cancer, death, disintegration, and so forth—and feelings of loss of control increase that anxiety. Anxiety is exacerbated further by the reaction of peer groups, who, with their own disturbing fantasies about someone who looks different, may try to master their fears aggressively, by laughing, teasing, or making derisive comments. Developmental delays in all areas of functioning are not uncommon in these children.

Adolescence itself is stressful [28,29]. It is a time when there is a restructuring of personality and when physical changes of the maturing body must be integrated into the body image and into the sense of self. It is a time when developing feelings of sexual arousal often are frightening. All these changes contribute to a sense of loss of control, making adolescence perhaps the most difficult time for patients to develop skin disease [27]. The developmental task of the adolescent is to separate emotionally from the parents and define individual identity and personality. Support and identifications are transferred from the parents to the peer group. Peers and media idols are deemed perfect, and any deviation from this "ideal" of perfection is viewed with embarrassment, shame, and even self-disgust, with loss of self-esteem [26,28,29]. These negative feelings about the self are projected onto others, so that adolescents anticipate that others share their disdain and inevitably judge, criticize, and reject. For example, even mild acne may feel like the end of the world, a feeling that is exacerbated by the cruel comments of siblings and peers who, like younger children, are trying to master their own anxiety about what they see. During this time, body image problems emerge, which may cause a distorted perception of the severity of skin lesions [27]. Emotional regression and academic difficulties may ensue.

The emotional impact of skin disease that starts in, or continues into, adulthood depends not only on the factors discussed previously but also on the specific disease and the restrictions that it may impose. There may be occupations or leisure-time activities that are precluded, restrictions in dress, and expenditures in time and money that are substantial, all of which may generate resentment and interfere in relationships [30–37].

Patients who feel good about themselves are better able to adjust and are flexible and imaginative in developing coping strategies. Those less fortunate expend emotional energy in defending against anxiety, anger, and resentment about the condition. They may deny that a problem exists, be noncompliant with treatment, or express symptoms of anxiety and depression. Fantasies about dirt, contamination, or contagion and feelings of embarrassment, shame, guilt, and loss of control are common and may result in social, occupational, or sexual inhibition. At the same time, the anticipation of rejection [38] arouses rejecting behavior in others, affirming for these patients their unacceptability.

## Nature of the disease

### Psoriasis

Dermatoses that have an impact on other family members or the community at large likely have an even greater emotional impact on the sufferer. For example, psoriasis, which usually has its onset in adult life, not only is unsightly and uncomfortable but also results in the constant shedding of scales and requires treatments that often are messy, time-consuming, and expensive. Many reports attest to the distress caused by psoriasis [30–33,38,39]; this article presents the sorts of issues that come up when working with psoriasis patients. Anxiety [34], depression [35], and suicidal ideation [36] occur in significant numbers of patients, and frightening fantasies as to cause and prognosis are common, as are feelings of stigmatization and anticipation of rejection [38]. The constant shedding of scales, and the need for their removal, is a daily reminder of the ongoing problem— a stigma—and a shameful recognition that the patient is "dirty," out of control, and unacceptable, feelings that may have an unconscious connection to sexual guilt and may be reinforced by the fact that people often avoid physical contact [40]. These patients may feel that they shame their families, causing trouble and extra work, and are a financial burden or, perhaps, the disease may be experienced as punishment. Depressed and chronically angry, patients may feel unfairly "chosen" and, in defense against this anger, may narcissistically feel entitled to, and use the disease to justify expectation of, special treatment.

A comparison of subjective and objective evaluations of disease severity reveals differing perceptions between physicians and patients; in one study, a response to treatment failed to improve the level of psychologic distress. The concept of being different, damaged, or stigmatized was integrated into the self-concept of these patients, so persisted, despite the dermatologic response [37]. Although in the author's experience, lesions on the head and neck or genital area generate the greatest emotional response [10], one study surprisingly refutes this [34].

*Atopic dermatitis*

Atopic dermatitis differs from psoriasis in that the onset, in the most severe and problematic cases, is in early infancy [41]. Whereas for many patients atopic dermatitis is mild and time limited, creating little emotional difficulty, for some it may be severe and intractable, with remissions and exacerbations throughout life that have an impact on every aspect of patients' lives.

Itching that often is intractable is the cardinal symptom of atopic dermatitis [42], so that the affected infants are uncomfortable, restless, and inconsolable. Scratching may be paroxysmal and intense, exacerbating the itch, leading to exudation and bleeding. Anxiety is handled less well than in patients who are nonatopic [43,44], and heightened anxiety leads to increased itching and scratching. As with psoriasis, treatments tend to be messy, time consuming, and expensive.

The feelings experienced by the mothers of these infants are complex. Having given birth to babies who are not "perfect," mothers may feel ashamed; lesser than their peers, whose children are perceived as unblemished; and guilty because their baby suffers. They may ask, "What have I done to deserve this?" and, because they cannot soothe their babies, they may begin to question their ability to parent [45], comparing themselves unfavorably with their own mothers, who are idealized and for whom they had never felt good enough. The anxiety generated in these mothers is picked up readily by their infants, who become even more frantic. To abort the possibility of a downward spiral, in which the anxiety of each feeds on the other, these mothers will do almost anything to prevent scratching. They and the infants are exhausted from lack of sleep; mothers feel inadequate and ineffective, and their time becomes monopolized by the infants, as they try constantly to soothe. Siblings feel unimportant and neglected, and marital relationships may suffer [46,47].

Afraid to upset their babies, and in compensation for their feelings of guilt, mothers may be overindulgent and reluctant to set limits, so that infants' social and emotional development is delayed [7,28,47–50]. Alternatively, in defense against feelings of guilt and shame, mothers may reject the infants emotionally, denying appropriate and empathic touching and generating in the infants a tendency toward later unmodulated anger, the capacity to somatize (express emotional content in somatic form), and self-esteem and body image issues [8–11]. Many studies suggest that atopic patients have difficulty with the management of anger, of which they may not be consciously aware [27,47,51]. Intense focus on affected infants also may lead to feelings of "specialness" that may result in narcissistic personality development and also may cause the body to be overvalued, with a later tendency toward hypochondria [41].

Because of the characteristic physical and emotional developmental delays seen in severe cases [26,47,48], once patients enter school there likely are academic and social difficulties. Frightening fantasies about patients' looks and behavior may lead peers to tease and reject, behavior that may cause patients to regress further, becoming more babyish and increasing their social isolation. As a defense against those feelings, patients may become pushy and aggressive, repelling the very peers from whom they long for acceptance.

There is a wealth of evidence to support the fact that atopic dermatitis is aggravated by stress [49–55], primarily through increased itching [56], so the stresses that are a part of adolescence (discussed previously) may precipitate flares at a time when being different is more problematic and self-esteem more fragile—a time when youngsters strive to maintain control of their bodies, feelings, and environment. This control is difficult particularly if crusting, bleeding, and exudation are evident, changes that may arouse anxiety as to what they mean—for example, Is the body disintegrating? Is it contagious? Is it the result of some forbidden, often sexual, thought or activity? There often is certainty that patients are seriously flawed and that no partner could wish to be with them and profound feelings of self-disgust that may lead to social inhibition and academic failure. For girls, the onset of menses brings an added stress, because in about 50% of women, premenstrual symptoms may trigger flares [57].

For many adult patients, the difficulties that emerge in adolescence continue into adulthood. The associated negative feelings then intrude into every aspect of patients' lives, creating the possibility of social and occupational inhibition, relationship difficulties, and lack of personal and sexual fulfillment.

*Acne*

Although often triggered by stress [58,59], acne itself causes considerable stress [60,61], and in our culture, where adolescents are bombarded continually with images of media idols who have seemingly perfect bodies and complexions, a culture in which parents often have unrealistic expectations of their children, the onset of acne can be devastating [25,26]. Not able to compete with the perfection of the idealized personalities or peers, even minimal lesions may serve to confirm for adolescents their worst fears [26]. Youngsters feel ugly, dirty, and flawed and have impoverished self-esteem and self-conscious feelings that everyone is looking and criticizing, with a certainty that the lesions proclaim to the world some dark secret about the self [26]. Because of the age-appropriate physical changes and the early arousal of sexual feelings, guilt about sexuality often is a part of the picture, and the outbreak may be experienced as a loss of control and as a punishment. These feelings may cause youngsters to become clinically depressed, avoid social situations, and refuse to go to school. Suicidal ideation or attempted suicide may occur [27,57–61].

Parents may focus on children's skin, experiencing the acne as a narcissistic injury, and putting pressure on adolescents, who, perhaps in identification with an affected parent, feel helpless, believing that they already are condemned. This feeling of helplessness may result in a failure to comply, which in turn may result in a painful power struggle with the parents. Parental pressures invariably are counterproductive, only intensifying adolescent resistance. Alternatively, the fear that by breaking out they are disappointing the parents may make the negative feelings even more intense.

The stress of integrating into the body image age-appropriate adolescent physical changes may lead to fragility of that image, with development of body dysmorphic disorder. This condition is characterized by pronounced anxiety and a distorted or exaggerated perception of the skin changes. In an effort to regain control of a situation that is not well understood, patients may pick off lesions with the half-held belief that this magically will make them disappear [62,63]. Anxiety may drive patients to pick compulsively, knowing, yet not knowing, that things will not improve, but unable to control the activity. Shame often follows because of the inability to control.

Picking the skin can have many different meanings in the inner life of individuals and varies from patient to patient, but it is not uncommon for patients to use the disfigurement produced to affirm that they are "no good" and neither conform to peer standards nor meet parental expectations. It also may be used as an excuse to avoid situations or relationships for which impoverished self-esteem or beliefs about the condition makes patients feel inadequate.

Acne may persist into adult life or, in women, may have its onset in adult life. The inter- and intrapersonal issues are similar to those in other chronic dermatoses and, in adults, a problem that is believed adolescent may raise disquieting fantasies of immaturity or belief that something is seriously wrong. One study shows that patients between ages 30 and 39 were those affected most negatively and, in the majority of cases, effective treatment improves self-esteem, body image, and social assertiveness [64]. It also helps to remove the need to pick [26,62,63], which seems to be a powerful reason for isotretinoin to remain available [65].

*Hair loss*

Since the beginning of time, hair has had great psychologic significance for men and women, and certain unconscious themes appear repeatedly in classical mythology, in anthropologic studies, and in patients whom seen in treatment [66,67].

Physiologically, the growth of hair parallels the course of physical development, increasing at puberty, and waning in senility. Thus, a profusion of hair in men has come to symbolize strength and virility and loss of hair a symbolic castration [68,69]. This theme can be found not only in the Biblical story of Samson, in classical literature, and in the history of certain North American native tribes [69] but also in our own time, when the shorn head of the marine recruit is a cogent reminder of his powerlessness in the military hierarchy, whereas British lawyers and judges wear elaborate wigs to signify their power. That the perception of excessive hair loss frequently is the focus of body dysmorphic concerns in men and women attests to its significance in the inner lives of patients [66].

At a superficial level, for women, hair traditionally is a measure of physical beauty, but here, too, references in literature and in mythology suggest deeper and often sexual meanings to the pelage [68–71]. It was, after all, by their long hair that the Sirens lured the sailors onto the rocks and the hair of the mythical Medusa that was believed to have great sexual power [70]. In women, beauty often is equated with power, and much in literature supports this contention [72,73]; as with men, loss of hair implies, at some level, a loss of sexual power.

Because there are media and cultural pressures for women to have long, beautiful, and silken hair, women who have hair loss, regardless of the cause, may feel less attractive and less feminine, particularly if self-esteem is dependent on outward appearance [73]. Many also describe shaming feelings of "nakedness" and "exposure," feelings that seem to support deeper sexual meanings for the hair and its loss. For many men also, hair loss arouses feelings of embarrassment and self-consciousness, again because the men feel lesser, no longer matching up to the current ideal view of masculinity. Sometimes the loss is experienced as a sign that men are aging and, therefore, no longer sexually attractive. The current trend of professional athletes and their followers to shave their heads could be interpreted as a defense against this fear of impending loss of masculine sexual power, used as a means of taking control to allay anxiety.

**Impact of skin disease on families**

The emotional impact of children who have chronic skin disease on their families depends largely on the self-esteem and emotional stability of the parents [24,72]. Stable parents who feel good about themselves are less likely to harbor ambivalence toward the patients. They support each other in accepting and respecting the patients, not needing to expend emotional energy in defending against their negative feelings.

They are able to seek and accept appropriate advice and more able to set appropriate limits, treating the patients just as they treat any sibling, whom they also may involve in care-taking activities, when appropriate. They also are alert to the possibility of stigmatization, seeking to educate those in the patients' environment, and they are flexible and without resentment in seeking vacation spots, hobbies, and activities favorable to the patients' condition. In a less favorable environment (discussed previously), siblings feel neglected and left out; may have a fantasy that patients are the favorite; may act out, creating problems at home and in school; and express anger and resentment to, and about, patient and parents. Tension between parents frequently is a part of the picture.

When patients are adults, the family dynamics essentially are similar to those described previously.

**Impact on society**

All of the factors discussed play a part in determining the impact that patients who have visible skin disease have on any particular society, although the level of sophistication of the society also plays a part. But even for those who are sophisticated, emotional responses not always are congruent with intellectual understanding; primitive and illogical fears lurk within the unconscious minds of most people.

Fantasies about dirt and contagion are common. Guilt because one is spared the suffering or anxiety because of an unconscious identification with the sufferer may lead to inappropriate behaviors. Unconscious anxiety about known infections, and particularly sexually transmitted diseases, may cause risk-taking behaviors because of a defensive denial of the risk. Vitiligo is perhaps a special case, particularly in those who have darker skin in whom the lesions, which frequently are on exposed areas, are more obvious. Often, fear of infection is uppermost as is, not uncommonly, fear of leprosy because of the pronounced color contrast [74,75]. This may result in others being unwilling to touch and patients spurned.

More sophisticated individuals, who have the benefit of insight, may have access to their inner lives and, with some awareness, may recognize the concerns in their inner lives, and in recognizing them, may be able to act appropriately, rather than having to act out those concerns in inappropriate behavior.

## Summary

This article discusses some major early factors that influence the evolving psychologic development, which in turn helps determine the emotional impact that chronic or disabling skin disease may have on patients' lives.

If the emotional environment, encompassed by the infant-caretaker relationship, is less than optimal, the stability of the body image may be compromised, self-esteem diminished, and affect less well handled and the somatic expression of emotional content may ensue. Each of these is important in dermatology, as is the nature of the disease and the capacity of families and of society to adapt. Psoriasis, atopic dermatitis, and acne are used as examples.

## References

[1] Exodus 15:26. King James version. Nashville (TN): Bibles Incorporated International; 1974.
[2] Garison FH. An introduction to the history of medicine. Philadelphia: W.B. Saunders; 1923. p. 69.
[3] van de Kerkhof PCM. Psoriasis. In: Bolognia JL, Jorizzo JL, Rapini RP, editors. Dermatology. London: Mosby; 2003. p. 125–49.
[4] Finlay AY, Khan GK. Dermatology life quality index (DLQI): a simple practical measure for routine clinical use. Clin Exp Dermatol 1994;19:210.
[5] Chren MM, Lasek RJ, Sahay AP, et al. Measurement properties of Skindex-16: a brief quality of life measurement for patients with skin disease. J Cutan Med Surg 2001;5:105–10.
[6] Chamlin SI, Frieden IJ, Williams ML, et al. Effects of atopic dermatitis on American children and their families. Pediatrics 2004;114:607–11.
[7] Ben-Gashir MA, Seed PT, Hay RJ. Quality of life and disease severity are correlated in children with atopic dermatitis. Br J Dermatol 2004;150:284–90.
[8] Hartman H, Kris E, Loewenstein RM. Comments on the formation of psychic structure. Psychoanal Study Child 1946;2:11–38.
[9] Krueger DW. Psychoanalytic perspective on body image. In: Cash TF, Pruzinsky T, editors. Body images. New York: Guilford Press; 2002. p. 32.
[10] Weiss SJ. Parental touching: correlates of a child's body concept and body sentiment. In: Barnard KE, Brazelton TB, editors. Touch: the foundation of experience. Madison (CT): International University Press; 1990. p. 425–58.
[11] Meissman W. The self and the body, Vol. 1. The body self and the body image. Psychoanalysis and Contemporary Thought 1997;20:419–48.
[12] Ginsburg IH. Psychosocial effects of skin disease on the patient. In: Koo JYM, Lee CS, editors. Psychocutaneous medicine. New York: Marcel Decker; 2003. p. 215–31.
[13] Levine S, Stanton ME. The hormonal consequences of mother-infant contact in primates and rodents. In: Brown CC, editor. The many facets of touch (Johnson and Johnson round table series), Vol. 10. Skillman (NJ): Johnson and Johnson Baby; 1984. p. 51–65.
[14] Korner AF. The many facets of touch. In: Brown CC, editor. The many facets of touch (Johnson and Johnson round table series), Vol. 10. Skillman (NJ): Johnson and Johnson Baby; 1984. p. 107–13.
[15] Phillips KA. Body dysmorphic disorder: the distress of imagined ugliness. Am J Psychiatry 1991;148:1138–49.
[16] Koblenzer CS. Dermatitis artefacta. Clinical features and approaches to treatment. Am J Clin Dermatol 2000;1:37–55.
[17] Beebe B, Lachman FM. Infant research and adult treatment. Hillside (NJ): Analytic Press; 2002. p. 95–119 [monograph].
[18] Anzieu D. The skin ego. New Haven (CT): Yale University Press; 1989. p. 3–35 [monograph].
[19] Greenspan SI. The development of the ego. In: Greenspan SI, Pollock GH, editors. The course of life, Vol. 1. Infancy. Madison (CT): International University Press; 1989. p. 121–4.
[20] Hofer MA. The mother-infant interaction as a regulator of infant physiology and behavior. In: Rosenblum LA, Moltz H, editors. Symbolism in parent-offspring interactions. New York: Plenum Publishing Corp.; 1983.
[21] Taylor GJ. Psychosomatic medicine and contemporary psychoanalysis. Madison (CT): International University Press; 1987. p. 149 [monograph].
[22] Malm M, Carlberg M. The port-wine stain—a surgical and psychological problem. Ann Plastic Surg 1988;20(6):512–9.
[23] Earle EM. The psychological effects of mutilating surgery in children and adolescents. Psychoanal Study Child 1979;34:527–46.
[24] Koblenzer CS. The psychological and social impact of skin disease. In: Pierini A-M, Garcia-Diaz de Pierini R, Bustamante RE, editors. Pediatric dermatology. Amsterdam: Elsevier; 1995. p. 3–12.
[25] Bergman T, Freud A. Children in the hospital. New York: International University Press; 1965.
[26] Koblenzer CS. Psychodermatology of girls and women. In: Parish CP, Brenner S, Ramos-e-Silva M, editors. Women's dermatology. New York: Parthenon Publishing Group; 2001. p. 10–27.
[27] Koblenzer CS. Psychotherapy for intractable dermatoses. J Am Acad Dermatol 1995;32:606–12.
[28] Sklansy MA. The pubescent years. In: Greenspan SI, Pollock SH, editors. The course of life, vol IV.

[29] Beiser HR. Ages eleven to fourteen. In: Greenspan SI, Pollock SH, editors. The course of life, vol IV. Adolescence. Madison (CT): International University Press; 1991. p. 99–118.
[30] Ginsburg IH, Link BG. Feelings of stigmatization in psoriasis. J Am Acad Dermatol 1989;20:53–63.
[31] Ginsburg IH, Link BG. Psychosocial consequences of rejection and stigma feelings in psoriasis patients. Int J Dermatol 1993;32:587–91.
[32] Picardi A, Abeni D, Melchi CF, et al. Psychiatric morbidity in dermatologic outpatients: an issue to be recognized. Br J Dermatol 1995;132:236–44.
[33] Hill L, Kennedy P. The role of coping strategies in mediating subjective disabilities in people who have psoriasis. Psych Health Med 2002;7:261–9.
[34] Richards HL, Fortune DG, Main CJ, et al. The contribution of perception of stigmatization to disability in patients with psoriasis. J Psychosom Rs 2001;50:11–4.
[35] Gupta MA, Gupta M, Schork NJ, et al. Depression modulates pruritus perception: a study of pruritus in psoriasis, atopic dermatitis, and chronic idiopathic urticaria. Psychsom Med 1994;56:36–40.
[36] Krueger G, Koo JYM, Lebwohl M, et al. The impact of psoriasis on quality of life. Arch Dermatol 2001;137:236–44.
[37] Fortune DG, Richards HL, Kirby B, et al. Successful treatment of psoriasis improves psoriasis-specific but not more general aspects of patients' well-being. Br J Dermatol 2004;151:1219–26.
[38] Leary MR, Rapp BR, Exuni ML, et al. Interpersonal concerns and psychological difficulties in psoriasis patients: effects of disease severity and fear of negative evaluation. Health Psychol 1998;17:530–6.
[39] Schmid-Ott G, Kneusebeck HW, Jaeger B, et al. Validity study for the stigmatization experience in atopic dermatitis and psoriasis. Derm Venereal 1999;79:443–7.
[40] Koblenzer CS. The psychologic aspects of atopic dermatitis. In: Bieber T, Leung DYM, editors. Atopic dermatitis. New York: Marcel Decker; 2002. p. 519–39.
[41] Hanafin JM, Rajka G. Diagnostic features of atopic dermatitis. Acta Derm Venereol (Stockh) 1980;92(Suppl):44–7.
[42] Buske-Kirschbaum A, Gierens A, Hollig H, et al. Stress induced immunomodulation is altered in patients with atopic dermatitis. J Neuroimmunol 2002;129:161–7.
[43] Buske-Kirschbaum A. Gieben—altered responsiveness of the hypothalamic-pituitary-adrenal axis and the sympathetic adrenomedullary system to stress in patients with atopic dermatitis. J Clin Endocrinol Metab 2002;87:4245–51.
[44] Pauli-Pott U, Darui A, Beckermann D. Infants with atopic dermatitis: maternal hopelessness, child-rearing attitudes and perceived infant temperament. Psychother Psychosom 1999;68:39–45.
[45] Howlet S. Emotional dysfunction, child-family relationships and childhood atopic dermatitis. Br J Dermatol 1999;141:381–4.
[46] Koblenzer CS, Koblenzer PJ. Chronic intractable atopic eczema. Its occurrence as a physical sign of impaired parent-child relationships and psychologic developmental arrest: improvement through parent insight and education. Arch Dermatol 1988;124(11):1673–7 [review].
[47] Daud LP, Garraldu ME, David JJ. Psychosocial adjustment in pre-school children with atopic eczema. Arch Dis Child 1993;69:647–54.
[48] Faulstich ME, Williamson DA. An overview of atopic dermatitis: towards a biobehavioral integration. J Psychosom Res 1985;19:647–54.
[49] Gil KM, Keef FJ, Sampson HA, et al. The relation of stress and family environment to atopic dermatitis symptoms in children. J Psychosom Res 1987;31:673–84.
[50] Linnet J, Jemec GBE. Anxiety, aggression, and body ideal in adult atopic dermatitis patients. Dermatology Psychosomatics 2001;2:124–9.
[51] Ginsburg IH, Prystowsky JH, Kornfeld DS, et al. The role of emotional factors in adults with atopic dermatitis. Int J Dermatol 1993;32:656–60.
[52] Wahlgren CF. Pathophysiology of itching in urticaria and atopic dermatitis. Allergy 1992;47:68–75.
[53] Benea V, Muresian D, Manolache L, et al. Stress and atopic dermatitis. Dermatology Psychosomatics 2001;2:205–7.
[54] Wilson ME, Megel ME, Fredrichs AM, et al. Physiologic and behavioral responses to stress, temperament and incidence of infection and atopic disorders in the first year of life: a pilot study. J Pediatr Nurs 2003;18:257–66.
[55] Buske-Kirschbaum A, Hellhammer DH. Endocrine and immune responses to stress in chronic inflammatory skin disorders. Ann N Y Acad Sci 2003;992:231–40.
[56] Kiriyama K, Sugiura H, Uehara M. Premenstrual deterioration of skin symptoms in female patients with atopic dermatitis. Dermatology 2003;206:110–2.
[57] Gupta MA, Gupta AK. Psychiatric and psychological co-morbidity in patients with dermatologic disorders: epidemiology and management. Am J Clin Dermatol 2003;4:833–42.
[58] Zouboulis CC, Bohm M. Neuroendocrine regulation of sebocytes—a pathogenetic link between stress and acne. Exp Dermatol 2004;13(Suppl 4):31–5 [review].
[59] Tan JK. Psychosocial impact of acne vulgaris: evaluationg the evidence. Skin Therapy Lett 2004;9:1–3.
[60] Koblenzer CS. Neurotic excoriations and dermatitis artefacta. Dermatol Clin 1996;14:447–55.
[61] Phillips KA, Taub SL. Skin-picking as a symptom of body dysmorphic disorder. Psychopharm Bull 1995;31:279–88.
[62] Lasek RJ, Chren M. Acne vulgaris and the quality of life in adult dermatology patients. Arch Dermatol 1998;134:454–8.

[63] Kellett SC, Gawkrodger DJ. The psychological and emotional impact of acne and the effect of treatment with isotretinoin. Br J Dermatol 1999;140:273–82.

[64] Berg C. Unconscious significance of hair. Int J Psychoanal 1936;17:73–88.

[65] Koblenzer CS. Trichotillomania. In: Stein DS, Christenson GA, Hollander E, editors. Trichotillomania. Washington, DC: Psychiatric Press; 1999. p. 125–45.

[66] Frazer JA. The golden bough, vol. 11. New York: Macmillan; 1923. p. 102.

[67] Freeman D. Thunder, blood and nicknaming God's creatures. Psychoanal Q 1968;37:355–99.

[68] Freud S. Medusa's Head. In: Strachey J, editor. Standard edition of the complete works of Sigmund Freud, vol. 18. London: Hogarth Press; 1955. p. 273–4.

[69] Barahal HS. The psychopathology of hair-plucking (Trichotillomania). Psychoanal Rev 1940;27:291–310.

[70] Cash TF. The psychology of physical appearance: Aesthetics, attributes, and images. In: Cash CF, Pruzinsky T, editors. Body images: development, deviance and change. New York: Guilford Press; 1990. p. 51–79.

[71] Cash TF. The psychological consequences of androgenetic alopecia: a review of the research literature. Br J Dermatol 1999;141:398–405.

[72] Kent G. Psychological effects of vitiligo: a critical incident analysis. J Am Acad Dermatol 1996;35:895–8.

[73] Jackson LA. Physical attractiveness. A sociocultural perspective. In: Cash TF, Pruzinsky T, editors. Body image: a handbook of theory, research and clinical practice. New York: Guilford Press; 2002.

[74] Ginsburg IH. Psychosocial effects of skin disease on the patient. In: Koo JYM, Lee CS, editors. Psychocutaneous medicine. New York: Marcel-Dekker, Inc.; 2003.

[75] Mosher DB, Fitzpatrick TB, Ortonne JP, et al. Disorders of pigmentation. In: Fitzpatrick TB, Eisen AZ, Wolff K, et al, editors. Dermatology in general medicine. New York: McGraw-Hill; 1987. p. 794–876.

# Psychosomatic Factors in Dermatology: Special Perspectives for Application in Clinical Practice

Emiliano Panconesi, MD

*Department of Dermatology, University of Florence, Florence, Italy*

Nothing is more profound than that which appears superficial.

—Hegel

A dermatologist's work would be incomplete if he/she did not consider and examine the whole patient, not only the physical body with the skin and mucosae, but also the individual's mind (the psyche or the psychologic aspects, "the soul"). The term originally proposed by Heinroth in 1818 for such a situation is "psychosomatic"—a term that is only relatively precise, but that presents the advantage of clear understanding; later, Jacobi widened the field with the term "somatopsychic." The former term refers to the influence of the mind on the body, and the latter refers to the influence of corporeal phenomena on the mind, although actually the two must be considered clinically indistinguishable. Today, there is a whole area of psychosomatic medicine, including, of particular interest to dermatologists, psychosomatic dermatology. It is not necessary or opportune to use separate neologisms, such as "psychocutaneous medicine," "emotional dermatoses," "psychocutaneous disease," or "psychodermatology," because psychosomatic medicine is a branch of medicine with a unified epistemologic basis correlated with the various organs and systems.

To cite a historical example, their use of the term "psychosomatic" indicates that the founders of the *Journal of Psychosomatic Medicine* (1939) had a similar opinion, just as Weiss and English [1] must have had, shown by their choice of the title *Psychosomatic Medicine* for their book, in which they noted that the creation of the *Journal of Psychosomatic Medicine* and the emphasis on the topic had been reported enthusiastically in the *Journal of the American Medical Association* in an article that underlined the true origin of the psychosomatic idea in the studies of Freud (and his followers, who more or less agreed with him). One of the many possible references to his thought is Freud's significant idea that no neurosis would be produced without some form of somatic connivance. In a study on epistemology in psychosomatic dermatology, Panconesi and Argentieri [2] agreed with the authors who followed Freud, including those of the Chicago Psychoanalytic School, who concluded that "all medicine must become (meaning *is*) psychosomatic medicine." This is a sort of reply, over the centuries, to Plato's phrase (presented as an epigraph in the book by Weiss and English): "this is the great error of our times ... physicians see the body separate from the soul."

These theories that make headway and develop and diversify in the field of psychology/psychiatry do not make operational contact in other clinical specialities, in either research or clinical activities. This situation seems to be due to various factors, in particular the hybrid status of psychosomatic epistemology, which is part of medicine with its empirical tradition and at the same time refers to psychology, with all the related hermeneutic difficulties. Experience (that of the author and many others) shows, however, that the somatist's (the dermatologist in this case) simple referral of the patient to a psychiatrist/psychologist is often unacceptable to the patient

E-mail address: epanconesi@dada.it

(who has chosen the dermatologist to solve his or her problems) and may even be risky (owing to the "delicate" patient's feeling that one has made an unfair, improper diagnosis of mental disturbance).

This problem could be managed by formalized collaboration through consultation-liaison psychiatry, a treatment method examined in depth by Koblenzer [3], who emphasized possible strategies for its practical application. She pointed out that it is helpful for the dermatologist to find a psychologist/psychiatrist colleague with whom he or she relates well to discuss or refer patients for specific psychologic problems. This collaboration provides the patient with the necessary dermatologic expertise and treatment and appropriate specialized psychologic/psychiatric management, while bypassing the various risks of all-out referral, such as labeling the patient as mentally ill and the specialists being played one against the other. In her discussion of the method, Koblenzer [3] pointed out that the consultation-liaison clinic is the ideal situation for such integrated care, and that such clinics operated successfully in many cities (Florence, Paris, Ghent, Amsterdam, Stanford), with varying organizational situations and different immediate objectives, but all aimed at total, integrated care of patients. The specified ideal organization requires space in a dermatology clinic, with regular liaison sessions, including a minimum staff of one psychiatrist and one dermatologist. The optimal situation is a team approach, however, including a clinical psychologist (to administer psychologic tests) and psychiatric social workers, and facilities for biofeedback training and other modalities. When the patient has been completely evaluated, treatment is continued by the dermatologist, who consults when necessary with the psychiatrist, who may begin biofeedback training, if indicated, or psychotherapy, in which case the psychiatrist consults with the dermatologist, who in the meantime continues the necessary dermatologic treatment. The advantage of establishing the liaison clinic in the regular dermatology clinic is that the patient sees that his or her choice of specialist, the dermatologist, is recognized, and evaluations, laboratory tests, and treatments are done there in the clinic with all dermatology patients who undergo various other examinations (eg, allergologic tests) or treatments (eg, phototherapy).

Koblenzer [3] pointed out that the aims of the various liaison clinics differ. The clinic in Stanford had a specific educational approach—to teach young dermatologists how to recognize and discover psychologic problems in patients. The clinic in Florence performed more fully developed activities, with a staff of dermatologists, psychologists, and psychiatrists who did separate dermatologic and psychiatric evaluations, with psychodiagnostic tests and treatments including biofeedback training, psychotherapy, and liaison consultation. All the data were stored for future reference and comparative studies, leading to therapeutic projection and the establishment of an index of psychosomaticity [4], a practical guide to assist dermatologists and psychologists/psychiatrists in their evaluation of dermatologic patients with psychosomatic and somatopsychic problems. Economic and organizational problems make it extremely difficult to establish such an integrated clinic, but the individual dermatologist can dedicate more time to needy patients and individuate one or more psychiatrist colleagues with whom consultation-liaison is possible for specific cases.

The times were not yet ripe when Freud performed the first biologic and histologic studies on biologic psychosomatics. The pioneer studies were those of Lewis (1930), who described the phenomenon of the triple response observed in human skin in response to an injury, with morphologic manifestations of wheals, local erythema, and flare reactions in response to external stimuli (and release or injection of histamine). In 1946, Selye proposed his general adaptation syndrome, introducing the concepts of stress and stressors, identifying them also with many substances (eg, endocrines, steroids, catecholamines), especially neuropeptides, that were identified in blood and tissue, even in the skin and mucosae. Since then, continuously more sophisticated research has supplied an enormous mass of data of unquestionable scientific importance.

The rapid proliferation of important findings, as often happens in science, led in the field of dermatology to expectations that soon information would be available that would provide valid epistemologic definitions of clinical pertinence for classification purposes in the field of psychosomatics, information that would allow dermatologists to individuate with scientific precision the various psychosomatic factors that influence specific dermatologic presentations. This expectation is not yet a reality. Dermatologists still must resort to practical, operational strategies.

## Research on the individuation of psychosomatic factors in diagnostic and clinical dermatology

Research in psychosomatics began in the Department of Dermatology and Venereology at the University of Florence, Italy, in the 1950s and developed at various levels. Laboratory studies in the metabolic and endocrinologic sectors of clinical pharmacology that involved investigation of hypophyseal and surrenal substances studied by Selye were fairly easy to organize. It was not possible until the 1970s, however, to organize and conduct research in medical psychology, with the collaboration of experts in that field, on site. These experts all worked on a volunteer basis because the administration could not include them in the budget. It was important that the work be done on site in the department of dermatology because the subjects, inpatients and outpatients, had to undergo dermatologic examination (when necessary with laboratory tests, including allergologic tests, mycologic and bacteriologic examinations, and histologic investigations) and psychologic investigation (attentive anamnesis and, when necessary, specific psychodiagnostic tests, such as the Rorschach test, which require specially trained personnel). Many of these subjects would not have accepted referral to dedicated psychiatric institutions because they felt branded by the idea or did not believe they needed such evaluation.

At the author's institution, a psychosomatic dermatology team (three to five dermatologists and three to five psychologists and psychiatrists) was organized that met regularly once a week with an agenda that included consultation liaison. The dermatologists all were University or National Health Service personnel, and the psychologists/psychiatrists (all volunteers) were on call to examine and talk with inpatients and outpatients at the request of the outpatient service and the ward physicians. The dermatologists and psychiatrists/psychologists all wore similar white hospital coats with a name badge, without reference to their specific specializations, to avoid emphasis on the presence of a psychiatrist, which some patients might not have welcomed. Inpatients who required follow-up after their release from the hospital continued therapy with the same personnel through the dermatologic outpatient clinic. The weekly meeting served for programming research projects, consultation and discussion regarding particular cases, and teaching undergraduates and residents the aims and tactics of psychosomatic investigations.

This collaboration led to numerous publications over the years as the study of psychosomatic dermatology became more profound and better recognized, accepted, and authorized by public institutions (in Europe, most individuals have access to some form of public health service, and acceptance by such national health services, public hospitals, and state universities to underwrite the costs of specific programs and services is paramount). In a relatively short time (mid-1950s–1970s), this group acquired remarkable experience and collected a large quantity of data. Another source of information was participation in meetings and congresses in Europe and the United States, although during those years and into the 1980s, with few exceptions, psychosomatic dermatology was generally ignored in US universities and at major dermatology congresses. Finally, in the early 1980s, there were signs that psychosomatic medicine was becoming a topic of interest in the United States. The *Clinics in Dermatology* published an issue dedicated to the subject [5], and shortly before the publication of this issue, the *New York Times* published a brief article on the skin and emotions [6]. This was *une ideé qui était dans l'air* or, as Parish wrote in his Foreword to the *Clinics in Dermatology* issue, "a rekindling of interest in psychosomatic medicine is currently in progress" [5].

## Specific cutaneous conditions and symptoms with psychosomatic associations

The *Clinics in Dermatology* issue [5] was based on the author's then more than 25 years of experience and the body of the existing literature on the subject; clinical pictures represented the most significant mind-body relationships, with reference to the current acquisitions in the field of psychoneuroendocrinoimmunology, including pruritus and prurigo, urticaria, contact dermatitis, atopic dermatitis, rosacea, acne, alopecia (in particular alopecia areata), telogen effluvium, vitiligo, purpura, seborrheic dermatitis, and psoriasis; cosmetologic alterations; and psychiatric syndromes with dermatologic expression, such as self-inflicted lesions, trichotillomania, and certain so-called phobias (eg, dysmorphophobia, glossodynia, delusions of parasitosis, venereophobia/syphilophobia, AIDS-phobia). Myriad observations refer to numerous different psychosomatic factors, where psychic problems seem to predispose, trigger, accompany, or exacerbate various dermatologic patterns, and to somatopsychic factors, where various dermatologic conditions or symptoms seem to trigger or exacerbate psychologic/psychiatric problems (Tables 1 and 2). This information remains valid today.

Research, the literature, and the author's own experience lead the author to reconfirm today that there is no physical pathology that does not influence the mind and vice versa. While waiting to be able to individuate other methods of classification—harmonizing etiopathogenetic criteria in the two fields of

Table 1
Dermatologic conditions that may involve somatopsychic rebound in childhood, adolescence, and adulthood

| Children | Adolescents | Adults |
| --- | --- | --- |
| Ichthyosis | Acne | Rosacea |
| Alopecia | Alopecia | Alopecia |
| Epidermolysis bullosa | — | Seborrheic dermatitis |
| Nevi | — | Psoriasis |
| Angioma | — | Skin aging |

research, one related to psychology and the other to clinical dermatology, the only modus vivendi that is acceptable is to base one's considerations on epistemologic empiricism, but closely related to the statistics of clinical observations of the various groups of conditions studied.

Box 1 lists cutaneous conditions reported to have a high incidence or evidence of psychoemotional (psychic factors influence the body) factors. Table 1 presents cutaneous conditions with frequent, strong somatopsychic rebound (somatic conditions influence the psyche). Box 2 lists psychiatric conditions or syndromes with clinical dermatologic expression

Table 2
Examples of psycho–somatic and somato–psychic influence in dermatologic affections

| Body (*soma*) | Influence | Mind (*psyche*) |
| --- | --- | --- |
| Acute urticaria | ← | Emotions |
| Chronic relapsing urticaria | ← | Anxiety |
| Psoriasis | ↔ | Stress |
|  | → | Depression |
| Atopic dermatitis | ← | Deep psychic conflicts |
| Androgenetic alopecia | → | Psychic problems |
| Telogen effluvium | ↔ | Stress |
| Alopecia areata | ← | Stress |
|  | ← | Psychic conflict |
|  | → | Psychic problems |
| Trichotillomania (hair-pulling tic) | ← | Psychic disease |
| Acne in adolescence | → | Psychic problems |
| Acne in adults | ← | Psychic problems/disease |

**Box 1. Dermatologic conditions with high incidence of psychoemotional factors**

Hyperhydrosis
Dyshydrosis
Pruritus
Urticaria
Lichen simplex
Atopic dermatitis
Acne
Rosacea
Telogen effluvium
Alopecia areata
Psoriasis
Seborrheic dermatitis
Perioral dermatitis
Lichen planus
Herpes
Nummular eczema

(correlated with psychogenic factors that are revealed clinically prevalently on the skin or mucosae).

The aforementioned paths of thought and method are useful in individuating psychosomatic (and somatopsychic) factors in the individual patient who presents to the dermatologist, with the dermatologist deciding case by case regarding the necessity for collaboration (or even close consultation-liaison) with a psychologist or psychiatrist. It is important for the dermatologist to find one or more psychologist/psychiatrist colleagues with whom he or she relates well to discuss cases and to whom the dermatologist

**Box 2. Psychiatric syndromes with dermatologic expression**

*Self-inflicted dermatologic lesions*
  Dermatitis artefacta
  Neurotic excoriations
*Trichotillomania*
*Hypochondriasis (the so-called phobias)*
  Venereophobia
  Dysmorphophobia
  Bromhidrosiphobia
  Glossodynia
*Delusions of parasitosis (Ekbom's disease)*

can refer patients for specifically psychologic problems, even while continuing to manage the dermatologic aspects. Such consultation-liaison also can be performed in private practice, as the author has done since the 1970s. The greatest advantage to such collaboration is that the patient receives the necessary dermatologic expertise and treatment and appropriate specialized psychologic/psychiatric management. The schematic information presented in Table 2 provides generic clues of what the dermatologist might need to look for or at in deciding when some form of psychologic/psychiatric assistance might be helpful or necessary in treating the patient.

The criteria used relate well to the opinions on psychosomatic medicine expressed by the psychiatrists Kaplan and Sadock [7]. In their *Handbook of Psychiatry* for students, which refers to the general classifications established in the *Diagnostic and Statistical Manual of Mental Disorders, Fourth Edition* (DSM-IV), they dedicate a chapter to "Psychosomatic Disorders," although the DSM-IV seems to ignore psychosomatics. The subtitle of the chapter is "Psychosomatic Factors Affecting Medical Conditions." Bypassing the prevailing position imposed by the DSM-IV, these authors offer their definition, *ad usum Delphini* (the student): "The term psychosomatic disorder refers to a physical condition[1]...While many disorders are influenced by stress, conflicts or generalized anxiety, some are more influenced than others" [7].

Regarding pathogenetic theories, basically the author agrees with Kaplan and Sadock's [7] "nonspecific theory:" any prolonged stress, or even strong emotion or conflict, can cause pathophysiologic changes that provoke pathologic disorders or alterations. Most individuals have a "shock organ" (or even more than one) that is genetically (or otherwise predisposed because of trauma or other stimulus) vulnerable to stressors ("meiopragia" is the term used in the past to refer to such organ vulnerability). Some subjects are cardiac reactors (stress provokes cardiac damage), others are gastric reactors, and others are skin reactors.

The advances in psychoneuroendocrinoimmunology based on neuropeptide research led the author and colleagues to state that the future had begun [8,9], but since then the arrival of new information in this field has been slow. Dermatologists are waiting for scientific data that show clearly the various factors operative in this field, individuating their specific mechanisms of influence in psyche–skin (skin–psyche) relationships.

Gabbard [10] reported on some new neurobiologic perspectives that he attempted to connect directly with psychodynamic psychotherapy. His article closed with a short list of clinical implications and limits of the studies presented, including the fact that psychotherapy and pharmacologic treatment can have similar influences on the brain in certain conditions, but that studies on changes in the brain during psychotherapy still need further investigation and confirmation.

## Summary

This article has been a series of notes, with references to certain milestones in the long march to bring the mind and body closer together through individuation of the factors involved in their intrinsic automatic relationship. It is hoped that with this understanding of psychosomatics the dermatologist can understand and treat his or her patients better.

## References

[1] Weiss E, English OS. Psychosomatic medicine. Philadelphia: Saunders; 1949.
[2] Panconesi E, Argentieri S. Epistemological aspects of psychosomatic dermatology. J Dermatol Psychosom 2000;1:53–5.
[3] Koblenzer CS. Psychocutaneous disease. Orlando (FL): Grune & Stratton; 1987.
[4] Panconesi E. Lo stress, le emozioni e la pelle: spunti di dermatologia psicosomatica per lo specialista e per il medico pratico. Milan: Masson; 1990.
[5] Panconesi E, editor. Stress and skin diseases: psychosomatic dermatologyClin Dermatol 1984;2(4):1–282.
[6] Blumenthal D. Skin and emotions—one's mental state affects the body; stress can precipitate or aggravate, skin disorders. New York Times Magazine September 30, 1984:62.
[7] Kaplan HI, Sadock BJ. Handbook of psychiatry. Baltimore: Williams & Wilkins; 1996.
[8] Lotti T, Hautmann G, Panconesi E. Neuropeptides in skin. J Am Acad Dermatol 1995;33:482–96.
[9] Panconesi E, Hautmann G, Lotti T. Neuropeptides and skin: the state of the art. J Eur Acad Dermatol Venereol 1994;3:109–15.
[10] Gabbard GO. A neurobiologically informed perspective on psychotherapy. Br J Psychiatry 2000;177: 117–22.

---

[1] In the author's opinion, this should read "The term psychosomatic disorder refers to a *pathologic* condition caused or aggravated by *psychologic and psychopathologic* factors."

# Stigma Experience in Skin Disorders: An Indian Perspective

Santosh K. Chaturvedi, MD, MRCPsych[a],*, Gurcharan Singh, MD[b], Nitin Gupta, MD[c]

[a]*National Institute of Mental Health and Neurosciences, Bangalore 560029, India*
[b]*Department of Dermatology and Sexually Transmitted Disease, Sri Devaraj Urs Medical College, Tamaka, Kolar 563101, India*
[c]*South Staffordshire Healthcare NHS Trust, Margaret Stanhope Centre, Burton upon Trent, Staffordshire DE130RB, UK*

Stigma is inherently integrated in different aspects of Indian life, especially with certain diseases. Since time immemorial, tuberculosis, cancer, leprosy, and mental illnesses were stigmatizing, until HIV infection became prevalent over the last two decades. Stigma in Indian society is also related from ancient times to certain castes and the lower socioeconomic strata of people. Illnesses in these sections of society are even more stigmatizing. Stigma is related to tradition and philosophy, and to appearance. Skin color and complexion, and other qualities in its appearance, influence public opinion and attitudes, especially prejudice. Skin diseases that alter skin complexion or color, texture, or appearance in any way induce negative emotions in others. This leads to social isolation, seclusion, discrimination, and ostracizing of such persons from their neighborhood or community. This stigma experience in relation to skin diseases has been prevalent in Indian societies since ancient times, as evident from ancient Indian writings and scriptures. The great ancient Indian physician Sushruta in his medical treatise *Sushruta Samhita* (600 BC) gives a fairly good description of leprosy, which was prevalent in India from olden days. A fatalistic attitude prevailed and leprosy was considered a curse of God, a myth, sanctified by religious beliefs and surrounded by superstitious fears, dread, and ostracism of the patient, leading to mental suffering, social dislocation, and serious socioeconomic difficulties for the patient [1].

Stigma is a society's negative evaluation of particular features or behavior. There is a great deal of variability in approaches to define stigma. Goffman [2] defined stigma as an "attribute that is deeply discrediting" that reduces the bearer "from a whole and usual person to a tainted, discounted one." Stafford and Scott [3] defined stigma as "a characteristic of persons that is contrary to norm of a social unit," where a norm is defined as "shared belief that a person ought to behave in a certain way at a certain time." Healthy looking skin is the normal, and skin disorders, which change the color or appearance of the skin, attract attention and usually disgust and social reactions. Social labeling and social stigma are interrelated. The culmination of stigma process occurs when designated differences lead to various forms of disapproval, rejection, exclusion, and discrimination [4]. Varied dimensions of stigmatized medical conditions include the nature of the illness, its history, and attributed characteristics; sources of creation and perpetuation of stigma; the nature of the population who are perceived to carry the illness; the kind of treatment and practitioners sought for the condition; and how individuals with stigmatized medical conditions, including skin disorders, cope with societal insults that endanger their personal identity, social life, and economic opportunities [5].

Studies on psychosocial aspects of dermatologic disorders in India have neither addressed stigma directly, nor in much detail. There are some studies on the prevalence and type of stigma, which is in relation to leprosy. There are a few studies that have

* Corresponding author.
  *E-mail address:* skchatur@yahoo.com
  (S.K. Chaturvedi).

discussed social consequences and impact thereof, psychosocial reactions, and adjustment issues. There are some studies, reviewed later, which have determined the prevalence and nature of psychosocial problems with skin disorders in the Indian subcontinent. It is mere speculation that the psychologic reactions in patients with skin disorder can to some extent reflect the social impact of their skin disorders.

**Psychosocial aspects of skin disorders in India**

There are a few studies on psychiatric and psychologic aspects of skin disorders from the Indian settings. Sharma and coworkers [6] studied and compared the psychiatric morbidity in five chronic and disfiguring diseases: (1) psoriasis, (2) chronic urticaria, (3) leprosy, (4) vitiligo, and (5) lichen simplex chronicus. The overall prevalence of the psychiatric morbidity was found to be 39%; common symptoms were depression (13%), anxiety (11%), suicidal ideations (16%), and somatization (13%). Interpersonal conflict was noted in 10% and suicidal attempts in 3%. Psychiatric morbidity was significantly higher in the psoriasis (53%) than vitiligo (16%) patients. A total of 23% of psoriasis and 10% of vitiligo patients reported depression. Sleep disturbance was significantly more often reported by psoriasis patients (57%) than vitiligo patients (20%).

In another study, Agrawal and coworkers [7] conducted a survey in Nepal to study the clinical profile of 210 psoriasis patients and also to assess their beliefs about their disease. The strongest belief of the patients in the causation of psoriasis was germs or virus (75%). Most patients believed that psoriasis had a major consequence on their lives (81%) and that psoriasis was a serious condition (83%). Women were significantly more likely to believe that their psoriasis had severe consequences on their lives.

Pulimood and coworkers [8] found a prevalence rate of 9% using the International Classification of Diseases – 10th revision diagnostic criteria, more commonly in patients receiving long-term high-dose steroids. Psychiatric morbidity was associated with a longer duration of hospital stay and more frequent admissions. The commonest illnesses were depressive episodes (34%) and adjustment disorders (29%). Bagadia and coworkers [9] found a prevalence rate of 37% on using a screening instrument, and 49% with a clinical interview.

The psychiatric and psychosocial morbidity of some of the common skin disorders in India are discussed next.

*Psoriasis*

The psychiatric comorbidity in patients of psoriasis greatly affects their quality of life and the course of the disease. Psychiatric comorbidity (anxiety and depression [10]) and poor quality of life, more so in women [11], have been reported. Patients reported avoiding communal baths, wearing uncomfortable clothes to cover diseased parts, inhibition of sexual relationship, suicidal ideation, and economic constraints in pursuing treatment and ineffectiveness of topical therapies. These behaviors can be considered to emerge from prevailing social norms and restrictions. A comparative study [12] of psoriasis and leprosy patients revealed higher presence of psychiatric morbidity in psoriasis (48%).

Chaudhury and coworkers [13] observed that patients with psoriasis had a psychiatric morbidity of 24% (predominantly with alcohol dependence) and scored significantly high on presence of anxiety, depression, trait presence of alexithymia, and stressful life events as compared with healthy controls and those with fungal infections. Deshpande and coworkers [14] noted a high degree of psychiatric morbidity (65%), mainly anxiety and depressive disorders. No study has attempted directly to address the issue of stigma in psoriasis patients, although social issues were addressed by some [9,11,15].

*Vitiligo*

In India, vitiligo is a common pigmentary disorder of great social and cosmetic concern. Since ancient times, patients of vitiligo have suffered the same physical and mental abuses as leprosy of that age and they were considered to have "*Sweta Kushta*," meaning white leprosy. It is particularly disfiguring in people with dark skin and causes such a severe social stigma in Indian society that patients are considered unmarriageable [16], and women developing vitiligo after marriage have marital problems perhaps culminating in divorce. The first Prime Minister of India, Pandit Jawaharlal Nehru, ranked vitiligo as one of the three major medical problems of India, the other two being leprosy and malaria. In India, vitiligo, commonly known as "leukoderma," is unfortunately associated with certain myths, superstitions, and adverse religious beliefs. In some Indian religious texts where reincarnation is believed, it is said that a person who had done "*Guru Droh*" (meaning "had insulted teacher") in his or her previous life suffers from vitiligo in the present life. People suffering from vitiligo in India may have more and quite unique psychosocial problems than in other countries [17]. In a study [17] in North India, 150 patients of vitiligo had a mean Dermatology Life Quality Index score higher than that obtained by Finlay and Khan [18], indicating greater impact on their quality of life. Indian people have a pigmented skin predisposing them to prominent observable effects of hypopigmentary disorders like vitiligo. The psychosocial milieu of the developing countries being different from that of the developed countries, the stigma associated with hypopigmentation or depigmentation is possibly more severe in colored races inhabiting most of the developing world [19,20].

*Leprosy*

Leprosy is still a major public health problem in India, even though the prevalence rate has come down from 57.6 cases per 10,000 population (1981) to 2.7 cases per 10,000 populations (September 2003) [21]. Reduction in prevalence rate alone, however, is not sufficient because the social consequences of the disease on the life of patients are often severe and persist even after its cure. Leprosy is a highly stigmatized disease. Misconceptions about leprosy including beliefs that it is contagious, incurable, and hereditary or a consequence of divine punishment all contribute to stigma in many societies. Many studies done in India have confirmed the high prevalence of psychiatric morbidity in persons affected by this condition. Kumar and Verghese [22] found psychiatric morbidity in the community to be 99 per 1000 in comparison with 63 per 1000 in the general population. Most of the studies on psychologic aspects of leprosy have stressed the role of social stigma [22,23]. Psychiatric morbidity was noted to be positively correlated with physical disability; knowledge about disease and social, emotional, and health maladjustment; but not with duration of illness [24]. Gender bias has been observed and social impact on daily life has been more in females than males as revealed by isolation from daily activities, such as restrictions on participation in familial functions and touching children [25,26]. Behere [27] observed that 58% expressed suicidal ideas, 8% had made suicidal attempts, and there was a negative correlation between psychologic symptoms and duration of illness, indicating that some adaptation occurs with time and maybe intervention.

Leprosy is probably associated with maximum degree of deformity, disability, and social stigma [28]. Because of medical advances, there has been a considerable reduction in the stigma in the last 50 years. It is only in the last few years, however, that the social dimension is being increasingly recognized as critical to the process of rehabilitation of these patients and being incorporated into the various leprosy control programs [29].

Since the early 1980s, there have been studies on leprosy patients emphasizing the presence of psychiatric morbidity [12,23,27,30]. Patients had more negative attitudes toward their illness, most commonly illness evokes public fear and hate, illness is degrading and humiliating, they should be segregated from society, and illness is incurable and is a consequence of sins. Segregation from family (by being inpatients) accentuated the negative attitudes and associated stigma [23]. Subsequently, 100 displaced or migratory leprosy patients in a center in North-West India were studied [31,32] for presence of psychiatric morbidity and its correlates. A very high prevalence rate was found (76%), depression and anxiety being the illnesses encountered. The authors attributed this high psychiatric morbidity to the fact that the migrated patients had been stigmatized and subjected to rejection. Presence of social support (in the form of living in a sheltered supportive environment [ie, "ashram"]), however, contributed to lesser presence of psychiatric morbidity by offering social and emotional security. The authors emphasized the need for focus on other aspects of rehabilitation, apart from vocational rehabilitation. Kopparty and co-workers [33] observed that 20% reported socio-economic problems, this being 10 times more common in those with deformities. The extent of social problems depended on the degree of visibility and severity of the disease. The most common social problem faced was denial of participation of the family in community affairs. Additionally, they faced avoidance by friends, relatives, and neighbors, and experienced diminished marital prospects. Acceptance was the major coping strategy adopted by those families having deformed patients, whereas avoidance was adopted by those with nondeformed patients. This study demonstrated the social problems (and associated stigma) experienced not only by patients but also their families.

Further addressing this aspect of impact on families, 77 school-going children aged 5 to 15 years and staying in an ashram were examined for any behavioral changes or psychopathology [34]. None, however, manifested with any behavioral changes necessitating a referral to mental health services, indicating a probable protective affect of the ashram and importance of appropriate support and rehabilitation of the leprosy-affected families.

There have been very few studies that have examined the attitudes and knowledge of the patients, families, and the community. In a community study

[35] conducted in two different high-prevalence states of India (Andhra Pradesh and Orissa), 1199 community members were assessed on knowledge and attitude related to leprosy. It was seen that a high knowledge level did not necessarily generate positive attitudes. Overall, there was a general negative attitude despite 35% to 50% of respondents demonstrating a high level of knowledge. Segregation from social events and responsibilities, and rejection in marital relationships, were the commonest negative attitudes seen. Bharath and coworkers [24] noted that psychiatric morbidity correlated positively with knowledge about illness and social, emotional, health maladjustment. Nearly two thirds believed that they were being avoided or rejected by their neighbors and the larger society. This perceived social stigma was seen to be influencing their social functioning and psychologic well-being. It has been additionally reported that patients with leprosy can be subject to two kinds of stigma: social stigma and self-stigma leading into socially imposed isolation and self-imposed isolation [36]. In this review, Srinivasan [36] cites a study wherein there was a higher prevalence of self-stigmatization (30%) as compared with social stigmatization (8%) in patients with leprosy-related disabilities. Despite available literature highlighting stigma in leprosy, its related social dimensions are complex, multifaceted, and context-dependent and need to be studied further in greater detail.

Acne is probably the commonest dermatologic disorder and is associated with significant degree of disability and psychosocial distress [37,38]. Its psychosocial aspects have not been reported, however, in Indian literature to date.

In comparative studies on psychiatric morbidity in India, prevalence of depression was 23% and 10% in psoriasis and vitiligo, respectively, in one study [39], whereas another study demonstrated higher psychiatric morbidity (34%) in vitiligo as compared with psoriasis (25%) [15]. Thomas [40] and Bharath [41] did not find any difference in the psychiatric symptomatology and personality profile between patients with leprosy and other skin conditions. Leprosy patients had poorer social adjustment and perceived their neighbors to be rejecting them [41].

## Quality of life

The measurement of the impact of skin diseases on patients' quality of life is important. It is important to be able to measure this effect for clinical, therapeutic, and health service research, for political purposes and potentially to form clinical decisions [42]. The lives of the families of patients with skin disease may be affected. They may experience severe symptoms, especially itch, pain, and discomfort, and can become profoundly psychologically disturbed. Simple aspects of daily living, such as shopping or looking after the home or garden, may become difficult. The choice of clothes may be restricted and these may need to be washed or replaced more frequently. Social activities, such as going out with friends or taking part in sports, swimming, or other physical activities, may become difficult, often because of a reluctance to allow others to see the diseased skin coupled with a fear of what others may think of the appearance. The itch, appearance, or the literal "handicap" of not being able to use the hands at a keyboard because of painful fissures may interfere with work, and the exhaustion of treatment and disturbed sleep may reduce concentration and make studying difficult. Personal relationships may be difficult to form or may be adversely affected. Their skin disease may also impact their sexual lives. The treatment of skin disease may unfortunately have an initial effect of making quality of life worse because of the difficulty of using topical creams and ointments. To a deeply hurtful extent, ignorant or prejudiced attendants bar many patients with psoriasis and other widespread skin diseases from public swimming baths and patients are excluded from work with the public because employers are concerned about the possible reaction of their customers [42]. A study on people's perception of leprosy noted that people believed that the leprosy-afflicted should stay in leprosy colonies away from the society and most reported reluctance to employ the leprosy-afflicted as domestic help [43]. It is important that stigma issues also be included as an important dimension for quality of life. Evidence of the growing awareness of the value of measuring quality of life in India has been seen in recent publications [44,45]. Prasad and coworkers [17] examined the levels of quality of life impairment of patients with vitiligo. Patients who had successful treatment had a lower impairment of their quality of life than those patients in whom treatment failed.

## Stigma in skin disease: Indian context

Skin diseases are highly prevalent in developing countries like India and failure of display as a result of visibility of skin diseases causes considerable anguish and distress to patients, because society treats them in the same way as anyone else who appears to be different. Moreover, chronicity of skin disorders punctuated by periods of remissions and exacerbations and associated treatment difficulties can have an adverse impact on various aspects of a person's life (social functioning, school, employment, finances, recreation, and interpersonal relationship). Skin diseases of cosmetic concern like alopecia, melasma, and vitiligo are associated with significant psychologic morbidity resulting in loss of self-esteem, embarrassment, and depression.

Stigma about leprosy has been prevalent since ancient times. Stigma about leprosy has four components [46]: (1) physical, (2) psychologic, (3) social, and (4) moral. Leprosy damages skin, face, hands, and feet, which are means of communication, and segregates the patient, because they do not fulfill the identity norms imposed by society [41]. Mhaswade [47] found anxiety and depression in leprosy patients to be related to social variables, such as stigma and ignorance, and reversible with intervention. There are no studies correlating the frequency and nature of psychiatric morbidity to the extent of social stigma, attitude, or knowledge. Knowledge about leprosy among leprosy patients has range from 8% [48] to 93% [41]. Leprosy is associated in minds of many Indian people with beggars. It is not that beggars get leprosy, but that the attendant stigma and consequent unemployment reduces ordinary people to the level of having no alternative but to beg [41]. Leprosy commonly causes physical disabilities, which generate social stigma [49].

There are certain religious or holy cities that used to be the abode of discarded leprosy patients, who had to survive as beggars. Hindu scriptures mention giving alms to such persons as a noble act. Many patients with vitiligo also resort to this because of public misconception of vitiligo as leprosy. Stigmatization by the general public and their negative attitudes toward leprosy negatively impacts on patients' mental health. The patients' perception of the stigma further impacts their mental health [50]. A study on 140 leprosy patients in Bangladesh found depression to be greater in those patients who reported "I have been physically attacked by people," "I feel people regard me as strange," and "I have been refused the purchase of something by a shopkeeper," actual experiences of discrimination based on stigma associated with depression in leprosy patients [50]. VanBrackel [51] conducted a review of literature to examine work done on measuring stigma related to leprosy. Studies that measure stigma were broadly categorized into two groups: studies that assessed the effects of stigma on the person affected, and surveys that assess community attitudes or practices. In a study of social stigma among leprosy patients [52] attending a leprosy clinic in Gwalior, 26% cases reported social stigma, 43% cases showed social stigma from their neighbors, and 63% cases had stigma for touch. The social stigma was more prevalent in illiterates and low socioeconomic group patients. A total of 69% of cases were in need of social rehabilitation. Males were more victims of social stigma than females. Another study in Nagpur found that women suffered more isolation and rejection from the society [53]. Vlassoff and coworkers [54] reported that although both men and women were negatively affected in terms of their family and marital lives, women suffered more isolation and rejection. Psychologically, women seemed more vulnerable because they were deprived of personal contact with others in the domestic environment where they were accustomed to receiving their greatest emotional rewards. Women reported that indifference to them by other family members, or seeming negation of their presence, caused them the greatest suffering.

Marital relations and occupation have also been reported to be affected by leprosy. In one study [55], 67% attributed leprosy as the only reason for not getting a partner for marriage. Divorcing a leprosy-afflicted spouse is one of the manifestations of social stigma attached to leprosy. It mostly depends on the community's decision resulting from the physical and social threat perceived [56]. Leprosy uprooted some patients from their residences, who subsequently settled in a leprosy village or settlement. The occupational status of 46% patients was adversely affected because of leprosy; they became dependents or beggars. The social prejudice and deformities caused by leprosy have played key roles in socioeconomic deterioration of patients. Because of the fear of infecting the family members, women sufferers keep themselves aloof and constantly worry about divorce. Fear of social ostracism prevents the disclosure of disease to the community [25]. Surprisingly, discriminative attitudes were more common in joint than nuclear families. There have been different trends of social problems among the caste groups. Whereas the lower caste groups experienced more severe economic problems, the upper caste groups faced more social problems [57]. The integrated approach to community-based primary health care was found to be effective in reducing leprosy stigma in society [58]. Ironically, the stigma shown toward leprosy was higher among doctors and health educators when compared with the rest of the multidisciplinary team members [59]. Stigma has an impact on decisions to seek help [60]. The review on leprosy-related stigma

[51] concluded that leprosy stigma is still a global phenomenon, occurring in both endemic and nonendemic countries. Despite enormous cultural diversity, the areas of life affected are remarkable similar. They include mobility, interpersonal relationships, marriage, employment, leisure activities, and attendance at social and religious functions.

Vitiligo is a common pigmentary disorder of major social and cosmetic concern in India [61]. This disorder does not result in restriction of capacity to work or expectancy of life, but it causes cosmetic disfigurement leading to psychologic trauma to the patients. The reported incidence of vitiligo in various dermatologic clinics in India now varies from 0.5% to 1% [62]. The male/female ratio in vitiligo was observed in this study to be nearly equal, meaning that this disease has no predilection for any sex. Various workers also noted similar observations [63,64]. Further, the incidence of vitiligo was 43% in the 0- to 20-year age group as compared with a low incidence of only 10% in individuals over 40 years of age, which means more young people are getting afflicted with this disorder. Because of social stigma in the community, young women tend to report earlier because of matrimonial anxiety.

## Dealing with social stigma

Irreversible impairments and deformities are the main causes of the complex of negative social reactions attached to leprosy and stigma. Deformities and disabilities led to deterioration in their functional capabilities and their psychologic state of mind [55]. Prevention of disabilities can be achieved by prevention of impairments and disabilities and prevention of worsening of disabilities, but often these do not accompany the services offered toward medical cure at the grass root level [49]. Basic level health workers who have been imparted simple task-oriented training can easily implement self-care learning by leprosy patients and prevention of disabilities services using aids [65]. These services are effective in preventing worsening of deformities of the hands and healing of trophic foot ulcers. The major advantage of such a community-based program is to eliminate the social stigma in the patients' families and the education of the community [49].

Mental health care for patients, regulation of discriminatory action, and education that decreases social stigma among the general population, especially those who might often have contact with leprosy patients, are necessary to improve mental health of leprosy patients [50]. This probably holds true for many of the dermatologic disorders that are associated with distress, disability, and impaired quality of life. A conceptual issue that needs to be addressed in studies on dermatologic illnesses is "self" versus "social" stigmatization. Studies in general have looked at the self-beliefs, cognitions, and attitudes of the individual in determining stigma. In leprosy, attempts have been made to address the beliefs and attitudes of both patient and society. Stigmatization of persons with leprosy causes the emotional harm of social, economic, and spiritual deprivation. Individual counseling has benefits in addressing these psychosocial problems but is a slow process and effects few people at any one time. Floyd-Richard and Gurung [66] described their experience of group counseling of stigmatized persons, which addressed common issues to more than one person at a time, encouraging the unity of sufferers, developing compassion for others, understanding the common effects of stigmatization, and beginning to overcome its harmful effects. Another important variable to be considered in evaluating stigma is disability and behavior of the individual, which could be seen as being a product of the clinical features of the illness, associated psychologic morbidity, and underlying attitudes. Mahatma Gandhi's contribution in this regard is worth a mention. The Mahatma had a Christ-like compassion for leprosy patients, his approach to leprosy was essentially spiritual, and he included leprosy work as an integral part of his activities [1].

## Summary

Dermatologic disorders, even though not life threatening, generally have a major impact on patients' daily activities, psychologic and emotional state; and social relationships. The intensity of impact of skin disease on an individual person is extremely variable, however, and depends on the natural history of the disorder; the patient's demographic characteristics, personality, character, and value; the patient's life situation; and the attitudes of society. Social stigma toward dermatologic disorders in the Indian society is quite widespread, especially toward leprosy. The national leprosy control program is quite intensive and addresses comprehensive treatment and medicosurgical facilities for rehabilitation, supporting voluntary agencies working in the field of leprosy welfare and rehabilitation, public education, and mass publicity programs [1]. It is difficult to speculate if this stigma in Indian society is different from other cultures and societies. Over the years, stigma toward leprosy certainly seems to have reduced. It is evident that this stigma is an important dimension or determinant of quality of life. Dermatologists are expected to consider quality of life issues along with social aspects, nature of disorder, efficacy, and tolerability of various therapeutic options to optimize relief and comfort to their patients.

To get rid of social stigma we have to have self confidence first.

—Cheng Li Wang, China

## References

[1] Ministry of Welfare. Encyclopedia of social work in India, vol. 3. Ministry of Information & Broadcasting, New Delhi (India): Government of India; 1987. p. 300–12.
[2] Goffman E. Stigma: notes on the management of spoiled identity. Englewood Cliffs (NJ): Prentice Hall; 1963.
[3] Stafford MC, Scott RR. Stigma deviance and social control: some conceptual issues. In: Ainlay SC, Becker G, Coleman LM, editors. The dilemma of difference. New York: Plenum; 1986.
[4] Bruce GL. The stigma process: reconceiving the definition of stigma. Presented at the 128th Annual Meeting of American Public Health Association. November 15, 2000, Boston, Massachusetts.
[5] Ablon J. The nature of stigma and medical conditions. Epilepsy Behav 2002;3(6S2):2–9.
[6] Sharma N, Koranne RV, Singh RK. A comparative study of psychiatric morbidity in dermatology patients. Indian J Dermatol 2003;48:137–41.
[7] Agrawal S, Garg VK, Agarwalla A, et al. Psoriasis in Eastern Nepal: clinical profile and patients' beliefs about the disease. Indian J Dermatol 2003;48:78–82.
[8] Pulimood S, Rajagopalan B, Rajagopalan M, et al. Psychiatric morbidity among dermatology inpatients. Natl Med J India 1996;9:208–10.
[9] Bagadia VN, Ayyar KS, Pradhan PV, et al. Life stress in dermatology outpatients. Archives of Indian Psychiatry 1998;4:47–9.
[10] Patil A, Sharma S, Dhavale HS. Coping with psoriasis: need for consultation-liaison. Indian J Dermatol 2002;47:143–6.
[11] Sumir Kaur A, Malhotra SK. Is quality of life in a psoriatic affected by the disease? Presented at the 32nd National Conference of Indian Association of Dermatologists, Venereologists & Leprologists. January 23–25, 2004, Mumbai, India.
[12] Bharath S, Shamsunder C, Raghuram R, et al. Psychiatric morbidity in leprosy and psoriasis: a comparative study. Indian J Lepr 1997;69:341–5.
[13] Chaudhury S, Das AL, John TR, et al. Psychological factors in psoriasis. Indian J Psychiatry 1998;40:295–9.
[14] Deshpande N, Desai N, Mundra VK. Psychiatric aspects of psoriasis. Archives of Indian Psychiatry 1998;4:61–4.
[15] Mattoo SK, Handa S, Kaur I, et al. Psychiatric morbidity in vitiligo and psoriasis: a comparative from India. J Dermatol 2001;28:424–32.
[16] Dogra S, Kanwar AJ. Skin diseases: psychological and social consequences. Indian J Dermatol 2002;47:197–201.
[17] Prasad D, Pandhi R, Dogra S, et al. Dermatology Life Quality Index Score in vitiligo and its impact on treatment outcome. Br J Dermatol 2003;148:373–4.
[18] Finlay AY, Khan G. Dermatology Life Quality Index: a simple practical measure for routine clinical use. Clin Exp Dermatol 1994;19:210–6.
[19] Handa S, Kaur I. Vitiligo: clinical findings in 1436 patients. J Dermatol 1999;26:653–7.
[20] Mattoo SK, Handa S, Kaur I, et al. Psychiatric morbidity in vitiligo: prevalence and correlates in India. J Eur Acad Dermatol Venereol 2002;16:573–8.
[21] Dhillon GPS. Leprosy elimination in India. Indian J Lepr 2004;76:119–25.
[22] Kumar JHR, Verghese A. Psychiatric disturbances among leprosy patients: an epidemiological study. Int J Lepr 1980;48:431–4.
[23] Chatterjee RN, Nandi DN, Banerjee G, et al. The social and psychological correlates of leprosy. Indian J Psychiatry 1989;31:315–8.
[24] Bharath S, Shamasundar C, Raghuram R, et al. Correlates of psychiatric morbidity in patients with leprosy. Indian J Lepr 2001;73:217–27.
[25] Kaur H, Ramesh V. Social problems of women leprosy patients: a study conducted at two urban leprosy centres. Lepr Rev 1994;65:361–75.
[26] Rao S, Garole V, Walawalkar S, et al. Gender differential in the social impact of leprosy. Lepr Rev 1996;67:190–9.
[27] Behere PB. Psychological reactions to leprosy. Lepr India 1981;53:266–72.
[28] Frist TF. Stigma and societal response to leprosy: experience of the last half century. Indian J Lepr 2000;72:1–3.
[29] Smith CM, Smith WCS. Current understanding of disability prevention. Indian J Lepr 2000;72:393–9.
[30] Ramanathan U, Srivastav I, Ramu G. Psychiatric morbidity in patients with leprosy. In: Brown SG, editor. XII International Leprosy Congress Proceedings. New Delhi: The Leprosy Mission; 1984. p. 810–1.
[31] Verma KK, Gautam S. Psychiatric morbidity in displaced leprosy patients. Indian J Lepr 1994;66:339–43.
[32] Verma KK, Gautam S. Effect of rehabilitation on the prevalence of psychiatric morbidity among leprosy patients. Indian Journal of Psychiatry 1994;36:183–6.
[33] Kopparty SNM, Kurup AM, Sivaram M. Problems and coping strategies of families having patients with and without deformities. Indian J Lepr 1995;67:133–52.

[34] Mahajan BB, Garg G, Gupta RR. A study of behavioural changes and clinical evaluation of leprosy in school going children of leprosy parents. Indian J Dermatol Venereol Lepr 2002;68:279–80.

[35] Raju MS, Kopparty SNM. Impact of knowledge of leprosy on the attitude towards leprosy patients: a community study. Indian J Lepr 1995;67:259–72.

[36] Srinivasan H. Disability and rehabilitation in leprosy: issues and challenges. Indian J Lepr 2000;72:317–37.

[37] Aktan S, Ozmen E, Sanli B. Anxiety, depression, and nature of acne vulgaris in adolescents. Int J Dermatol 2000;39:354–7.

[38] Finlay AY. The pathogenesis, disability and management of acne. Indian J Dermatol Venereol Lepr 1990; 56:349–53.

[39] Sharma N, Koranne RV, Singh PK. Psychiatric morbidity in psoriasis and vitiligo. J Dermatol 2001;28: 419–23.

[40] Thomas MJ. Psychiatric symptomatology and personality profiles of certain specific skin disorders [dissertation]. Bangalore (India): University of Bangalore; 1983.

[41] Bharath S. Pattern of psychiatric morbidity and psychosocial correlates in Hansen's disease: a controlled study [thesis]. Bangalore (India): University of Bangalore; 1987.

[42] Finlay AY. Quality of life indices. Indian J Dermatol Venereol Lepr 2004;70:143–8.

[43] Kaur H, Gandhi A. People's perception of leprosy: a study in Delhi. Indian J Lepr 2003;75:37–46.

[44] D'Souza M, Rakesh SV, Unni KES, et al. Quality of life in patients with psoriasis: a preliminary study from South India. Ann Dermatol Venereol 2002;129:1S752.

[45] Rakesh SV. Quality of life in patients with psoriasis: a dermato-psychological study [thesis]. Pondicherry (India): Pondicherry University; 2003.

[46] Gonzalez A. Stigma and leprosy. Int Lepr Congress Series 1978;11:466.

[47] Mhaswade BC. Leprosy: a case for mental health care. Lepr India 1983;55:310–3.

[48] Pal S, Girdahar BK. Knowledge and attitude among leprosy patients. Ind J Leprosy 1985;57:620–3.

[49] Ganapati R, Pai VV, Kingsley S. Disability prevention and management in leprosy: a field experience. Indian J Dermatol Venereol Lepr 2003;69:369–74.

[50] Tsutsumi A, Izutsu T, Islam MDA, et al. Depressive status of leprosy patients in Bangladesh: association of self perception of stigma. Lepr Rev 2004; 75:57–66.

[51] VanBrackel WH. Measuring leprosy stigma: a preliminary review of leprosy literature. Int J Lepr Other Mycobact Dis 2003;71:190–7.

[52] Kushwah SS, Govila AK, Upadhyay S, et al. A study of social stigma among leprosy patients attending leprosy clinic in Gwalior. Lepr India 1981;53:221–5.

[53] Zodpey SP, Tiwari RR, Salodkar AD. Gender differentials in the social and family life of leprosy patients. Lepr Rev 2000;71:505–10.

[54] Vlassoff C, Khot S, Rao S. Double jeopardy: women and leprosy in India. World Health Stat Q 1996;49: 120–6.

[55] Kumar A, Anbalagan M. Socio-economic experiences of leprosy patients. Lepr Rev 1983;55:314–21.

[56] Raju MS, Reddy JV. Community attitude to divorce in leprosy. Indian J Lepr 1995;67:389–403.

[57] Kopparty SN. Problems, acceptance and social inequality: a study of the deformed leprosy patients and their families. Lepr Rev 1995;66:239–49.

[58] Arole S, Premkumar R, Arole R, et al. Social stigma: a comparative qualitative study of integrated and vertical care approaches to leprosy. Lepr Rev 2002; 73:186–96.

[59] Premkumar R, Kumar KS, Dave SL. Understanding the attitude of multidisciplinary teams working in leprosy. Lepr Rev 1994;65:66–77.

[60] Nicholls PG, Weins C, Smith WCS. Delay in presentation in the context of local knowledge and attitude towards leprosy: the results of qualitative fieldwork in Paraguay. Int J Lepr Other Mycobact Dis 2003;71:198–209.

[61] Kar PK. Vitiligo: a study of 120 cases. Indian J Dermatol Venereol Lepr 2001;67:302–4.

[62] Das SK, Mazumdar PP, Chakraborty R. Studies on vitiligo. I: Epidemiological profile in Calcutta. India Genet Epid 1985;2:71–8.

[63] Sarin RC, Kumar AS. A clinical study of vitiligo. Indian J Dermatol Venereol Lepr 1977;33:190–4.

[64] Behl PN, Agarwal RS, Singh G. Aetiological studies in vitiligo and therapeutic response to standard treatment. Indian J Dermatol 1961;6:101.

[65] Ganapati R, Kingsley S, Pai VV, et al. A field model for prevention of leprosy disabilities: a step towards achieving a world without leprosy. Int J Lepr 2002; 70:289A.

[66] Floyd-Richard M, Gurung S. Stigma reduction through group counselling of persons affected by leprosy: a pilot study. Lepr Rev 2000;71:499–504.

# Psychosocial Aspects Of Aging Skin

Madhulika A. Gupta, MD, FRCPC[a,b],*, Barbara A. Gilchrest, MD[c]

[a]Department of Psychiatry, University of Western Ontario, London, Canada
[b]Mediprobe Research Inc, London, ON, Canada
[c]Department of Dermatology, Boston University School of Medicine, Boston, MA, USA

There is a steady rise in the number of individuals in the United States who are over 65, and the demand for rejuvenating products and procedures that delay or conceal the signs of skin aging is expanding rapidly [1,2]. Some of the major determinants of aging of the appearance include genetics, sun exposure, smoking, and activity of the facial muscles. The skin is a powerful organ of communication and projects various socially important attributes including social status, wealth, and sexuality, in addition to age [3–8]. Today's consumer culture sends a strong message about the need to get older without the signs of aging. The idea that chronologic age itself does not signal the beginning of old age [9] has become increasingly prevalent, with a high value placed by society on the maintenance of a youthful appearance and the reversal of some age-related bodily changes. In the media, average consumers are shown undergoing surgical and nonsurgical makeovers to rejuvenate their appearance, implying that ordinary individuals (not only movie stars and celebrities) readily can achieve a younger-looking body. This most likely places greater pressure on individuals to pursue such treatments and procedures and tends to trivialize the risks associated with the relatively major surgery that some of the procedures involve. It also is important to distinguish aging from age-related disease [10]. The failure to distinguish between the two has psychosocial consequences, as individuals often are lured into using products and procedures that claim to reverse the aging process. At present, the rejuvenating products and procedures essentially mask age-related changes and, therefore, may be considered palliative [10].

Data from the United States Census Bureau for 2000 [11,12] indicate that the 65-year and older population comprised 35 million people. The over-65 age group comprised 12% of the total United States population in 2000, and it is projected that by 2025 this age group will constitute more than 18% of the total population. In some of the most populous developing nations, the overall percentage of older individuals is smaller, even though the absolute numbers still are high. For example, in China, where 6.9% of the total population was in the over-65 age group in 2000, the projected increase in the over-65 age group by 2025 is to 13.7% [12]; and in India, where only 4.6% of the population was over age 65 in 2000, the projected increase by 2025 is to 7.8% [12]. An increase in the aging population and rapid globalization likely will result in an increasing worldwide demand for cutaneous rejuvenation products.

Over the past several decades, the cultural and social meanings of growing old have changed, and old age has started to acquire increasingly negative connotations [7–9]. Often, normal intrinsic aging is viewed as a medical and social problem that needs to be addressed by health care professionals. An increasing number of individuals, therefore, are turning to dermatologic procedures and products that may have a rejuvenating effect on the appearance. Another aging-related phenomenon with an important psychosocial component is the increasing emphasis on a youthful appearance, as greater numbers of individuals are becoming concerned about age-

* Corresponding author. 645 Windermere Road, London, ON N5X 2P1, Canada.
E-mail address: magupta@uwo.ca (M.A. Gupta).

related changes at a much younger age. For example, a recent study reports that more than 50% of women under age 30 report dissatisfaction with the appearance of their skin; some of their dissatisfactions for example, with "bags and darkness" under the eyes, freckles, patchy hyperpigmentation and fine wrinkles, are associated with aging of the skin [13]. This emerging phenomenon, wherein younger individuals may be seeking treatments for cutaneous rejuvenation, suggests that in many instances the psychosocial dimension is perhaps the most important aspect of the management of aging skin.

## Aging skin and interpersonal interactions

The body, especially the appearance of the face, greatly influences individual personal and social identity, and exterior surfaces of the body often become symbols of the inner self [14], an intuitive notion that is supported experimentally. A youthful appearance is associated with increased self-esteem and improved social relations [15]. In one study [16], 20 observers representing both genders rated photographs of 48 white women between ages 54 and 96 for physical attractiveness. Two essentially nonoverlapping groups of 16 women each who were on opposite ends of the attractiveness spectrum were selected from the 48 subjects [16]. The attractiveness ratings were affected strongly by cutaneous signs typically associated with aging (eg, wrinkling and sagging) by male and female judges [16]. Furthermore, the group of women rated as good-looking by the observers also reported greater satisfaction with their lives and described themselves as more socially outgoing. This further supports the view that an attractive appearance has a positive effect on social functioning. In a study of 20 subjects who had mild to moderately photodamaged skin [17] and who had entered a study to evaluate the efficacy of topical tretinoin for the treatment of photodamaged skin, it was observed that at baseline the subjects had high scores on the Interpersonal Sensitivity and Phobic Anxiety subscales of the Brief Symptom Inventory (BSI) [17]. The Interpersonal Sensitivity (BSI) [18] subscale measures a lack of ease during interpersonal interactions, and the Phobic Anxiety (BSI) [18] subscale provides an index of a persistent fear response to certain situations, including social situations, that leads to avoidance of the anxiety-provoking situations. High scores on these BSI subscales, therefore, suggest that the subjects who have photodamage were experiencing uneasiness during their interpersonal interactions. After 24 weeks of therapy, the Interpersonal Sensitivity (BSI) and Phobic Anxiety (BSI) scores decreased significantly ($P < 0.05$) in the topical tretinoin but not the control group that was receiving the inactive vehicle [17]. These finding were confirmed in another study [19] involving 40 subjects who had moderate to severe photodamage. In this study [19], a significant decrease in Phobic Anxiety (BSI) [18] ($P < 0.05$) was observed after 24 weeks of therapy with topical tretinoin, whereas an increase in Phobic Anxiety (BSI) ($P < 0.05$) was noted in the group receiving the inactive vehicle. These findings indicate that age-related changes affecting the skin cause increased social anxiety in some subjects, and this anxiety decreases with the treatment of photodamage [7,8]. Increased ease during interpersonal interactions usually translates into increased socialization and possibly increased physical activity. These lifestyle-related factors may have a protective effect on the overall physical health of older adults, especially those who have chronic health problems [20,21]. It is shown further that when older adults' feelings of personal control over their health are low, collective self-esteem (individual self-evaluation of social identify) may compensate and have a protective effect on overall health [21]. A strong and positive social identity facilitates accommodation to negative health-related circumstances in later life, especially when one is unable to alter these circumstances directly [21]. An improved appearance and its positive effect on socialization are likely to have a positive impact on the collective self-esteem of older adults. These findings suggest that the therapies for the cutaneous changes secondary to photodamage, and the changes associated with intrinsic aging, can have a significantly favorable impact on the overall heath and well-being of individuals, even if the treatments are palliative.

Facial appearance and expressions play a central role in the communication of emotions, in addition to signaling characteristics such as age [22]. The interpretation of facial expressions is an integral component of interpersonal communication and tends to be universal and constant across time and cultures [22]. The face is the focus of human communication and facial expressions have evolved as a means of nonverbal communication and as a way of enhancing verbal communication [22]. The repeated expression of emotion over time produces hyperfunctional facial lines [22]. The presence of these lines when the face is at repose may give a person an aged appearance or give an erroneous impression of emotions or personality characteristics. As the skin ages and the support of the underlying cutaneous structures is lost, more wrinkles and folds develop, and gradually the dynamic lines that communicate emotion change to static lines ingrained on the face at rest. The orientation and depth of these folds is influenced greatly by the underlying activity of the facial muscles [22]. These hyperfunctional lines are common in the forehead, between the brows, around the eyes, and in the area of the mouth [22]. For example, hyperfunctional forehead lines may give an impression of aging, and frown lines or deep vertical creases in the glabelar region give the impression of anger or dissatisfaction. It is suggested that these hyperfunctional lines can result in a "malfunction of the facial organ of communication" [22,23]. With aging, the corner of the mouth often droops, creating an appearance that may be misinterpreted as displeasure or sadness [22], or the drooping of the brow or sagging of the upper eyelid may result in the appearance of drowsiness and exhaustion [22]. Therefore, the internal emotion may be different from the message received by others, and the disparity between the internal mood and external appearance may culminate in a feeling of disconnect between the inner self and the face that individuals see in the mirror. This incongruity may be confirmed in social interactions, resulting in a sense of alienation. These miscues may affect reciprocal behavior further; for example, a frown is more likely to elicit a frown rather than a smile from another person, and negative responses usually reinforce negative behavior, resulting in greater social alienation [22]. The increasing presence of hyperfunctional facial lines with age, therefore, has implications beyond considerations of attractiveness, as they affect the perception of emotions and perceived personality traits of individuals; treatments to smooth the hyperfunctional facial lines may be warranted because of their positive social ramifications [22].

An aged appearance can elicit certain reactions from caregivers and influence the type of care individuals receive [7,8]. For example, it is observed that caregivers in nursing homes and hospitals sometimes disengage from patients emotionally when their grooming habits, hygiene, or appearance begin to deteriorate or when the patient appears aged [7,8,24]. Alternately, an improved appearance secondary to improved hair care and cosmetics is associated with increased interest by caregivers and even taken as evidence by caregivers that a patient's physical state is improving. It is likely that older individuals in the community, who are regularly in contact with professionals in the community for their heath care and other needs that enable them to maintain an independent lifestyle, also experience similar reactions. The beneficial effects of touch seem to increase with age [25]; however, the opportunity to be touched by friends and family tends to decrease significantly with age, in part because people often do not like touching the elderly [25]. An attractive appearance is more likely to elicit touching by caregivers and, in a circular fashion, nursing home residents who receive regular touch through massages, hugs, squeezes of the hand, and so forth, show fewer signs of senility and are more alert [25].

An aged appearance plays a central role in the interpersonal transactions of the business world. More than ever before, society today tends to equate beauty and productivity with youth [26,27], and older individuals face discrimination in the workplace. This is especially relevant for women, as the double standard of aging [8,28] continues to be an important factor. Most positive traits associated with masculinity, such as autonomy, power, and competence, increase with age, whereas feminine characteristics, such as gentleness and passivity, do not change with age [29]. Women tend to be valued more for their attractiveness than their competence, and attractiveness tends to decrease with age. Therefore, in contrast to older men, older women tend to face appearance-related problems in the workplace to a greater degree and at an earlier age. In a study [24] involving eight women ranging in age from the late 20s to 60s, photographs before and after cosmetic makeovers were attached to resumes and submitted to 120 major private employment agencies and large corporations. The physical appearance of the applicant was observed to play an important role in the hiring process at all skill levels, with the greatest difference noted on jobs requiring the lowest skill level. In this job category, the same individuals after the cosmetic makeover received 8% to 20% higher salary offers than those before.

## Aging skin and the psychologic state

An aged appearance can have a significant psychologic impact on individuals [7,8]. Pearlman [30] describes a transitional developmental phase, sometimes reaching the proportions of a crisis, that she has termed "late midlife astonishment" [30]. She describes a psychologic reaction to a sudden awareness of the stigmatization of aging, which may manifest as amazement, despair, a disruption of sense of self and identity, or feelings of heightened vulnerability, shame, depression, and severe loss of self-esteem [30]. Other factors, such as declining health and menopause, can further lead to a sense of diminished physical or sexual attractiveness [7,8,30]. Perlman observes that in late midlife it may not be possible to pass as younger than one's chronologic age, making the psychologic adjustment to aging more difficult [30]. This may be one reason why studies show that treatment of photodamaged skin with topical tretinoin [17,19] and cosmetic makeovers to cover the cutaneous signs of aging [7,16] are associated with an increased sense of well-being, increased ease during interpersonal interactions, and decreased anxiety [17,19].

Individuals who have severely narcissistic personalities may develop a major adjustment disorder in reaction to the cutaneous signs of aging [6–8]. Among such narcissistic individuals who have a desperate need to be admired, having a youthful appearance often is a precondition for self-acceptance and trusting that they are accepted by others, and an aged appearance can result in a significant emotional crisis, including a severe depressive reaction. The incidence of some psychiatric emergencies, such as suicide, increases with age [31], and rates of completed suicide are higher among men but rise in men and women in the latter decades of life and rise significantly after age 75 [31]. Older persons attempt suicide less often but are more successful in committing suicide [31]. It is possible that some of the psychosocial reactions to aged appearance, such as social isolation, decreased self-esteem, and depression, also make some older individuals more vulnerable to psychiatric emergencies, such as suicide [8].

A psychologic dimension that plays a critical role in the degree to which individuals are affected by cutaneous aging is an internal locus of control, which refers to the degree to which individuals see life's outcomes as dependent on their own abilities and efforts [7,8]. It was observed that patients who were concerned about their photodamaged skin and volunteered for studies [19] evaluating the efficacy of topical tretinoin also had obsessive-compulsive traits, indicated by high obsessive-compulsiveness scores on the BSI [18]. Obsessive-compulsiveness is associated with perfectionistic personality traits, a tendency to be excessively self-critical, and an inordinate need to be in control of one's life [18]. These personality traits probably predisposed these individuals to seek treatment for their wrinkles [19]. After 24 weeks of therapy with topical tretinoin, the subjects reported a decline in their obsessive-compulsiveness (BSI) scores, but those receiving the inactive vehicle reported an increase in this symptom dimension [19]. These findings also suggest that external life events that adversely affect an individual's internal locus of control, such as loss of livelihood or health, making them feel more vulnerable, also may heighten their concern about their aging appearance and predispose them to seek treatment for their aging skin [5].

## Aging skin and body image

The impact of aging skin on body image, which is defined as the mental representation of the body and its organs, may generalize to concerns about overall body image not related directly to the skin [7,8]. It is shown, for example, that concerns about the aging of the appearance often are associated with concerns about other aspects of body image, such as body weight. In a study of 71 men and 102 women recruited simply because they were present in a shopping mall [32], it was observed that the effect of aging on the appearance correlated directly, albeit weakly (r = 0.4; $P < 0.05$), with the Drive for Thinness subscale of the Eating Disorder Inventory (EDI) [33], even after the possible confounding effect of body mass index (BMI = $kg/m^2$) and chronologic age were partialled out statistically. This correlation was significant among men and women. The Drive for Thinness subscale of the EDI [33] measures an excessive preoccupation with dieting and exercise and an ardent desire to lose weight. Furthermore, among the women, the belief that having younger-looking skin is a prerequisite to good looks correlated with Drive for Thinness (EDI) [33] (r = 0.3; $P < 0.01$) and Body Dissatisfaction (EDI) [33] (r = 0.4; $P < 0.01$) after the effects of age and body mass index were partialled out statistically. The Body Dissatisfaction subscale of the EDI [33] measures dissatisfaction with body shape and weight and the concern that certain body regions, such as the abdomen, hips and thighs, are too fat. This finding was replicated in another randomly selected sample of nonclinical subjects [34]. Furthermore, in a prospective controlled study of patients undergoing treatment of photodamaged skin [19] with topical tretinoin or an inactive vehicle (control group), it was observed that the patients receiving the active treatment with topical tretinoin and not the control group reported a significant decline ($P < 0.01$) in Drive for Thinness (EDI) and Body Dissatisfaction (EDI) after 24 weeks. These findings highlight the impact of photodamaged skin on satisfaction with overall body image, including aspects of body image not necessarily related to aging.

A youthful look typically is associated with a slim and well-toned body, and some individuals may become excessively preoccupied with diet and exercise as they age [5]. In a small group of individuals who have other risk factors for the development of an eating disorder, the fear of aging precipitated by the cutaneous changes of aging can culminate in anorexia nervosa [5,35]. Eating disorders, such as anorexia nervosa and bulimia nervosa, are associated with a distortion of body image perception, which manifests mainly as a fear of fatness and drive for thinness. In some patients who have eating disorders, the body image concerns generalize to other aspects of appearance in addition to body weight, including concerns about the appearance of their skin. In some patients who have eating disorders, the concern about cutaneous body image may be grossly inconsistent with the norms for their age [13]. In a cross-sectional study [13] examining concerns about various aspects of skin appearance in 30-year-old patients who had eating disorders (n = 32) and nonclinical controls (n = 34), it was observed that 81% of the patients who had an eating disorder versus 56% of controls reported dissatisfaction with the appearance of their skin ($P = 0.03$). The cutaneous attributes that were of the greatest concern to the patients who had eating disorders were those that also are associated with aging and photodamage (eg, darkness under the eyes, freckles, fine wrinkles, and patchy hyperpigmentation [in addition to dryness and roughness of the skin, which often are secondary to an eating disorder]). One of the central psychopathologic factors underlying eating disorders, which have a peak incidence during the teenage years, is difficulty dealing with the developmental tasks of adolescence and young adulthood. It is possible that the greater concerns about aging skin in the sample that had eating disorders was an index of the overall difficulties experienced by these patients in dealing with growing up and growing old [8]. Patients who had body dysmorphic disorder (BDD) (previously termed dysmorphophobia) [36], which usually also begins during adolescence, present with an excessive preoccupation about their appearance. The defect is either imagined or slight and patients' concern is grossly out of proportion to any objective problem. BDD commonly is associated with concerns that are associated with aging skin, such as wrinkles, hair thinning, and vascular markings [36]. Therefore, some younger patients who have severe body image pathologies, such as eating disorders and BDD, may present to the dermatologist with concerns about aging skin. For example, in cosmetic surgery and dermatology settings, reported rates of BDD range from 6% to 15% [36].

## Summary

A youthful and slim body has become a symbol of financial success, social acceptance, and interpersonal happiness. The idea that chronologic age itself does not signal the beginning of old age has become increasingly prevalent and there is a steady rise in the number of older individuals who are becoming avid consumers of products and procedures that delay or conceal the signs of aging. A greater number of individuals is becoming concerned about aging-related skin changes at a much younger age (eg, under age 30). Some younger individuals who have serious body image pathologies, such as eating disorders and BDD, seek treatments for minimal age-related changes of the skin.

Some of the major psychosocial factors associated with skin aging include social anxiety, isolation, and, occasionally, a more serious emotional crisis, such as depression, in severely narcissistic individuals for whom a youthful appearance is a precondition for self-acceptance. Alternately, older individuals who have a positive self-perception of aging and a favorable body image are less likely to suffer from chronic diseases, as they are more likely to practice preventive behaviors, such as diet, exercise, and adherence to medications. Caregivers sometimes disengage emotionally from individuals who appear less attractive as a result of aging and this may affect the quality of support and care they receive adversely. Older individuals, especially older women, may face age-related discrimination in the workplace. It is important, therefore, for dermatologists to provide effective treatments for cutaneous aging, albeit palliative, while ensuring that patients have a realistic view of what treatment has to offer.

## References

[1] Gilchrest BA. Skin aging 2003: recent advances and current concepts. Cutis 2003;72(3 Suppl):5–10 [discussion: 10].
[2] Hurza GJ. Rejuvenating the aging face [editorial]. Arch Dermatol 2004;140:1383–6.
[3] Koblenzer CS. Psychologic aspects of aging and the skin. Clin Dermatol 1996;14:171–7.
[4] Kligman AM. Psychological aspects of skin disorders in the elderly. Cutis 1989;43:489–501.
[5] Gupta MA. The aging face: a psychocutaneous perspective. Facial Plast Surg 1995;11:86–90.
[6] Kligman AM, Graham JA. The psychology of appearance in the elderly. Dermatol Clin 1986;4:501–7.
[7] Gupta MA. Aging skin and quality of life. In: Rajgopalan R, Sheretz EF, Anderson RT, editors. Care management of skin diseases: life quality and economic impact. New York: Marcel Dekker; 1998. p. 245–51.
[8] Gupta MA, Gupta AK. Psychological impact of aging and the skin. In: Koo JYM, Lee CS, editors. Psychocutaneous medicine. New York: Marcel Dekker; 2003. p. 365–73.

[9] Hirshbein LD. Popular views of old age in America, 1900–1950. J Am Geriatr Soc 2001;49:1555–60.
[10] Hayflick L. "Anti-aging" is an oxymoron. J Gerontol Biol Sci 2004;59A:573–8.
[11] US Census Burea. Older Americans Month: May 2004 new information. US Census Burea Public Information Office: Multimedia. Available at: http://www.census.gov/pubinfo/www/multimedia/Older2004.html. Accessed January 2, 2005.
[12] US Census Bureau. International database summary demographic data. Available at: http://www.census.gov/ipc/www/idbsum.html. Accessed January 2, 2005.
[13] Gupta MA, Gupta AK. Dissatisfaction with skin appearance among patients with eating disorders and non-clinical controls. Br J Dermatol 2001;145:110–3.
[14] Oberg P, Tornstam L. Body images among men and women of different ages. Aging Society 1999;19:629–44.
[15] Kligman AM, Koblenzer C. Demographics and psychological implications for the aging population. Dermatol Clin 1997;15:549–53.
[16] Graham JA, Kligman AM. Physical attractiveness, cosmetic use and self-perception in the elderly. Int J Cosmet Sci 1985;7:85–97.
[17] Gupta MA, Goldfarb MT, Schork NJ, et al. Treatment of mildly to moderately photoaged skin with topical tretinoin has a favorable psychosocial effect: a prospective study. J Am Acad Dermatol 1991;24:780–1.
[18] Derogatis LR, Spencer PM. The Brief Symptom Inventory (BSI), administrative, scoring and procedures manual-I. Baltimore: Clinical Psychometric Research, Johns Hopkins University; 1982.
[19] Gupta MA, Schork NJ, Ellis CN. Psychosocial correlates of the treatment of photodamaged skin with topical retinoic acid: a prospective controlled study. J Am Acad Dermatol 1994;30:969–72.
[20] Levy BR, Myers LM. Preventive health behaviors influenced by self-perceptions of aging. Prev Med 2004;39:625–9.
[21] Bailis DS, Chipperfield JG. Compensating for losses in perceived personal control over health: A role for collective self-esteem in healthy aging. J Gerontol Psychol Sci 2002;57B:531–9.
[22] Finn JC, Cox SE, Earl ML. Social implications of hyperfunctional facial lines. Dermatol Surg 2003;29:450–5.
[23] Khan JA. Aesthetic surgery: diagnosing and healing the miscues of human facial expression. Opthal Plastic Reconstr Surg 2001;17:4–6.
[24] Waters J. Cosmetics and the job market. In: Graham JA, Kligman AM, editors. The psychology of cosmetic treatments. New York: Praeger; 1986. p. 113–24.
[25] Field T. Touch. Cambridge (MA): MIT Press; 2001. p. 19–32
[26] Rodeheaver D. Labor market progeria. Generations: Journal of the American Society on Aging 1990;14(3):53–8.
[27] Koblenzer CS. Psychosocial aspects of beauty: how and why to look good. Clin Dermatol 2003;21:473–5.
[28] Sontag S. The double standard of aging. In: Williams J, editor. Psychology of women. New York: Academic Press; 1979. p. 462–78.
[29] Saucier MG. Midlife and beyond: issues for aging women. J Couns Dev 2004;82:420–5.
[30] Pearlman SF. Late mid-life astonishment: disruptions to identity and self-esteem. Women Ther 1993;14:1–12.
[31] Sadock BJ, Sadock VA. Suicide, violence and other psychiatric emergencies. In: Sadock BJ, Sadock VA, editors. Kaplan & Sadock's pocket handbook of clinical psychiatry. 3rd edition. Philadelphia: Lippincott Williams & Wilkins; 2001. p. 261–74.
[32] Gupta MA, Schork NJ. Aging-related concerns and body image: possible future implications for eating disorders. Int J Eat Disord 1993;14:481–6.
[33] Garner DM, Olmstead MP. Eating disorder inventory manual. Lutz (FL): Psychological Assessment Resources; 1984.
[34] Gupta MA. Concern about aging and drive for thinness: a factor in the biopsychosocial model for eating disorders? Int J Eat Disord 1995;18:351–7.
[35] Gupta MA. Fear of aging: a precipitating factor in late onset anorexia nervosa. Int J Eat Disord 1990;9:221–4.
[36] American Psychiatric Association. Diagnostic and statistical manual for mental disorders (DSM IV-TR). 4th edition, text revision. Washington, DC: American Psychiatric Association; 2000.

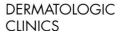

# Psychologic Trauma, Posttraumatic Stress Disorder, and Dermatology

Madhulika A. Gupta, MD, FRCPC[a,b,*], Ruth A. Lanius, MD, PhD[c], Bessel A. Van der Kolk, MD[d]

[a]*Department of Psychiatry, University of Western Ontario, London, Ontario, Canada*
[b]*Mediprobe Research Inc, London, ON, Canada*
[c]*Traumatic Stress Program, Department of Psychiatry, University of Western Ontario, London, ON, Canada*
[d]*Boston University School of Medicine, Brookline, MA, USA*

Psychologic stress has been long recognized as associated with the onset or exacerbation of a wide range of dermatologic disorders [1,2]. The term, stress, is used to address three major areas in the dermatologic literature: natural or manmade catastrophic events (eg, major earthquakes or a plane crash); psychologic stress, which focuses on patients' subjective evaluations of their ability to cope with demands posed by certain experiences (eg, stress caused by the social stigma associated with a skin disorder or stress secondary to the unexpected death of a loved one); and biologic measures, such as stress-induced activation of the hypothalamic-pituitary-adrenal axis function after exposure of patients to mental arithmetic. Psychologic trauma, by definition, means that the human capacity to cope is overwhelmed and that normal homeostatic mechanisms no longer are operative. Trauma represents a more severe form of stress. Family violence and child abuse are the most common causes of posttraumatic stress disorder (PTSD). Traumatic events include, but are not limited to, natural or manmade disasters; war; torture or concentration camp experiences; severe accidents;

the development of severe and life-threatening illness; and violent personal assault, such as rape, sexual assault, and physical abuse, which all may be associated with PTSD. The literature on psychologic trauma and dermatology has examined the role of the lack of tactile nurturance and maternal deprivation during the developmentally critical periods of early childhood. Maternal deprivation and neglect may lead to symptoms by a different pathophysiologic process than traumatic experiences, such as family violence and child abuse. Skin disorders also are associated with catastrophic events, such as earthquakes and plane crash, which are rare compared with family violence and child abuse, and conversion symptoms [3] or somatoform dissociation [4], which may occur when traumatic life experiences result in PTSD [3].

Some of the major features of PTSD include psychophysiologic reactions, such as (1) intrusive re-experiencing and intense physiologic reactivity to situations and stimuli that are reminiscent of the trauma; (2) hyperarousal and hypervigilance associated with trauma; and (3) avoidance and emotional numbing. Emotional numbing may present as depressive or dissociative states when a patient's responsiveness to the external world is diminished and the patient experiences emotional or physical numbing and anesthesia. PTSD probably is under-recognized in dermatology. This article reviews some of the salient literature on psychologic trauma and dermatology.

* Corresponding author. 645 Windermere Road, London, ON N5X 2P1, Canada.
E-mail address: magupta@uwo.ca (M.A. Gupta).

0733-8635/05/$ – see front matter © 2005 Elsevier Inc. All rights reserved.
doi:10.1016/j.det.2005.05.018

*derm.theclinics.com*

## Emotional neglect during early development

The skin is a primary organ of communication between infants and their environment, and the interaction between the skin and the environment has a lasting physical and psychologic impact on physical growth and psychologic development [5–7]. Psychosocial dwarfism is a recognized sequel of maternal deprivation [2,8], mainly as a result of a lack of tactile nurturance. Severe maternal deprivation is associated with failure to thrive and sometimes death, even when adequate food and shelter are provided [9]. Spitz observes that lack of a nurturing mother-child relationship in an institutional setting is associated with the development of certain syndromes, such as rocking, fecal play, and infantile eczema [9]. In this institutionalized population, 15% of the infants had infantile eczema, most likely atopic dermatitis, compared with 2% to 3% prevalence in the population at large [2,9]. Inadequate caressing and soothing physical contact are shown to be associated with atopic dermatitis in other studies [10–12]. The pathophysiology of this association is attributed to "psychogenic factors playing a crucial aggravating role" in the pathogenesis of a skin disorder "where allergic factors seem to be important" [10]. Massage therapy is shown to have a beneficial effect on childhood atopic dermatitis [13].

Alternately, children's need to be held and physically nurtured may be neglected in cases where they have severe skin disease. The chronic skin conditions of children also place emotional and physical demands on the family [12,14], which in turn may affect their capacity to nurture the child. This is a clinical situation that is more likely to be encountered in a dermatologist's office, and the possible long-term impact of relative deprivation of tactile nurturance may be prevented by counseling parents or caretakers.

Communication through the skin during early development plays a critical role in the development of body image. Through contact with mothers' skin, infants, over the course of development, begin to recognize their boundaries. Body image, defined as the mental representation of the body and its organs, initially develops in response to the empathic reflections of the caregiver, which in early life are communicated mainly by physical sensations, such as caressing, touch, and secure holding [15]. Caregivers' touch outlines the original boundary of a body's surface, thereby describing a shape to an infant's otherwise shapeless and boundless space. When there is neglect and the environment does not provide consistent or adequate nurturance by holding and touch, body image may become unstable or fragmented [15]. When the foundations of body image are weak, a person may become obsessionally or even delusionally preoccupied about skin and other aspects of the appearance, especially during stressful situations, even in the absence of significant skin disease. Children who have a recurring and potentially cosmetically disfiguring skin disorder and who do not get adequate nurturance during early development, therefore, may be at greater risk for the development of body image pathology.

## Abuse

The direct dermatologic manifestations of physical and sexual abuse are some of the most common and easily recognized forms of injury [16], and a detailed discussion of the acute and direct dermatologic effects of sexual and physical abuse is outside the scope of this article. The skin lesions that are associated with physical and sexual abuse, however, all have a wide spectrum of possible differential diagnosis [16,17]. For example, lichen sclerosus et atrophicus and genital condyloma in children are associated with sexual abuse; however, sexual abuse is not the underlying cause in many cases. In a recent study of 21 cases of child death resulting from repeated physical assault or neglect, 67% had evidence of blunt injuries to the skin and soft tissues [18]. Dermatologic symptoms in cases of sexual abuse are diverse and dermatologists often are uneasy about addressing this issue with patients [17]. A history of sexual abuse often is obtained only after a psychiatric referral or long-term psychotherapy [17]. It is important to obtain a careful history from patients and caretakers and other collateral history, if possible, whenever abuse is suspected.

In one study, 239 female patients attending a gastroenterology clinic [19] were assessed for history of sexual and physical abuse and a 30 commonly occurring nongastrointestinal physical symptoms. The odds ratio of having a rash or skin itching in patients who had an abuse history versus those who did not have an abuse history was 2.18 ($P = 0.007$) [19]. Other cutaneous symptoms for which the odds ratios were not statistically significant included sensitive skin and excessive sweating [19]. There are case reports of the association of chronic urticaria [20] and herpes zoster in a medically healthy child [21] who had covert sexual abuse.

Cutaneous symptoms and dermatologic disorders not associated directly with sexual or physical abuse may appear as a long-term consequence of abuse [17].

It is important for dermatologists to be aware of this link, as a there is a clear temporal association between cutaneous symptoms and psychologic trauma and, in many instances, patients may not be immediately aware of a possible association of their symptoms with psychologic trauma. When dermatologic symptoms emerge as a long-term symptom of abuse, patients usually have at least some of the psychophysiologic features of PTSD [3] (discussed later).

## Catastrophic life events

In the case of catastrophic life events, (1) the acute dermatologic symptoms resulting from the immediate damages caused by the event, such as unhygienic conditions, and (2) the development of stress-mediated dermatologic symptoms, which typically appear later, should be recognized [22]. Six months after a major earthquake in the Marmara region of Turkey, which was associated with approximately 17,000 deaths and the displacement of approximately 500,000 people, all outpatient registrations at a dermatology clinic were evaluated [22]. Postearthquake patient registrations were compared with a control group of patient registrations during a similar 6-month period before the earthquake. During the first 3 months after the earthquake, patient registrations indicated mainly infections and infestations, such as superficial fungal infections, viral dermatoses, insect bites, and scabies in comparison with the control group [22]. This outbreak was attributed to the damage in infrastructure and compromised hygienic conditions immediately after the earthquake. In contrast, patient registrations during the second 3-month period (ie, months 4 through 6 postearthquake) indicated that the incidences of erythematous- squamous skin diseases (eg, psoriasis, pruritus, eczemas, and neurocutaneous dermatoses) were significantly higher [22]. The investigators observed that the skin disorders with a higher incidence during months 4–6 postearthquake can be explained by the emotional and psychologic stress-related factors implicated in the onset or exacerbation in most of these dermatoses [22]. It is possible that in some instances, the documentation of more stress-related and relatively chronic dermatoses at a later date indicates the more acute and immediately treatable conditions occurring after and likely attributable to that catastrophic event, are more likely to get attention than chronic conditions. For example, a case study of a woman who had no prior history of urticaria reports she developed extensive urticaria within hours after the October 1987 Los Angeles earthquake [23]. The patient was "severely emotionally distressed" after the earthquake. In another study, 25 days after a smaller earthquake in another region of Turkey [24] that was associated with 1000 deaths, dermatologic symptoms were observed most frequently in individuals who were homeless. Symptoms consisted mainly of infections and infestations [24], followed by allergic and contact dermatitis, atopic dermatitis, and urticaria and skin disorders known as "psychogenic," such as psoriasis, alopecia areata, neurotic excoriations, and vitiligo. These psychogenic or stress reactive skin disorders were observed in 1.3% of the survivors [24]. In a Japanese study [25] of patients who had atopic dermatitis 1 month after the Great Hanshin Earthquake of 1995 that killed over 5500 people injuring approximately 40,000, 34%–38% of patients in the mild to severely affected regions, respectively, experienced exacerbations of atopic dermatitis, which is recognized as a stress-reactive dermatosis, in contrast to 7% of patients from areas that did not suffer damage from the earthquake. Subjective distress reported by the patients was the most responsible factor for increased symptoms of atopic dermatitis postearthquake [25]. A study of 553 individuals 6 years after a cargo plane crashed in their community reports that one of the six most frequently reported clinical complaints attributed to the plane crash were skin-related and endorsed by 73 individuals [26]. Concentration and sleep difficulties, which are classically associated with trauma and PTSD [3], were reported by 77 and 88 patients, respectively. It is not clear from the report [26] which symptoms were comorbid. The dermatologic diagnoses made by the subjects' general practitioners were as follows: contact eczema and/or other eczema, dermatophytosis, constitutional eczema, seborrheic eczema, and other skin or subcutis diseases. The general practitioners, who had known the patients before the plane crash, rated the odds that the skin problem was associated with the psychologic trauma of the plane crash to be realistic in 11.1% of subjects and possible in 33.3%. The literature on catastrophic traumatic life events, therefore, suggests that dermatologic symptoms emerge as a direct physical effect of the trauma and secondary to the psychosocial impact of the traumatic event, which may emerge several months after the catastrophic event. Clinically, trauma and abuse survivors tend to present with multiple somatic complaints. Symptoms seem to commonly involve musculoskeletal pain, fatigue, and a range of other nonspecific complaints, usually involving the neurologic, cardiopulmonary, gastrointestinal, and genitourinary systems, which typically are chronic and associated with significant psychosocial disability.

## Posttraumatic stress disorder

Some or all features of PTSD [3,27,28] may be associated with a range of traumatic experiences (discussed previously). The PTSD-associated responses include (1) the intrusive re-experiencing of the trauma, which may manifest in several ways, including nightmares, flashbacks, and somatic sensations; (2) autonomic hyperarousal, where the body continues to react to certain physical and emotional stimuli as if there were a continuing threat of annihilation, even when there is no threat; and (3) numbing of responsiveness, which may manifest in some cases as a dissociative reaction. Some of these core symptoms of PTSD and examples of their dermatologic manifestations are discussed.

### Intrusive re-experiencing of trauma

Childhood maltreatment can result in classically conditioned associations between abusive stimuli and negative emotions [29]. These classically conditioned responses are not encoded as autobiographic memories, rather as simple associations between certain stimuli (eg, the touch of the clinician, which may be reminiscent of a perpetrator's touch when the patient was being sexually abused) and a seemingly inappropriate response of fear and helplessness on part of patients. Such traumatic memories are not remembered per se, rather evoked or triggered by events that are similar to the original abuse situation. Later in life, exposure to abuse-reminiscent stimuli and memories may produce strong and negative affects, which, given the nonverbal nature of the conditioning, may not be understandable to the former victims, let alone others, including dermatologists who are taking care of the symptom. Traumatic memories also may be re-experienced on a sensory level, as sensory flashbacks or body memories, which are fragments of the sensory component of the traumatic experience [28,29]. These fragmented sensory components may manifest as visual, auditory, olfactory, or kinesthetic sensations or sensations in the skin or waves of cutaneous sensations that the patients typically claim to be representative of the original traumatic event as demonstrated in the case reports below.

### Case report 1

A 54-year-old woman had a long history of experiencing "waves of heat" throughout her body and a feeling that her hands and forearms were "hot." She had been investigated extensively by various internists, including several dermatologists, and no specific cause was identified for her symptoms. She also had a history of self-abuse and recently was referred for psychiatric evaluation because she had a compulsion to slash her face. Several months later, over the course of psychotherapy, the patient remembered that her mother often threatened to place her inside a hot oven as punishment,and, in fact, had forced her to put her hands inside a heated oven on a few occasions. Once the patient was able to work through her severe childhood abuse, her symptoms no longer were an issue for her.

### Case report 2

A 26-year-old married woman was referred for recurrent complaints of a swelling inside her mouth and tongue, which had been investigated extensively by ear, nose, and throat specialists; immunologists; and several dermatologists, and no definitive diagnosis was made. The patient reported that she experienced a fullness in her mouth and throat, typically when she was engaged in a consensual sexual relation with her husband, and had to be rushed to the emergency department on three previous occasions, where she was given adrenalin. After several months of therapy, the patient recalled a history of severe childhood sexual abuse, including recurrent oral sexual abuse when the perpetrator thrust his penis into her mouth. During these times, the patient often felt like she was choking to death. The oral symptoms remitted and the patient was symptom free for more than 3 years, once she was able to work through some of her severe childhood trauma.

### Autonomic hyperarousal

Autonomic hyperarousal may manifest as a range of cutaneous symptoms, including strong flushing reactions, periods of profuse perspiration and night sweats for which no basis can be found, and waves of pruritus. It is well recognized that the skin, like the heart, reacts strongly and reliably to stress, as evidenced by the extensive literature on stress and skin conductance. In PTSD, the baseline autonomic response tends to be elevated, which is consistent with the state of hypervigilance that is characteristic of PTSD. Furthermore there is an elevated skin conductance response to the presentation of neutral and aversive stimuli in PTSD [30]. The bodies of traumatized individuals continue to react to certain physical and emotional stimuli as though they are facing imminent danger to their survival. The essential function of autonomic arousal in the face of a threatening situation is to alert the organism to potential danger, and this is lost in traumatized patients in whom the somatic stress-related reactions can be triggered easily by stimuli that are reminiscent of the trauma. The patient, therefore, is not able to rely on these bodily sensations to warn them against real threat. This autonomic arousal may make patients more vulnerable to flare-ups of stress-reactive dermatoses, such as atopic dermatitis, urticaria, and psoriasis.

*Case report 3*

A 45-year-old railroad worker eventually had to quit working for the railroad because he found the crossing accidents increasingly distressing. He returned to college and ran a successful computer repair business until he was involved in a serious head-on collision, when his car was hit by a drunk driver and immediately caught fire. The patient and his passengers left the accident scene without any serious physical injuries; however, from that night on, the patient reported sleep difficulties, vivid nightmares, and flashbacks about the accident. He woke up from sleep with the "smell of burning rubber and smoke" and was overcome by chills and profuse sweating. He also tended to sweat profusely from time to time during the day (eg, when he heard a fire engine that reminded him of the accident scene). The patient was not able to make the association between his daytime sweating and the triggers and had seen a dermatologist for his hyperhidrosis before he was referred for psychiatric assessment. The patient's night sweats improved significantly after his acute autonomic hyper-reactivity was managed with a low dose of antipsychotic medications. The patient continues to receive psychotherapy for his trauma.

*Case report 4*

A 36-year-old woman presented with a long history of relatively intractable psoriasis. She sought a psychiatric consultation because of a long history of panic attacks and her increasing use of alcohol to self-medicate. The patient also described an abusive home environment and her sister leaving home at age 15 because their father was abusing her sexually. The patient later remembered her father entering the bedroom that she and her sister shared but had little recollection of what happened after that. She discussed the possibility of her also being abused by the father and reestablished contact with her sister, who gave corroborative history. The patient's panic attacks diminished significantly, as did her alcohol intake, and her psoriasis became more responsive to standard dermatologic therapies as she started working through her childhood trauma issues with psychotherapy and pharmacotherapy with antidepressant drugs.

*Numbing of responsiveness and difficulties with regulation of internal emotional states*

Severe childhood trauma and maltreatment often interfere with the capacity of individuals to control and tolerate strong, especially negative, emotional states without resorting to avoidance strategies, such as substance abuse, external tension-reducing behavior (which can manifest as self-injury to the integumentary system), and dissociation, defined as a disruption in the usually integrated functions of consciousness, memory, identity, and perception [3] and the lack of integration of the somatoform components of experiences, functions, and reactions [4]. Dissociation also is associated with an increased threshold for pain perception [31], which may be a physical manifestation of the dissociative process. Moderately painful sensations from the skin and its appendages, therefore, may help dissociative individuals to ground themselves [32]. It is well recognized that the experience of stigmatization in certain disorders, such as psoriasis, can be a source of distress for patients who often become hypervigilant of negative responses and remarks from others. In patients who have difficulty regulating their internal emotional states, this added emotional burden may cause them to resort to substance abuse or self-injury to the skin, which may in turn exacerbate their underlying psoriasis.

Self-induced injury to the body, without the intent of suicide, frequently is associated with a history of severe sexual, physical, and emotional abuse in early life [33–38]. The integumentary system frequently is the focus of the tension-reducing behavior not only because of its easy access but also because of the primary role of the skin in early attachment, which is typically disrupted when abuse occurs in early life. Some commonly encountered forms of self-injury in dermatology include repetitive superficial wrist lacerations, self-inflicted cigarette burns, and compulsive picking of skin lesions (as in the case of acne excoriée, onychophagia, onychotillomania, trichotillomania, and dermatitis artefacta) [1,39,40]. Eating disorders, such as anorexia nervosa and bulimia nervosa, often also emerge as mechanisms for affect regulation and may coexist with these dermatologic symptoms. Trichotillomania and dermatitis artefacta [32,39,41–47] often occur in conjunction with severe trauma, which can result in a dissociated state, including multiple personality disorder [48]. As a result of the dissociation, in many cases of trichotillomania and dermatitis artefacta, patients do not recall that they self-induced their lesions and often are misdiagnosed as malingerers.

*Case report 5*

A 32-year-old woman presented with severe acne excoriée. The self-excoriated acne lesions were interfering with her professional life as a college teacher. Her history revealed that she had experienced ongoing sexual abuse by her father and was asked to leave the house at age 16 when she attempted to resist her father. The patient supported herself through college and had little contact with her family. Approximately 2 years previously she had been abused in a romantic relationship by a man and felt devastated by this major breach of trust. Shortly after this, she started picking her skin and this aggravated her acne. The patient often did not remember picking her acne. She initially was treated with antidepressants, which helped her somewhat, and over the course of therapy she shared her trauma experiences. She was able to recognize that her recent experience had triggered PTSD in relation to her severe childhood abuse. The patient's acne excoriée has improved significantly since she started to work on her childhood trauma.

*Case report 6*

An 11-year-old girl presented with acute onset of trichotillomania. During most instances, the patient did not recall self-inducing her lesions. The patient was assessed with her family and it was revealed that her mother had a baby 6 months previously, and this was a major adjustment for the patient, who had been an only child. In addition, the parents were having marital difficulties and had separated on a few occasions and were contemplating a divorce. The patient's maternal grandmother, who had raised her during her early childhood, had died suddenly a few months previously. Although this patient did not present with a history of abuse, she presented with a history of significant losses over a short time period. The traumatic experiences most likely caused her to dissociate, and the trichotillomania served as a grounding and tension-releasing mechanism.

Trauma and PTSD often are associated with conversion symptoms or somatoform dissociation [3,4] (referred to has hysteria in earlier literature). These present as symptoms or deficits affecting the voluntary motor or sensory functions and often are referred to as pseudoneurologic [3]. Symptoms of psychologic and somatoform dissociation tend to be correlated positively [4]. Some of the cutaneous sensory symptoms or deficits include loss of touch or pain sensation for which no medical basis can be determined [3]. These conversion symptoms may emerge as body memories during a flashback (discussed previously) [28]. Autoerythrocyte sensitization or psychogenic purpura is a rarely reported and poorly understood dermatologic syndrome that has been attributed to a conversion reaction [49–52], as the purpuric lesions often are associated with an intense emotional experience, including trauma.

## Summary

Psychologic trauma refers to events that are outside the range of normal human experience and, therefore, traumatic for almost anyone. As psychologic trauma represents a more severe form of stress, it may be associated with an exacerbation of the stress-reactive dermatoses, such as psoriasis, atopic dermatitis, alopecia areata, and urticaria. The skin is a vital organ of communication and plays a central role in early attachment. Inadequate caressing and soothing skin contact during early development can affect the overall physical and mental development of the infant and is associated with infantile eczema. Dermatologic symptoms, such as eczema and pruritus also are some of the more commonly encountered physical complaints in adult survivors of abuse and neglect and in individuals who experience catastrophic events, such as earthquakes. When trauma results in the development of PTSD, traumatic memories may be re-experienced at a sensory level as cutaneous sensory flashbacks or body memories, which are fragments of the sensory component of the traumatic experience. The autonomic hyperarousal in PTSD can be associated with a range of dermatologic symptoms, including bouts of profuse sweating or flare-up of a stress-reactive dermatosis, such as psoriasis. The difficulties in the regulation of internal emotional states that are encountered in PTSD can lead to tension-reducing behaviors, which can manifest as excessive stimulation or self-injury to the integumentary system and present as trichotillomania, dermatitis artefacta, neurotic excoriations, and so forth. The numbing of responsiveness and dissociative responses also can present with a range of medically unexplained cutaneous sensory symptoms, such as numbness, pruritus, and pain. When psychologic trauma is associated with PTSD, it can result in dermatologic symptoms that may persist long after the traumatic event has subsided. Furthermore, when dissociation is a prominent feature of the PTSD, patients initially may not recognize that their dermatologic symptom is trauma related.

# References

[1] Gupta MA, Gupta AK. Psychodermatology: an update. J Am Acad Dermatol 1996;34:1030–46.

[2] Koblenzer CS. Psychocutaneous disease. Orlando (FL): Grune & Stratton; 1987.

[3] American Psychiatric Association. Diagnostic and statistical manual of mental disorders, fourth edition, text revision. Washington, DC: American Psychiatric Association; 2000.

[4] Nijenhuis ERS. Somatoform dissociation: phenomena, measurement and theoretical issues. New York: W.W. Norton; 2004.

[5] Evoniuk GE, Kuhn CM, Schanberg SM. The effect of tactile stimulation on serum growth hormone and tissue ornithine decarboxylase activity during maternal deprivation in rat pups. Comm Psychopharmacol 1979;3:363–70.

[6] Field TM, Schanberg SM, Scafidi F, et al. Tactile/kinesthetic stimulation effects on preterm neonates. Pediatrics 1986;77:654–8.

[7] Field T. The effects of mother's physical and emotional unavailability on emotion regulation. Monogr Soc Res Child Dev 1994;59:208–27.

[8] Schanberg SM, Kuhn CM. Maternal deprivation: an animal model of psychosocial dwarfism. In: Usdin F, Sourkes TL, Youdim MBH, editors. Enzymes and neurotransmitters in mental disease. New York: Wiley; 1980. p. 374–9.

[9] Spitz RA. The first year of life: a psychoanalytic study of normal and deviant development of object relations. New York: International Universities Press; 1965.

[10] Rosenthal MJ. Psychosomatic study of infantile eczema. I. The mother-child relationship. Pediatrics 1952;10:581–92.

[11] Williams DH. Management of atopic dermatitis in childres: control of the maternal rejection factor. AMA Arch Dermatol Syph 1951;63:545–60.

[12] Howlett S. Emotional dysfunction, child-family relationships and childhood atopic dermatitis. Br J Dermatol 1999;140:381–4.

[13] Schachner L, Field T, Hemandez-Reif M, et al. Atopic dermatitis symptoms decreased in children following massage therapy. Pediatr Dermatol 1998;15:390–5.

[14] Balkrishnan R, Housman TS, Grummer S, et al. The family impact of atopic dermatitis in children: the role of the parent caregiver. Pediatr Dermatol 2003;20:5–10.

[15] Kreuger DW. Body self and psychological self. New York: Brunner/Mazel; 1989.

[16] Mudd SS, Findlay JS. The cutaneous manifestations and common mimickers of physical child abuse. J Pediatr Health Care 2004;18:123–9.

[17] Harth W, Linse R. Dermatological symptoms and sexual abuse: a review and case reports. J Eur Acad Dermatol Venereol 2000;14:489–94.

[18] Pollanen MS, Smith CR, Chiasson DA, et al. Fatal child-abuse maltreatment syndrome. A retrospective study in Ontario, Canada, 1990–1995. Forensic Sci Int 2002;126:101–4.

[19] Leserman J, Li Z, Drossman DA, et al. Selected symptoms associated with sexual and physical abuse among female patients with gastrointestinal disorders: the impact on subsequent health care visits. Psychol Med 1998;28:417–25.

[20] Marley J. Child sexual abuse and the skin. J Fam Pract 1990;31:356.

[21] Gupta MA, Gupta AK. Herpes zoster in the medically healthy child and covert severe child abuse. Cutis 2000;66:221–3.

[22] Bayramgurler D, Bilen N, Namli S, et al. The effects of 17 August Marmara earthquake on patient admittances to our dermatology department. J Eur Acad Dermatol Venereol 2002;16:249–52.

[23] Stewart JH, Goodman MM. Earthquake urticaria. Cutis 1989;43:340.

[24] Oztas MO, Onder M, Oztas P, et al. Early skin problems after Duzce earthquake. Int J Dermatol 2000;39:952–8.

[25] Kodama A, Horikawa T, Suzuki T, et al. Effect of stress on atopic dermatitis: investigation in patients after the Great Hanshin earthquake. Allergy Clin Immunol 1999;104:173–6.

[26] Donkcr GA, Yzermans CJ, Spreeuwenberg P, et al. Symptom attribution after a plane crash: comparison between self-reported symptoms and GP records. Br J Gen Pract 2002;52:917–22.

[27] Van der Kolk BA, Van der Hart O, Burbridge J. Approaches to the treatment of PTSD. In: Williams MB, Sommer JF, editors. Simple and complex posttraumatic stress disorder: strategies for comprehensive treatment in clinical practice. Binghamton (NY): Hawthorne Press; 2002. p. 23–45.

[28] Van der Kolk BA, Fisler R. Dissociation and the fragmentary nature of traumatic memories: overview and exploratory study. J Trauma Stress 1995;8:505–25.

[29] Briere J. Treating adult survivors of severe childhood abuse and neglect: further development of an integrative model. In: Myers JFB, Berliner L, Briere J, et al, editors. The APSAC handbook on child maltreatment. 2nd edition. Newbury Park (CA): Sage Publications; 2002. p. 175–204.

[30] Peri T, Ben-Shakhar G, Orr SP, et al. Psychophysiologic assessment of aversive conditioning in posttraumatic stress disorder. Biol Psychiatry 2000;47:512–9.

[31] Van der Kolk BA, Greenberg MS, Orr SP, et al. Endogenous opioids, stress induced analgesia, and posttraumatic stress disorder. Psychopharmacol Bull 1989;25:417–21.

[32] Gupta MA, Gupta AK, Chandarana PC, et al. Dissociative symptoms and self-induced dermatoses: a preliminary empirical study. J Eur Acad Derm Venereol 2000;14(Suppl 1):278 [abstract].

[33] Briere J, Gil E. Self-mutilation in clinical and general population samples: prevalence, correlates and function. Am J Orthopsychiatry 1998;68:609–20.

[34] Van der Kolk BA, Perry JC, Herman JL. Childhood origins of self-destructive behavior. Am J Psychiatry 1991;148:1665–71.
[35] Winchel RM, Stanley M. Self-injurious behavior: a review of the behavior and biology of self-mutilation. Am J Psychiatry 1991;148:306–17.
[36] Romans SE, Martin JL, Anderson JC, et al. Sexual abuse in childhood and deliberate self-harm. Am J Psychiatry 1995;152:1336–42.
[37] Wiederman MW, Sansone RA, Sansone LA. Bodily self-harm and its relationship to childhood abuse by women in a primary care setting. Violence Against Women 1999;5:155–63.
[38] Saxe GN, Chawla N, Van der Kolk B. Self-destructive behavior in patients with dissociative disorders. Suicide Life Threat Behav 2002;32:313–20.
[39] Gupta MA, Gupta AK. Dermatitis artefacta and sexual abuse. Int J Dermatol 1993;32:825–6.
[40] Gupta MA, Gupta AK, Haberman HF. The self-inflicted dermatoses: a critical review. Gen Hosp Psychiatry 1987;9:45–52.
[41] Fabisch W. Psychiatric aspects of dermatitis artefacta. Br J Dermatol 1980;102:29–34.
[42] Farrier JN, Mansel RE. Dermatitis artefacta of the breast: a series of case reports. Eur J Surg Oncol 2002;28:189–98.
[43] Singh AN, Maguire J. Trichotillomania and incest. Br J Psychiatry 1989;155:108–10.
[44] Lochner C, du Toit PL, Zungn-Dirwayi N, et al. Childhood trauma in obsessive-compulsive disorder, trichotillomania and controls. Depress Anxiety 2002;15:66–8.
[45] Boughn S, Holdom JJ. The relationship of violence and trichotillomania. J Nurs Scholarship 2003;35:165–70.
[46] Lochner C, Seedat S, Hemmings SMJ, et al. Dissociative experiences in obsessive-compulsive disorder and trichotillomania: clinical and genetic findings. Compr Psychiatry 2004;45:384–91.
[47] Begotka AM, Woods DW, Wetterneck CT. The relationship between experiential avoidance and the severity of trichotillomania in a nonreferred sample. J Behav Ther Exp Psychiatry 2004;35:17–24.
[48] Shelley WB. Dermatitis artefacta induced in a patient by one of her multiple personalities. Br J Dermatol 1981;105:587–9.
[49] Yucel B, Kiziltan E, Aktan M. Dissociative identity disorder presenting with psychogenic purpura. Psychosomatics 2000;41:279–81.
[50] Ratnoff OD, Agle DP. Psychogenic purpura: a re-evaluation of the syndrome of autoerythrocyte sensitization. Medicine 1968;47:475–500.
[51] Agle DP, Ratnoff OD, Wasman M. Studies in autoerythrocyte sensitization: the induction of purpuric lesions by hypnotic suggestion. Psychosom Med 1967;29:491–503.
[52] Agle DP, Ratnoff OD, Wasman M. Conversion reactions in autoerythrocyte sensitization: their relationship to the production of ecchymoses. Arch Gen Psychiatry 1969;20:438–47.

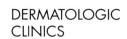

# Depression and Skin Disease

Richard G. Fried, MD, PhD[a,*], Madhulika A. Gupta, MD, FRCPC[b,c], Aditya K. Gupta, MD, PhD[c,d]

[a]Yardley Dermatology Associates, 903 Floral Vale Boulevard, Yardley, PA 19067, USA
[b]Department of Psychiatry, University of Western Ontario, London, ON, Canada
[c]Mediprobe Research Inc, London, ON, Canada
[d]Division of Dermatology, Department of Medicine, University of Toronto, London, ON, Canada

Depression is observed commonly in dermatology patients. Psychiatric disturbance and psychosocial impairment is reported in at least 30% of patients who have dermatologic disorders [1–6]. Recognition of depression and appropriate intervention are essential for effective management of skin conditions. Depression often is conceptualized broadly as either initiating or worsening skin disease or, alternatively, having its onset or exacerbation as a consequence of skin disease. Specifically, it can function as a biologic and psychosocial stressor that elicits or exacerbates skin disease. Conversely, the physical symptoms and daily demands of living with a skin disease, coupled with potential psychosocial effects (ie, stigmatization, discrimination, rejection, and so forth) can elicit or exacerbate depression.

Depression is a negative emotional state that affects everyone to some degree. It can rob individuals of happiness and substantially diminish quality of life. It can be conceptualized as a continuum that ranges from mild sadness and lack of vivre to intense misery, despair, and intense desire to die. In addition, often it disrupts functional capacity, resulting in poorer vocational, social, and intimate functioning. Decreased energy levels, impaired attention and concentration, somatic complaints, and preoccupation with bodily concerns make personal hygiene and compliance with treatment regimens more difficult.

Whether or not depression precedes skin disease or occurs as a consequence of skin disease may seem like a chicken-or-egg dilemma. A reciprocal cycle of deleterious perpetuation can evolve in which sadness worsens skin disease and the consequent burden of worsening skin exacerbates depression. Major depression and dysthymic disorder are the most common mood disorders encountered in dermatology patients. The Diagnostic and Statistical Manual of Mental Disorders–4th edition (DSM-IV) criteria for dysthymia and major depressive episode are listed in Boxes 1 and 2 [7].

Psychodermatologic disorders are separated broadly into two major groups: (1) cutaneous associations of psychiatric disorders, such as neurotic excoriations, acne excorie, skin manipulation associated with delusions of parasitosis, and excessive concerns about cutaneous body image or odors that are not consistent with objective clinical dermatological evaluation, and (2) the large group of dermatologic disorders, such as psoriasis, rosacea, atopic dermatitis (AD), chronic idiopathic urticaria, alopecia areata (AA), and acne that are exacerbated by psychosocial stress and are comorbid with a wide range of psychiatric disorders, including major depressive disorder.

Depression in dermatology patients often is multifactorial in its cause. Genetic factors, psychosocial stressors, age of patients at onset of skin disease, body areas involved, physical discomfort (ie, pruritus, pain, or burning), and clinical severity all are potential contributors. The degree of depression not always directly correlates directly with clinical

\* Corresponding author.
E-mail address: dermshrink@aol.com (R.G. Fried).

> **Box 1. Diagnostic and Statistical Manual of Mental Disorders – 4th edition criteria for dysthymia**
>
> Dysthymia is characterized by an overwhelming yet chronic state of depression, exhibited by a depressed mood for most of the day, for more days than not, for at least 2 years. (In children and adolescents, mood can be irritable and duration must be at least 1 year.) The person who suffers from this disorder must not have gone for more than 2 months without experiencing two or more of the following symptoms:
>
> 1. Poor appetite or overeating
> 2. Insomnia or hypersomnia
> 3. Low energy or fatigue
> 4. Low self-esteem
> 5. Poor concentration or difficulty making decisions
> 6. Feelings of hopelessness
>
> *Data from* American Psychiatric Association. Diagnostic and Statistical Manual of Mental Disorders. 4th edition. Washington DC: American Psychiatric Association; 1994.

> **Box 2. Diagnostic and Statistical Manual of Mental Disorders – 4th edition criteria for major depressive episode**
>
> Five or more of the following symptoms must have been present during the same 2-week period and represent a change from previous functioning; at least one of the symptoms is either depressed mood or anhedonia (ie, loss of interest or pleasure in activities that the patients usually found pleasurable).
>
> 1. Depressed mood most of the day, nearly every day, as evidenced by subjective report of sadness or objective evidence, such as tearfulness. In children and adolescents, the presentation may be different, as the most prominent finding may be irritable mood.
> 2. Markedly diminished interest or pleasure in all, or almost all, activities nearly every day.
> 3. Significant weight loss (when not dieting) or weight gain (eg, in either case, a change of >5% of body weight in a month) or decrease or increase in appetite nearly every day. In growing children this may present as a failure to make the expected weight gains.
> 4. Insomnia or hypersomnia nearly every day.
> 5. Psychomotor agitation or retardation nearly every day.
> 6. Fatigue or loss of energy nearly every day.
> 7. Feelings of worthlessness or excessive or inappropriate guilt (which may be delusional) nearly every day (not merely guilt or self-reproach about being sick).
> 8. Diminished ability to think or concentrate, or indecisiveness, nearly every day (either by subjective account or as observed by others).
> 9. Recurrent thoughts of death (not just fear of dying), recurrent suicidal ideation without a specific plan, or a suicide attempt or a specific plan for committing suicide.
>
> *Data from* American Psychiatric Association. Diagnostic and Statistical Manual of Mental Disorders. 4th edition. Washington DC: American Psychiatric Association; 1994.

severity. Therefore, no presumptions regarding psychiatric impact can be made based on clinical severity alone.

Readers are encouraged to keep several general concepts in mind as the prevalence of depression occurring in association with specific skin disorders is reviewed: (1) there is a need to maintain clinical vigilance for depression in dermatology patients, because its occurrence is common; (2) when depression is present, psychiatric intervention in the form of psychotherapy or psychotropic medications may be necessary adjuncts to dermatologic therapy to achieve adequate emotional health for compliance with treatment regimens; (3) treating depression may decrease the physical and emotional burden on individuals, allowing greater benefit from dermatologic intervention; and (4) vigilance for active suicidality is necessary because dermatologic disease is associated with a greater risk for suicide.

### Depressive equivalents

Cutaneous symptoms, such as pain, burning, and other dysesthesias without identifiable organic basis, can be manifestations of underlying depression. These symptoms are referred to as depressive equivalents or masked depression. Alternatively, depressed patients may present with excessive concern and preoccupation about a minor dermatologic problem, such as minimal hair loss, enlarging pores, fine wrinkles, and so forth. They often express feelings of low self-worth and unattractiveness in association with the relatively minor dermatologic problem. These preoccupations can consume a great deal of time and energy leading to dramatic impairments in psychosocial functioning. More severe depression can be associated with mood congruent delusions. These can include morbid preoccupation with delusions of ill health, such as having cancer or a sexually transmitted disease, delusions of skin deterioration, and malodorous or rotting skin.

**Subclinical depression**

There is a substantial group of patients who fail to meet all the DSM diagnostic criteria for depression but probably are suffering from some degree of depressive disorder. They often meet some, but not all, the criteria necessary to make a formal diagnosis of depression. Common symptoms include a subtle decrease in energy and enthusiasm, mild fatigue, a narrowing of leisure interests, obsessive preoccupations, and decrease in sexual desire. Patients who have subclinical depression do not perceive themselves as depressed; usually they deny persistent feelings of sadness. They may report that food does not taste quite as good, flowers do not smell quite as sweet, and sexual interest and gratification have diminished. These individuals seem blasé, lacking enthusiasm about daily life events. Individuals who have subclinical depression simply feel that life inevitably loses some of its shine. This constellation of symptoms can lead to weight gain, poor compliance with treatment regimens, and increased psychosocial stress, all of which can impede effective treatment outcomes. Patients who have subclinical depression often respond favorably to cognitive-behavioral psychotherapy and psychotropic medications. Only in retrospect, after their symptoms have improved, do most affected individuals recognize that they were in fact depressed.

**Suicide and parasuicidal behavior**

Suicide, defined as intentional self-inflicted death, is a feared outcome of depressive disease. Approximately 50% of all persons who kill themselves are depressed, and 15% of depressed patients eventually kill themselves [8]. It is reported that approximately 35,000 individuals commit suicide every year in the United States and 250,000 attempt it [8]. Woman attempt suicide four times more frequently than men, but men are three times more successful. The suicide rate in the United States is 12 per 100,000 [8]. Among men, the suicide rate peaks after age 45 and among women, after age 65. Overall suicide rates increase with age. Currently, the most rapid rise in suicide rates is among males 15 to 24 years of age. This is of concern, because acne has its peak occurrence during this age period. Rates of suicidal ideation and attempts are high among cosmetically disfiguring skin diseases, even though these diseases are not life threatening. A 5.6% to 7.2% prevalence of active suicidal ideation is observed among psoriasis and acne patients, higher than the 2.4% to 3.3% prevalence observed in general medical patients. Substance abuse in association with a skin disease also increases suicide risk [8].

Parasuicidal behavior is defined as repeated self-harm or self-injury. In dermatology practices, parasuicidal behavior frequently is encountered (eg, in patients who have dermatitis artifacta or present with superficial lacerations of the wrist or other evidence of self-cutting behavior). Patients who have major depressive disorder and borderline personality disorder are at increased risk for parasuicidal behavior. Parasuicidal behavior should be viewed as a serious indicator of elevated risk for suicide even if the behavior is believed to be attention seeking in nature.

**Developmental considerations**

Given the common ectodermal origins of the epidermis and the central nervous system, it is suggested that some dermatologic and psychiatric disorders may have a common origin. Ongoing tactile stimulation of the skin is necessary for normal psychosocial development. The touch of the caregiver, consisting of secure holding, hugging, and consistent caressing, is essential for mental health and social development and bonding [9]. Failure to develop this early and primary caregiver infant bond is associated with depressive disease in later life.

Onset of skin disorders, such as acne and psoriasis, during critical psychosocial periods can be especially devastating. Skin disease during adolescence and young adulthood can lead to greater emotional impact in contrast to disease having a later onset in adulthood [10], when the patient is not dealing with the intense and chaotic social demands of adolescence and young adult life.

**Diagnosing depression in the dermatologic patient**

The diagnostic criteria for dysthymia and major depressive disorder (see Boxes 1 and 2) can serve as a useful and standardized guideline to aid in the diagnosis of depression. In addition, depression can manifest as excessive anxiety, extreme frustration over minor matters, increased irritability, and outbursts of anger.

Premenstrual dysphoric disorder [7] (also referred to as premenstrual syndrome) can be associated with a markedly depressed mood, intense anxiety, lability of mood, and a flare of acne during the last week of the luteal phase of the menstrual cycle. It is difficult to ascertain if the occurrence of acne is solely the result of the hormonal changes that elicit the premenstrual dysphoric disorder or is fueled partially by the physical correlates of the negative emotions.

**Specific dermatologic disorders**

*Cutaneous associations of depressive disease*

Delusions of parasitosis, bromhidrosis, and delusions of disfigurement related to the skin may be a feature of a major depressive disorder with psychotic features [7]. Body image distortions related to the skin, such as body dysmorphic disorder (dermatologic nondisease) [11] also can be associated with depression. These patients present with extreme distress and preoccupation with dermatologic complaints that are not consistent with objective findings (eg, complaints about minimal hair loss or very minimal acne) can be the presenting feature of a major depressive disorder [7]. Various cutaneous dysesthesias, such as a burning sensation in the scalp or tongue can be a somatic feature of depressive disease. Self-induced dermatoses, such as neurotic excoriations and acne excoriee, are examples of repetitive self-excoriation. The excoriations may be initiated by itch or other cutaneous dysesthesias or may be the result of persistent urges to excoriate an acne lesion or another irregularity of the skin [12]. Depressive disease and significant psychosocial stressors are reported in 33% to 98% of patients who have neurotic excoriations [13,14]. Other self-inflicted dermatoses, such as dermatitis artifacta and trichotillomania, are disorders associated with a wide range of psychopathologies, including obsessive-compulsive disorder, borderline personality disorder, and major depressive disorder. Depression and self-injury may lead to more extensive excoriations in patients who have AD, exacerbation of psoriatic lesions secondary to Koebner's phenomenon, and manipulation of acne as seen in acne excoriee.

*Depression and primary dermatologic disorders*

*Psoriasis*

Depressive psychopathology in psoriasis may be primary or secondary to the impact of the disease on the quality of life of the patient. Psoriasis-related stress is associated with greater psychiatric morbidity [15]. Psoriasis patients who feel stigmatized in social situations have higher depression scores. Adult psoriasis patients who experienced greater touch deprivation in social situations as a result of their psoriasis had higher depression scores than those who did not perceive deprivation of social touch [16]. A wide range of psychologic characteristics are reported in various cross-sectional surveys [17], including high depression, high anxiety, and obsessionality or difficulties with verbal expression of emotions [18–21], especially anger [20,21]. Early-onset psoriasis is associated with greater difficulties with expression of anger [21], a personality trait that may render patients more vulnerable to stress and depression. Severity of pruritus, which can be one of the most bothersome features of psoriasis, correlates directly with the severity of depressive symptoms [22,23] in psoriasis. The severity of depressive symptoms and the occurrence of suicidal ideation are shown to correlate with psoriasis severity [24]. A 7.2% prevalence of suicidal ideation was observed among severely affected psoriasis inpatients versus a 2.5% suicidal ideation occurrence reported in less severely affected psoriasis outpatients [25].

*Atopic dermatitis*

School-aged children who have moderate to severe AD are at a greater risk for developing psychologic difficulties, which can affect their academic and social development adversely [26]. Higher anxiety and depressive symptoms [27–31] are reported in atopic patients, and anxiety may be a feature of an underlying primary depressive disorder in some patients who have AD. Adult patients who have AD often were chronically anxious and felt ineffective in handling anger in comparison to controls [28,31]. Pruritus severity was related directly to severity of depressive symptoms [22] in atopic patients. Psychiatric factors, however, do not always correlate with severity and chronicity of disease. A study of 10 atopic patients showed no correlation between the severity of psychopathology and chronicity of the skin disorder [32]. Chronic intractable eczema in a child may be a sign of a disturbed parent-child relationship [33]; however, a major depressive disorder should be ruled out before family problems are implicated [34]. The majority of patients who have AD probably have neither a depressive disorder nor severely dysfunctional families.

*Urticaria and angioedema*

A wide variety of personality characteristics is described in earlier literature [35,36], most frequently reported being difficulties involved with expression of anger and hostility in association with the need for approval. Thirty-four patients who had chronic idiopathic urticaria had lower depression scores than 34 patients who had idiopathic generalized pruritus [37]. Pruritus severity in urticaria, however, increased with increasing severity of depressive symptoms [22].

*Alopecia areata*

Patients whose AA was exacerbated by stress also had higher depression scores, suggesting that comorbid depression may render the condition more stress reactive [38]; a 33% to 93% incidence of psychiatric illness is reported in patients who have AA [39]. Among 31 surveyed patients who had AA, 74% had a lifetime prevalence of one or more psychiatric disorders with a 39% prevalence of major depression and 39% prevalence of anxiety disorder [40]. Among 294 surveyed patients who had AA, the prevalence of major depression was 8.8%, generalized anxiety disorder 18.2%, and paranoid disorder 4.4%, with an overall 23.3% prevalence of at least one psychiatric disorder [41].

*Acne*

Higher anxiety levels in cystic acne are associated with higher blood catecholamine levels [42], which decrease with treatment of the acne, suggesting that the psychosocial impact of acne can be associated with significant physiologic stress for the patient. The stress resulting from the impact of acne on the quality of life can be disabling [43], comparable to the disability resulting from chronic disorders, such as diabetes and asthma. The impact of acne on quality of life often does not necessarily correlate strongly with the clinical severity of acne [44], as some patients who have even mild acne are severely psychosocially disabled by their disorder. Mild to moderate acne is associated with significant psychologic morbidity, including depression, suicidal ideation [25], and completed suicide [45]. A 5.6% prevalence of suicidal ideation was observed among patients who had noncystic facial acne [25]. Acne patients who experience problems at school or work and blame these problems on their acne may be clinically depressed [46]. Anxiety and anger are important factors in acne [44]; treatment of mild and moderate noncystic acne [47] and treatment of cystic acne with isotretinoin are associated with improvements in the psychologic-morbidity (ie, decreased anxiety and depression) [48]. In some instances of chronic acne, some of the psychologic morbidity may persist at the end of treatment after the acne has improved because of the impact of acne on psychosocial development and the long-term impact of acne [49,50]. This finding underscores the importance of treating even mild acne aggressively if the disorder is psychosocially distressing for the patient.

**Treatment**

Effective treatments are available for subclinical depression, dysthymic disorder, and major depressive disorder. Cognitive behavioral psychotherapy and antidepressant medication are effective modalities for the management of subclinical depression and dysthymic disorder. Major depressive disorder is less responsive to psychotherapy and often requires aggressive pharmacologic management. Clinicians may consider including an antidepressant medication to augment traditional dermatologic therapy in patients who have subclinical depression and dysthymic disorder. Referral to a skilled cognitive-behavioral therapist also can be helpful. A recent text on psychocutaneous medicine [51,52] provides an overview of the wide range of psychologic interventions and psychotropic medications that may be used in dermatology. Before prescribing psychotropic agents, clinicians should familiarize themselves with the approved indications and guidelines for prescribing each drug. Patients meeting the criteria for major depressive disorder and those who have suicidal ideation should be referred for immediate psychiatric evaluation.

**Discussion**

The disorders described previously can be classified accurately as psychophysiologic disorders. They can be elicited and worsened by psychologic factors and, in turn, living with them is associated with a higher prevalence of emotional disorders, such as depression and anxiety.

The relationship between depressive disease and skin disorders can be complex and multidimensional. The severity of depressive symptoms correlates directly with disease severity in psoriasis [24], but this is not a consistent finding in acne, where even mild to moderate acne is associated with depression scores similar to patients who have more severe psoriasis [25]. Prospective studies involving treatment of the acne, however, show that psychologic morbidity in mild and moderate noncystic acne [47] and more severe cystic acne [48] improve with treatment of the acne. Acne has a peak incidence during adolescence, a life stage when individuals normally are highly invested in their appearance and body image. The onset of acne can be the proverbial straw that breaks the camel's back, unmasking significant depression. Further support for concomitant psychosocial contributions to depression come from the finding that acne and other body image pathologies, such as eating disorders, may coexist [53,54]. Conditions such as acne excoriee frequently present with psychologic dynamics that are similar to those encountered in adolescents who have eating disorders [55].

Depression can modulate itch perception in a wide range of pruritic disorders, such as psoriasis, AD, and chronic idiopathic urticaria [22,23]. The severity of depression correlates with pruritus severity [22,23], and improvement in pruritus is associated with an improvement in depression scores in psoriasis [23]. These findings suggest that if depression is comorbid with pruritus, treatment of the depression may have a beneficial effect on the symptom of pruritus.

The impact of a skin disorder on patients' quality of life can result in significant psychologic and psychiatric pathology (eg, dysthymic disorder and major depressive disorder) (see Boxes 1 and 2). The depression and impaired quality of life can in turn have an adverse impact on the course of some stress-reactive dermatoses, such as psoriasis, rosacea, and AD. Group psychotherapy [56] can help patients cope with the stress of skin disease and possibly prevent the onset of depression.

Is important to recognize the presence of clinical depression in the acne patient. In some instances, depressive symptoms are far greater then those expected based on the objective cosmetic disfigurement caused by the acne. The seriousness of this impact is highlighted by the 5.6% prevalence of suicidal ideation in patients who have mild to moderate noncystic facial acne. This is comparable to the 5.5% prevalence of suicidal ideation among the more severely affected patients who have psoriasis [25].

The acne patients in this study [25] were mainly adolescents and young adults, a group already noted at higher risk for depression and suicidal ideation independent of whether or not they have acne.

An article on depression and skin disease would be incomplete without addressing the potential association of isotretinoin and depression. There are sporadic reports of depression, suicidal behavior, and other psychiatric reactions in patients treated with isotretinoin [57–59]. The majority of available objective data continue to support the efficacy and safety of isotretinoin. Isotretinoin does not seem to reliably cause depression or suicidality. The majority of studies suggest no association with negative psychiatric outcomes and some suggest that people treated with isotretinoin actually have an improvement in their psychiatric status, as living with acne can be depressing. The idiosyncratic occurrence of depression may be real; thus, clinicians and parents should maintain vigilance for signs and symptoms of depression. Recent speculations that retinoids may have effects on brain function are not substantiated in larger studies.

Decisions regarding the use of isotretinoin are based, like all medical decisions, on the available objective scientific data and thorough evaluation of risks versus benefits. There is no question that untreated acne vulgaris, of any severity, has the strong potential for negative psychiatric sequelae, including depression, anxiety, functional impairment, and suicide. These realities must be weighed against the possibility of idiosyncratic depression and suicidality present with isotretinoin or any other systemic agent.

## References

[1] Gupta MA, Gupta AK. Psychodermatology: an update. J Am Acad Dermatol 1996;34:1030–46.
[2] Medansky RS, Handler RM. Dermatopsychosomatics: classification, physiology, and therapeutic approaches. J Am Acad Dermatol 1981;5:125–36.
[3] Koblenzer CS. Psychosomatic concepts in dermatology. Arch Dermatol 1983;119:501–12.
[4] Panconesi P. Psychosomatic dermatology. Clin Dermatol 1984;2:94–179.
[5] Koo JYM, Pham CT. Psychodermatology-practical guidelines on pharmacotherapy. Arch Dermatol 1992; 126:381–8.
[6] Gupta MA, Gupta AK. The use of psychotropic drugs in dermatology. Dermatol Clin 2000;18:711–25.
[7] American Psychiatric Association. Diagnostic and statistical manual of mental disorders. 4th edition. Washington, DC: American Psychiatric Publishing; 1994.
[8] Sadock BJ, Sadock VA. Kaplan and Sadock's pocket

book of clinical psychiatry. 3rd edition. Philadelphia: Lippincott Williams & Wilkins; 2001. p. 261–74.
[9] Krueger DW. Body self and psychological self. New York: Brunner/Mazel; 1989. p. 3–31.
[10] Gupta MA, Gupta AK. Age and gender differences in the impact of psoriasis upon the quality of life. Int J Dermatol 1995;34:700–3.
[11] Cotterill JA. Dermatologic non-disease: a common and potentially fatal disturbance of cutaneous body image. Br J Dermatol 1981;104:611–9.
[12] Gupta MA, Gupta AK, Haberman HF. The self-inflicted dermatoses: a critical review. Gen Hosp Psychiatry 1987;9:45–52.
[13] Freunsgaard K. Neurotic excoriations; a controlled psychiatric examination. Acta Psychiatr Scand 1984; 69(Suppl):1–52.
[14] Gupta MA, Gupta AK, Haberman HF. Neurotic excoriations: a review and some new perspectives. Compr Psychiatry 1986;27:381–6.
[15] Fortune DG, Main CJ, O'Sullivan TM, et al. Quality of life in patients with psoriasis: the contribution of clinical variables and psoriasis- specific stress. Br J Dermatol 1997;137:755–60.
[16] Gupta MA, Gupta AK, Watteel GN. Perceive deprivation of social touch in psoriasis is associated with greater psychological morbidity: an index of the stigma experience in dermatologic disorders. Cutis 1998;61: 339–44.
[17] Gupta MA, Gupta AK, Haberman HF. Psoriasis and psychiatry: an update. Gen Hosp Psychiatry 1987;9: 157–66.
[18] Vidoni D, Campiutti E, D'Aronco R, et al. Psoriasis and alexithymia. Acta Derm Venereol (Stockh) 1989; 146:91–2.
[19] Rubino IA, Sonnino A, Stefanto CM, et al. Separation-individuation, aggression, and alexithymia in psoriasis. Acta Derm Venereol (Stockh) 1989;146:87–90.
[20] Niemeier V, Fritz J, Kupfer J, et al. Aggressive verbal behavior as a function of experimentally induced anger in persons with psoriasis. Eur J Dermatol 1989;9: 555–8.
[21] Gupta MA, Gupta AK, Watteel G. Early onset (<age 40 years) psoriasis is associated with greater psychopathology than late onset psoriasis. Acta Dermato-Venereol 1996;76:464–6.
[22] Gupta MA, Gupta AK, Schork NJ, et al. Depression modulates pruritus perception: a study of pruritus in psoriasis, atopic dermatitis, and chronic idiopathic urticaria. Psychosom Med 1994;56:36–40.
[23] Gupta MA, Gupta AK, Kirkby S, et al. Pruritus in psoriasis: a prospective study of some psychiatric and dermatologic correlates. Arch Dermatol 1988;124: 1052–7.
[24] Gupta MA, Schork NJ, Gupta AK, et al. N. Suicidal ideation in psoriasis. Int J Dermatol 1993;32:188–90.
[25] Gupta MA, Gupta AK. Depression and suicidal ideation dermatology patients with acne, alopecia areata, atopic dermatitis and psoriasis. Br J Dermatol 1998;139:846–50.

[26] Absolon CM, Cottrell D, Eldridge SM, et al. Psychological disturbance in atopic eczema: the extent of the problem in school-age children. Br J Dermatol 1997; 137:241–5.
[27] Al-Ahmar HF, Kurban AK. Psychological profile of patients with atopic dermatitis. Br J Dermatol 1976; 95:373–7.
[28] White A, Horne DJ, Varigos GA. Psychological profile of the atopic eczema patient. Australas J Dermatol 1990;31:13–6.
[29] Linnet J, Jemec GB. An assessment of anxiety and dermatology quality-of-life in patients with atopic dermatitis. Br J Dermatol 1999;140:268–72.
[30] Hashiro M, Okumura M. Anxiety, depression and psychosomatic symptoms in patients with atopic dermatitis: comparison with normal controls and among groups of different degrees of severity. J Dermatol Sci 1997;14:63–7.
[31] Ginsburg IH, Prystowsky JH, Kornfeld DS, et al. Role of emotional factors in adults with atopic dermatitis. Int J Dermatol 1993;32:656–60.
[32] Ullman KC, Moore RW, Reidy M. Atopic eczema: a clinical psychiatric study. J Asthma Res 1977;14: 91–9.
[33] Koblenzer CS, Koblenzer PJ. Chronic intractable atopic eczema. Arch Dermatol 1988;124:1673–7.
[34] Allen AD. Intractable atopic eczema suggests major affective disorder: poor parenting is secondary [letter]. Arch Dermatol 1989;125:567–8.
[35] Rees L. An aetiological study of chronic urticaria and angioneurotic oedema. J Psychosom Res 1957;2: 172–89.
[36] Juhlin L. Recurrent urticaria: clinical investigations of 330 patients. Br J Dermatol 1981;104:369–81.
[37] Sheehan-Dare RA, Henderson MJ, Cotterill JA. Anxiety and depression in patients with chronic urticaria and generalized pruritus. Br J Dermatol 1990;123:769–74.
[38] Gupta MA, Gupta AK, Watteel GN. Stress and alopecia areata: a psychodermatologic study. Acta Dermato-Venereol (Stockh) 1997;77:296–8.
[39] Sandok BA. Alopecia areata: an apparent relationship to psychic factors. Am J Psychiatry 1964;121:184–5.
[40] Colon EA, Popkin MK, Callies AL, et al. Lifetime prevalence of psychiatric disorders in patients with alopecia areata. Compr Psychiatry 1991;32:245–51.
[41] Koo JYM, Shellow WV, Hallman CP, et al. Alopecia areata and increased prevalence of psychiatric disorders. Int J Dermatol 1994;33:849–50.
[42] Schulpis K, Georgala S, Papakonstantinou ED, et al. The psychological and sympatho-adrenal status in patients with cystic acne. J Eur Acad Dermatol Venereol 1999;13:24–7.
[43] Mallom E, Newton JN, Klassen A, et al. The quality of life in acne: a comparison with general medical conditions using generic questionnaires. Br J Dermatol 1999;140:672–6.
[44] Wu SF, Kinder BN, Trunnell TN, et al. Role of anxiety and anger in acne patients: a relationship with severity

[45] Cotterill JA, Cunliffe WJ. Suicide in dermatological patients. Br J Dermatol 1997;137:246–50.
[46] Gupta MA, Johnson AM, Gupta AK. The development of an Acne Quality of Life scale: reliability, validity, and the relation to subjective acne severity in mild to moderate acne vulgaris. Acta Derm Venereol 1998;78: 451–6.
[47] Gupta MA, Gupta AK, Schork NJ, et al. Psychiatric aspects of the treatment of mild to moderate facial acne: some preliminary observations. Int J Dermatol 1990;29:719–21.
[48] Rubinow DR, Peck GL, Squillace KM, et al. Reduced anxiety and depression in cystic acne patients after successful treatment with oral isotretinoin. J Am Acad Dermatol 1987;17:25–32.
[49] Layton AM, Seukeran D, Cunliffe WJ. Scarred for life? Dermatology on 1997;95(suppl):15–21.
[50] Kellett SC, Gawkrodger DJ. The psychological and emotional impact of acne and the effect of treatment with isotretinoin. Br J Dermatol 1999;140:273–82.
[51] Lee CS, Koo JYM. The use of psychotropic medications in dermatology. In: Psychocutaneous medicine. New York/Basel: Marcel Dekker; 2003. p. 427–51.
[52] Fried RG. Nonpharmacological treatments in psychodermatology. In: Psychocutaneous medicine. New York/Basel: Marcel Dekker; 2003. p. 427–51.
[53] Gupta MA, Gupta AK, Haberman HF. Dermatologic signs in anorexia nervosa and bulimia nervosa. Arch Dermatol 1987;123:1386–90.
[54] Gupta MA, Gupta AK. Dermatological complications. Eur Eat Disord Rev 2000;8:134–43.
[55] Sneddon J, Sneddon I. 'Acne excorie': a protective device. Clin Exp Derm 1983;8:65–8.
[56] Seng TK, Nee TS. Group therapy: a useful and supportive treatment for psoriasis patients. Int J Dermatol 1997;36:110–2.
[57] Gupta MA, Gupta AK. The psychological comorbidity in acne. Clin Dermatol 2001;19:360–3.
[58] Engel GL. The clinical application of the biopsychosocial model. Am J Psychiatry 1980;137:535–44.
[59] Scheich G, Florin I, Rudolph R, et al. Personality characteristics and serum IgE level in patients with atopic dermatitis. J Psychosom Res 1993;37:637–42.

# Acne, Depression, and Suicide

Peter R. Hull, MD, PhD(Med), FFDerm(SA), FRCPC[a],*, Carl D'Arcy, PhD[b]

[a]*Division of Dermatology, Department of Medicine, Royal University Hospital, University of Saskatchewan, 103 Hospital Drive, Saskatoon, SK, Canada S7N 0W8*
[b]*Applied Research, Department of Psychiatry, College of Medicine, Royal University Hospital, University of Saskatchewan, 103 Hospital Drive, Saskatoon, SK, Canada S7N 0W8*

The topic of acne and depression is completely overshadowed by the more pressing issue regarding the role played by isotretinoin in the causation of depression and its extreme outcome, suicide. This is an issue that has generated worldwide concern and has spawned several organizations dedicated to the investigation of duplicity by the manufacturer and to the assignment of legal culpability. This article systematically examines the literature on (1) the prevalence of depression and suicide in adolescents and young adults; (2) the psychologic impacts of acne on anxiety, depression, and suicide; and (3) the evidence for an association between isotretinoin and depression and suicide.

## Methods

The MEDLINE database (1966–January 2005. Available at http://medline.cos.com) was searched for literature using the following key words: acne, depression, mood disorder, suicide, depressive disorders, isotretinoin, Accutane, Roaccutane, retinoids, etretinate, acitretin, and vitamin A. In addition, an internet search of the Food and Drug Administration database files and the Reports of the Committee on Government House Reform (US House of Representatives) for isotretinoin and depression was also conducted.

## Prevalence of depression and suicide in adolescents and young adults

### Defining depression

Episodes of sadness or melancholy are quite normal emotions that all people experience. Common descriptive phrases for this expression of mood include feeling down, having the blues, unhappy, down-hearted, and low spirits. When the word "depression" is used in the context of depressive illness, a more distressed component is required. Synonyms here include despair; hopelessness; weeping; worthlessness; and, in general, an inability to find pleasure in those things that are normally pleasurable. When used to define disease, added features indicating severity, duration (persistence), and functional impairment are required.

The Diagnostic and Statistical Manual of Mental Disorders–IV (DSM-IV) [1] lists 10 depressive mood disorders ranging from major depressive episode, dysthymic disorder, bipolar I disorders, bipolar II disorders, substance-induced mood disorders, to adjustment disorder with depressed mood.

The DSM-IV criteria for the diagnosis of major depressive episode are listed next. At least five of the symptoms must be present during the same 2-week period. These symptoms must be a change from a previous level of functioning:

1. Depressed mood, nearly every day during most of the day.
2. Markedly diminished interest or pleasure in almost all activities.

* Corresponding author.
E-mail address: hullp@duke.usask.ca (P.R. Hull).

3. Significant weight loss (when not dieting), weight gain, or a change in appetite.
4. Insomnia or hypersomnia.
5. Psychomotor agitation or psychomotor retardation.
6. Fatigue or loss of energy.
7. Feelings of worthlessness or inappropriate guilt.
8. Impaired ability to concentrate or indecisiveness.
9. Recurrent thoughts of death, recurrent suicidal ideation.

Patients with major depressive disorder often have recurrent discrete episodes of depression that persist throughout their lifetime.

*Prevalence of depression*

Acne affects predominantly adolescents and young adults. Depressive symptoms in this group are often concealed or denied or may be masked by aggression or disruptive behavior. Large-scale national population studies give an indication of both the prevalence and incidence of depression [2]. Such population studies include the Canadian Community Health Survey of Mental Health and Well-Being [3]. Similar national survey data are available for the United States [4], Britain [5], Australia [6], and other countries. The Canadian Community Health Survey 1.2 used the detailed long form of the Composite International Diagnostic Interview for major depression to assess the occurrence of that disorder in the general population. The information gathered was from households, and anyone institutionalized is not included in the results. The interviews were conducted during 2002. The 12-month point prevalence of major depression for 15- to 19-year-old persons in Canada was found to be 8.1% for women and 3.3% for men. For those age 20 to 24 years, 9.8% of women and 5.9% of men were found to have had a major depressive episode in the last year [7]. The incidence for major depression in population studies is generally higher in younger age groups and within all age groups was generally higher in women than in men. In Australia, a similar population survey suggested that 5.2% of the population aged 13 to 17 met the criteria for self-reported depression [7].

In the United States, the National Comorbidity Survey indicated that 17% of Americans experience depression at some point during their lives and 5% are depressed in any given month [8,9]. Several epidemiologic studies reported that up to 8.3% of adolescents in the United States suffer from depression [10]. Depression in adolescence is associated with persistence into adult life and a high rate of suicide [11]. Suicide is the third commonest cause of death in adolescence and is frequently associated with drug and alcohol abuse, smoking, hopelessness, social withdrawal, isolation, negative self concept, violent behavior, and familial transmission [10,12–14]. In Canada, the rate of suicide for persons 15 to 19 years of age is 5.5 per 100,000 in women and 19.9 among men. For those 20 to 24 years of age the comparable rates are 3.6 and 24.9 [15]. The high frequency of depression and suicide in the adolescent and young adult population is significant when factoring in the influence of both acne and medication use, including oral contraceptives and isotretinoin.

## The emotional impact of acne, anxiety, and depression

The psychologic impact of acne can be profound. Acne patients may experience problems with self-esteem [16], self-confidence, body image, embarrassment, social withdrawal, anger, anxiety, and impaired social functioning including poorer academic achievement, unemployment [17], and decreased dating and participation in sports.

Although there is a paucity of well-controlled studies examining depression associated with acne [18], there are studies documenting this relationship. Anxiety and depression were assessed in a series of 34 patients with chronic acne (severe enough to justify the use of isotretinoin) using the Hospital Anxiety and Depression (HAD) scale [19]. Significant levels of anxiety were found in 44% of these patients and depression in 18%. On the basis of the HAD scores, this study indicated that the scores for the acne group of patients fell between those seen in psychiatric patients and patients with general medical diagnoses. Age–sex comparisons were not provided.

In a study of depression and suicide ideation, 72 adolescent and young adult patients with mild to moderate, noncystic acne were evaluated using the 52-item Carroll Rating Scale for Depression [20]. The Carroll Rating Scale for Depression is a validated self-administered rating instrument for depression. Active suicidal ideation was elicited in 5.6% of these patients responding with a "Yes" to the item "I have been thinking about trying to kill myself." The mean score for depression was greater than 10, a score indicating clinical depression. The comparators were other dermatologic conditions including alopecia areata, atopic dermatitis, outpatient psoriasis (less severe), and inpatient psoriasis (more severe). Only patients with severe psoriasis had higher scores for both depression and suicidal ideation.

In a larger study, patients with acne were identified from referral letters to the Dermatology Department at the Churchill Hospital in Oxford, England [21]. One hundred and thirty individuals older than 16 years were sent a questionnaire before being seen by the dermatologist. Two scales included in the questionnaire were the EuroQol and the Short Form 36. The EuroQol is a five-question instrument that asks about mobility, self-care, usual activities, pain or discomfort, and anxiety or depression. Of the 110 responders with acne (mean age of 22.1 with range of 16–39 years), 52.8% were assessed as having moderate to severe problems with anxiety or depression with 4% having a severe problem. The percentage of individuals in the control population group (aged 20–39 years) with moderate or severe anxiety or depression was 15.5%. In the acne group, there was no significant relationship between anxiety and depression and age, sex, duration of symptoms, or severity of acne. The Medical Outcomes Study Short Form 36 is a 36-question instrument assessing eight health domains and providing both a physical component summary and a mental health component summary. Short Form 36 scores for this same cohort of acne patients were compared with six other chronic diseases occurring in an age- and sex-matched general population [22]. The acne patients' mental health scores were worse than any of the other diseases. There was no correlation with the clinician-observed severity of acne.

A study from Turkey compared 61 acne patients with 38 volunteer controls using the HAD [23]. The mean HAD anxiety subscale and HAD depression subscale scores of the patients were significantly higher than those of the controls. The rates of subjects at risk for anxiety (26.2%) and for depression (29.5%) were significantly higher in the patient group than in the control group (0% and 7.9%, respectively). There were no significant sex differences, nor did the HAD depression subscale scores correlate with the severity of the acne. A cross-sectional survey of 2657 school children in Turkey found acne in 16.1% of the girls and 29.2% of the boys [24]. The HAD scores for anxiety and depression were not significantly different from the control group of students. The HAD scores also did not correlate with the severity of the acne.

Most of the case control studies presented here indicate that acne patients are more likely to have symptoms suggestive of clinically significant depression. One study also showed a significant association between acne and suicide ideation [20].

**Drug-induced depression**

Drug-induced depression is classified in the DSM-IV as a substance-induced mood disorder. The diagnostic features include a prominent and persistent disturbance in mood judged to be the physiologic effect of the substance (drug). The diagnosing clinician is asked to make a judgment on an individual level as to whether a drug caused the symptoms.

The etiologic relationship between any drug and depression is complex. If one considers the "component cause" model proposed by Rothman [25], then exposure to a particular drug is one component cause acting together with other component causes in a component field to produce an effect: depressive symptoms. The frequency of the effect depends on the prevalence of the other causal components and might apply to only a very small subset of the population. Drugs may theoretically act in a manner to be "sufficient cause" or "necessary cause," but probably mostly have a role rather as a weak and "contributing cause."

In a critical review of the literature, Patten and Barbui [26] found evidence linking corticosteroids, interferon-α, interleukin-2, gonadotropin-releasing hormone agonists, mefloquine, progestin-releasing implanted contraceptives, and propranolol to the etiology of atypical depressive syndromes. They concluded that although drugs could induce depressive symptoms, drug-induced depression seems to differ symptomatically from classical major depression. Interestingly, evidence was not presented linking isotretinoin or antidepressants to depression. The Food and Drug Administration did a rank order for depression of all drugs in the spontaneous reporting and adverse event reporting database. Isotretinoin ranked number 5 for serious depression and 10 for suicide attempts [27].

**Links between isotretinoin and depression and suicide**

*Establishing a causal connection*

Because depression, suicide, and acne are not infrequent disorders, particularly among adolescents and younger adults, to establish a relationship between isotretinoin treatment and depression and suicide it is important to establish that the risk of these psychiatric disorders is greater among users as opposed to nonusers or that there are unique subsets of subsets of isotretinoin users at increased risk of these disorders. The association should be consistently evident in studies using a variety of study designs. The articulation of a plausible mechanism of action would strengthen the argument for an association. A temporal pharmacokinetic effect of challenge, dechallenge, and rechallenge should be evident and some form of a dose-response relationship and a drug class effect. The absence of a strong competing hypothesis is also supportive of a connection. Rothman and Greenland provide a more formal extended discussion of causality [28]. Case reports, although useful for hypothesis generation and alerting one to potential effects and relationships, are of limited value in and of themselves for establishing a causal connection.

*Reviews*

There have been several recent reviews examining possible linkage between isotretinoin, depression, and suicide [29–34]. Most of these reviews conclude that at present there is no conclusive evidence that either supports such an association or rejects it.

*Spontaneous (case) reports in the medical literature*

There are relatively few spontaneous case reports in the literature of depression or suicide occurring in acne patients treated with isotretinoin. These are presented in Table 1 [35–52] and discussed in detail elsewhere [31]. In addition to these cases in the medical literature, case reports of depression or suicide have been reported to governmental adverse drug monitoring agencies, either directly or indirectly through the manufacturer, and are shown in Table 2 [53–57]. Without any increase in prevalence of depression or suicide a background rate of occurrence can be expected. The authors have estimated background rates for depression and suicide using available epidemiologic data for selected countries (Table 3). These estimates ignore the effects of acne in increasing the likelihood of both depression and suicide.

*Cohort studies*

In a nonrandomized, prospective study, 215 patients were treated with either isotretinoin (N = 174) or minocycline and topical retinoids (N = 41) [58]. The treatment given was determined by a dermatologist on the basis of acne severity. The 21-item Beck's Depression Inventory and the 26-item abbreviated version of the World Health Organization Quality of Life 100-item questionnaire were administered before treatment. At baseline, 8.4% of all patients had a Beck's Depression Inventory score of 10 or greater, indicating at least a moderate level of depressive symptoms. Patients on isotretinoin, whose scores were greater than 10, showed a significant decrease in their scores during treatment. Five of the 174 patients on isotretinoin complained of worsening mood and isotretinoin was stopped. Two of these five patients were examined by a psychiatrist and neither was deemed to have clinical depression (DSM-IV major depression episode criteria). Both were assessed as having coexisting psychologic stressors unrelated to either their acne or isotretinoin. Both were rechallenged with isotretinoin, with no reported problems. Three refused psychiatric evaluation. Two did not return for further follow-up and the third improved 2 weeks after stopping isotretinoin. The study weaknesses include the small number of patients, the lack of a randomization, and the incomplete data on those whose mood deteriorated and who left the study.

*Population-based studies*

A large case-control cohort study, sponsored by Hoffmann-La Roche, found no increased risk of depression in individuals treated with isotretinoin when compared with those treated with antibiotics [59]. This study used two validated databases (one Canadian, the other British) to compare the prevalence rates of neurotic and psychotic disorders, suicide, and attempted suicide between isotretinoin and antibiotic users. The study concludes that the use of isotretinoin is not associated with an increased risk of depression, suicide, or other psychiatric disorders. This study represents the first attempt formally to evaluate an association between isotretinoin use and depression and suicide. There are a number of weaknesses in the study design, however, most importantly in the identification of the study disease by relying on an incomplete set of diagnostic codes and not using drug data to maximize identification. Wysowski [60] has also commented on limitations of this study whose findings must be considered to be inconclusive.

A further study sponsored by Hoffmann-La Roche used a sequence symmetry method to evaluate a large nationwide United States prescription database [61]. The method infers causality based on the sequence of filled prescriptions. In this case, isotretinoin or minocycline followed by antidepressants (causal group) were compared with antidepressants followed by either isotretinoin or minocycline (noncausal group). The database contains prescription information from about 90 million patients, and during the period of the study (July 1, 1998–March 31, 2000)

Table 1
Spontaneous literature reports linking depression and suicide to isotretinoin use

| First author, year, [Ref.] | No. of patients and sex | Onset | Prior Depression | Isotretinoin use | Resolution of depression | Rechallenge |
|---|---|---|---|---|---|---|
| Cotterill, 1981 [35] | 1 (NS) | 5th mo | NS | No | Suicide | No |
| Hazen, 1983 [36] | 6 of 110 (NS) | >2 wk on Rx | 1 | NS | Rapid | NS |
| Lindemayr, 1986 [37] | 1M | 8 wk on Rx | NS | NS | Suicide attempt | NS |
| Burket, 1987 [38] | 1F | During Rx | 0 | No | Rapid | No |
| Scheinman, 1990 [39] | 7 of 700 (5F and 2M) | 14 wk on Rx (mean) | 2 | 2 (ND) | Within 1 wk | 1 (recurred in 3rd mo) |
| Hepburn, 1990 [40] | 1F | 2 mo on Rx | NS | NS | Suicide attempt | NS |
| Gatti, 1991 [41] | 1M | 1 mo after Rx | 0 | No | Suicide | No |
| Duke, 1992 [42] | 2 (1F and 1M) | 1 mo on Rx | 0 | No | Recovered (1 after 6 mo) | No |
| Bravard, 1993 [43] | 3 (1F and 2M) | 4, 2, 3 mo of Rx | 0 | NS | 2 suicides. Other after 1 mo. | NS |
| Byrne, 1995 [44] | 3 (2F and 1M) | During Rx | 0 | NS | >5 mo in 1 | No |
| Aubin, 1995 [45] | 1M | Day 1 | NS | NS | Suicide attempt | NS |
| Hull, 2000 [46] | 6 (NS) | Within 1 mo | NS | NS | NS | No |
| Robusto, 2003 [47] | 1F | Within 1 mo | 0 | No | Present 1 y after stopping isotretinoin | No |
| Van Broekhoven, 2003 [48] | 1M | Had been on isotretinoin for 9 mo | Bipolar disorder | No | Suicide | No |
| Millard, 1999 [49] | 6 (4F and 2M) | "Early in 3, later in 1" | 0 | NS | Recovered 4–6 wk | NS |
| Ng, 2001 [50] | 1M | 2 wk | 0 | No | Suicide attempt. Positive dechallenge. | Yes—depression recurred with increased dose. |
| Shehi, 2004 [51] | 1M | 3 d | Major depressive disorder | No | Improved in 3 d | No |
| Barak, 2005 [52] | 5 (3F and 2M) | 7.6 mo (mean) | Affective psychosis. Preceding cofactors present in all. | NS | Suicide attempts in 3 | >6 mo in 3 |

*Abbreviations*: F, female; M, male; ND, no depression; NS, not stated; Rx, prescription.

Table 2
Governmental adverse reaction agency reports of isotretinoin-related depression and suicide

| Country government agency, years, [Ref.] | Depression (% with contributing factors) | Suicide | Isotretinoin users |
|---|---|---|---|
| US FDA, 1982–2000 | 431 (69%[a]) | 37 (62%) | 5 million |
| Canada, 1983–1999 [53] | 10 | 0 | N/A |
| Australia, 1985–1998 [54] | 12 (16%) | 1 | N/A |
| Ireland [55] | 6 psychiatric events | 1 | N/A |
| Denmark, 1997–2001 [56] | 23 | 0 | 43126 |
| UK, 1999–2002 [57] | 79 | NS | 375,000[b] |

*Abbreviations:* N/A, not available; NS, not stated.

[a] 76 of 110 (69%) US patients hospitalized for depression and suicide ideation or attempt.

[b] 1983–2002.

there were approximately 5.6 million prescriptions for antidepressants. During this period, there were 2821 new incident prescriptions for isotretinoin with 1382 filling subsequent prescriptions for antidepressants and in 1439 patients the antidepressant was prescribed before the isotretinoin. The adjusted risk ratio was below 1, suggesting that isotretinoin does not have a depression-provoking effect. Antidepressant drug usage is used in this study as an indicator of major depression. It may be argued that a significant number of depressed patients may not have sought treatment or may have received nondrug treatment for their depression. In a study of 1709 randomly selected high school children in Oregon, mental health use in those diagnosed with major depressive disorder was only 60%, with individual psychotherapy being the most used form of treatment. Antidepressants were used in only 4.2% [62]. Other studies have also indicated that the most frequently used form of treatment for child-adolescent depression is outpatient psychotherapy, with only a relatively small percentage of young patients receiving antidepressant medication [63,64].

A third formal study by Hoffmann-La Roche has appeared in abstract form with further details supplied by Martin Huber, Global Head, Drug Safety Risk Management, Hoffman-La Roche, Nutley, New Jersey [65]. This was a retrospective study using a major, nationwide United States health plan database (United Health Care Research Database) and included 5130 first-time isotretinoin users and 25,600 age-, sex-, and health plan unit–matched controls. A 6-month screening period was included to identify pre-existing depression and the follow-up period extended to 30 days after the last dose of isotretinoin. A diagnosis of depression was ascertained using eight definitions including a claims database, office visits claims, and psychiatric drug dispensing claims. At screening the isotretinoin users had a higher rate of psychiatric illness compared with nonusers (13.5%

Table 3
Estimated background rates of depression and suicide to be expected among isotretinoin users for selected countries

| Country | Population aged 15–24 y (source) | Estimated no. of new isotretinoin users aged 15–24 y in 1 year | Estimated annual background no. of Depressed individuals among isotretinoin users aged 15–24 y [Ref.] | Suicides among isotretinoin users aged 15–24 y (suicides per 100,000)[a] |
|---|---|---|---|---|
| US | 39,183,891 (census 2000) | 340,000[b,c] | 28,220 [9] | 35 (10.2) |
| Canada | 4,009,190 (census 2001) | 34,880[c,d] | 2363 [83] | 4.5 (13.0) |
| Australia | 1,306,832 (census 2001) | 11,370[c,d] | 591 [7] | 1.5 (12.9) |
| Ireland | 641,522 (census 2002) | 5580[c,d] | 390[e] | 0.9 (16.1) |
| Denmark | 593,555 (statistical report 2004) | 5165[c,d] | 361[e] | 0.4 (7.5) |
| UK | 7,209,766 (census 2001) | 62,725[c,d] | 6760[f] | 4.2 (6.7) |

[a] Based on national suicide rates reported for each country on the World Health Organization website [81].

[b] Based on FDA reporting for 1999 [82] and assuming that 80% of isotretinoin users are aged 15–24 y.

[c] Assumed based on FDA [82] reporting approximately equal numbers of males and females receiving isotretinoin treatment.

[d] Estimated based on FDA data for the US [82] and assuming a similar level of prescription as in the USA.

[e] Based on an estimated 7% prevalence rate.

[f] Based on the National Statistics Report on Psychiatric Morbidity [5] among adults living in private households, 2000.

versus 9.5%). Depression (defined as a depression diagnosis or antidepressant dispensing) was also initially higher in the isotretinoin group, occurring in 9.1% compared with 5.7%. These data suggest that those prescribed isotretinoin had more severe acne and more negative emotions associated with their condition in comparison with others. Rates of depression, during and after isotretinoin use, were similar for both users and nonusers. In those patients having more than four physician visits (high medical care use), the rate of depression for isotretinoin users was 7.66 per 100,000 and 14.88 per 100,000 for nonusers. This study includes a large number of isotretinoin users and shows that patients with acne have significant rates of depression before starting isotretinoin. The study, however, did not validate the diagnosis of depression by patient chart review. These epidemiologic studies fail to show that isotretinoin acts as a necessary or sufficient cause in the occurrence of depression.

**Vitamin A and other retinoids and depression: is there a drug class effect?**

A drug class effect might be expected if isotretinoin produced depression by a pharmacologic effect on cerebral retinoid receptors. Symptoms of vitamin A toxicity generally require a daily dose in excess of 100,000 IU. Hypervitaminosis A results in many of the well-known side effects of isotretinoin, including raised blood lipids, dry skin, cracked lips, fatigue, hair loss, and teratogenicity. Hypervitaminosis A may also be associated with central nervous system effects, such as sleeping difficulties, loss of appetite, tiredness, irritability, ataxia, and increased intracranial pressure. Bauernfeind did not list depression as a symptom in 200 cases of hypervitaminosis [66]. Restak [67] described an 18-year-old female acne patient who developed a severe psychosis and depression following 6 months self-medication on high-dose (100,000–150,000 IU) vitamin A. She had no antecedent psychiatric problems. This episode preceded the development of pseudotumor cerebri. Both resolved rapidly when the vitamin A was stopped. A 54-year-old with no prior psychiatric history developed depression following ingestion of 12 times the normal dietary supplement of vitamin A over a 2-year period [68]. This patient recovered within 2 months of stopping the vitamin A. When high-dose oral vitamin A acid (100–200 mg/day) was used in early clinical studies in 30 patients, three patients developed "changes in psychologic state" [69].

*Etretinate*

Henderson and Highet [70] described three patients with psoriasis developing depression associated with etretinate treatment. There was no past history of depression. In all three patients, the depression resolved when the etretinate was withdrawn; in one patient it recurred on rechallenge. A 49-year-old man with symmetric erythrokeratodermia was treated with etretinate in a dose of 1 mg/kg/d [71]. After 1 month on treatment, he developed profound depression, fatigue, aggression, somnolence, and reduced work capacity. These symptoms resolved after stopping etretinate and did not recur when rechallenged at a dose of 0.5 mg/kg/d. To date, there are no case reports in the literature linking two other retinoids, bexarotene and acitretin, with depression.

**Mechanism of action**

Retinoid receptors are present in the brain and retinoic acid signaling has been extensively studied [72,73]. Retinoic acid plays a crucial role in brain development and the continued expression of retinoic acid receptors in the adult brain suggests ongoing function of this signaling pathway in adults. Retinoids exert their effects by binding to their nuclear receptors, the retinoic acid receptors ($\alpha$, $\beta$, or $\gamma$) and retinoid X receptors, to regulate gene transcription. Retinoic acid receptors are known to control a large number of genes, and retinoic acid can signal neural stem cells to become neurons.

It has been suggested that the hippocampal area of the brain may be an important region in the pathophysiology of major depressive disorder [74,75]. Loss of hippocampal volume has been associated with depression [76,77]. Volumetric imaging studies have indicated that early history of depression and a family history may contribute to the volume loss. This loss of volume may be related to retraction of the neuronal dendritic tree and with apoptosis of neuronal cells. Antidepressant drugs may stimulate neurogenesis and prevent volume loss [73]. In mice exposed to isotretinoin, hippocampal neurogenesis is suppressed and it has been suggested that this is a possible mechanism for isotretinoin-induced depression [78]. In a study only reported in abstract form, Bremner and coworkers [79] measured brain function with [F-18]-2-fluoro-2-deoxyglucose positron emission tomography before and after 4 months of treatment with isotretinoin (N = 13) and antibiotic (N = 15). Isotretinoin (but not antibiotic) treatment was associated with decreased brain metabolism in the orbitofrontal cortex (−21% change versus a +2% change for antibiotic; $P < .05$), a brain area thought to mediate symptoms of depression. There was no difference, however, in severity of depressive symptoms in the two groups before or after treatment.

The relatively low frequency of depression associated with isotretinoin suggests that the relationship is unlikely to be a direct pharmacologic effect. Other predisposing factors need to be identified and it could be speculated that this might include pre-existing hippocampal neuron loss.

## Summary

Both adolescents and acne patients have significant psychologic problems, including depression. There is no formal epidemiologic evidence from either treatment cohort studies or large-scale population studies for an association between isotretinoin use and depression. There is, however, case report evidence that isotretinoin may be associated with the development of depression. Cases showing positive dechallenge and rechallenge are important in pointing to an individual susceptibility. There should be further rigorously designed cohort and population-based epidemiologic studies, however, of this possible connection. Such studies should include a focus on possible contributing factors and pre-existing conditions.

In 2004, there were about 70 lawsuits in the United States alleging that isotretinoin had caused patients injury, including suicide, depression, birth defects, and gastrointestinal injuries [80]. Although such lawsuits may reveal much about the inner conflicts within a major pharmaceutical company concerning adverse effect disclosure, it is unlikely that they provide new and credible information about the relationship between isotretinoin and these adverse events. It is possible that public and political pressure will force the withdrawal of isotretinoin, at least from the United States markets. Such a move would deprive many thousands of patients with severe acne from benefiting from the unchallenged efficacy of the drug. It might also spawn an illicit market for isotretinoin, lacking the control of informed and concerned physicians.

Patients and their relatives must be informed about the occasional occurrence of depression in patients on isotretinoin and they should be encouraged to report depressive symptoms promptly. At each visit, the physician should inquire specifically about symptoms of depression and, if necessary, antidepressant treatment, referral to a psychiatrist, or discontinuation of isotretinoin should be considered.

## References

[1] American Psychiatric Association. Diagnostic and Statistical Manual of Mental Disorders–IV. 4th edition. Washington, DC: American Psychiatric Association; 1994.

[2] Patten SB. Incidence of major depression in Canada. CMAJ 2000;163:714–5.

[3] Statistics Canada. Canadian Community Health Survey of Mental Health and Well-Being. Available at: http://www.statcan.ca/English/freepub/82-617-XIE. Accessed June 21, 2005.

[4] Kessler RC, Berglund P, Demler O, et al. Lifetime prevalence and age-of-onset distributions of DSM-IV disorders in the National Comorbidity Survey Replication. Arch Gen Psych 2005;62:593–602.

[5] Singleton N, Bumpstead R, O'Brien M, et al for the Office of National Statistics. Psychiatric morbidity among adults living in private households, 2000. London: Her Majesty's Stationery Office; 2001.

[6] Commonwealth Department of Health and Aged Care and Australian Institute of Health and Welfare. National health priority areas report: mental health 1998 [cat. no. PHE13]. Canberra (Australia): Health and AIHW; 1999.

[7] Based on the authors' analysis of the data in the public use data file for the Canadian Community Health Survey of Mental Health and Well-being. Available upon application submission to Statistics Canada.

[8] Rey JM, Sawyer MG, Clark JJ, et al. Depression among Australian adolescents. Med J Aust 2001;175: 19–23.

[9] Kessler RC, McGonagle KA, Zhao S, et al. Lifetime and 12-month prevalence of DSM-III-R psychiatric disorders in the United States. Results from the National Comorbidity Survey. Arch Gen Psychiatry 1994;51:8–19.

[10] National Institutes of Health, US Department of Health and Human Services, National Institute for Mental Health. Depression in children and adolescents: a fact sheet for physicians. Available at: http://www.nimh.nih.gov/publicat/NIMHdepchildresfact.pdf. Accessed January 30, 2004.

[11] Wilcox HC, Anthony JC. Child and adolescent clinical features as forerunners of adult-onset major depressive disorder: retrospective evidence from an epidemiological sample. J Affect Disord 2004;82:9–20.

[12] Wu P, Hoven CW, Liu X, et al. Substance use, suicidal ideation and attempts in children and adolescents. Suicide Life Threat Behav 2004;34:408–20.

[13] Adams DM, Overholser JC. Suicidal behavior and history of substance abuse. Am J Drug Alcohol Abuse 1992;18:343–54.

[14] Rutter PA, Behrendt AE. Adolescent suicide risk: four psychosocial factors. Adolescence 2004;39:295–302.

[15] Statistics Canada. Suicides and suicide rate, by sex and by age group. Available at: http://www.statcan.ca/english/Pgdb/health01.htm. Accessed January 30, 2005.

[16] Shuster S, Fisher GH, Harris E, et al. The effect of skin

disease on self image [proceedings]. Br J Dermatol 1978;99(Suppl 16):18–9.
[17] Koo J. The psychosocial impact of acne: patients' perceptions. J Am Acad Dermatol 1995;32:S26–30.
[18] Tan JK. Psychosocial impact of acne vulgaris: evaluating the evidence. Skin Therapy Lett 2004;9:1–9.
[19] Kellett SC, Gawkrodger DJ. The psychological and emotional impact of acne and the effect of treatment with isotretinoin. Br J Dermatol 1999;140: 273–82.
[20] Gupta MA, Gupta AK. Depression and suicidal ideation in dermatology patients with acne, alopecia areata, atopic dermatitis and psoriasis. Br J Dermatol 1998;139:846–50.
[21] Klassen AF, Newton JN, Mallon E. Measuring quality of life in people referred for specialist care of acne: comparing generic and disease-specific measures. J Am Acad Dermatol 2000;43(2 Pt 1):229–33.
[22] Mallon E, Newton JN, Klassen A, et al. The quality of life in acne: a comparison with general medical conditions using generic questionnaires. Br J Dermatol 1999;140:672–6.
[23] Yazici K, Baz K, Yazici AE, et al. Disease-specific quality of life is associated with anxiety and depression in patients with acne. J Eur Acad Dermatol Venereol 2004;18:435–9.
[24] Aktan S, Ozmen E, Sanli B. Anxiety, depression, and nature of acne vulgaris in adolescents. Int J Dermatol 2000;39:354–7.
[25] Rothman KJ. Causes. Am J Epidemiol 1976;104: 587–92.
[26] Patten SB, Barbui C. Drug-induced depression: a systematic review to inform clinical practice. Psychother Psychosom 2004;73:207–15.
[27] Wysowski DK, Pitts M, Beitz J. An analysis of reports of depression and suicide in patients treated with isotretinoin. J Am Acad Dermatol 2001;45:515–9.
[28] Rothman KJ, Greenland S. Causation and causal inference. In: Rothman RJ, Greenland S, editors. Modern epidemiology. Philadelphia: Lippincott-Raven; 1998. p. 7–28.
[29] Bremner JD. Does isotretinoin cause depression and suicide? Psychopharmacol Bull 2003;37:64–78.
[30] Enders SJ, Enders JM. Isotretinoin and psychiatric illness in adolescents and young adults. Ann Pharmacother 2003;37:1124–7.
[31] Hull PR, D'Arcy C. Isotretinoin use and subsequent depression and suicide: presenting the evidence. Am J Clin Dermatol 2003;4:493–505.
[32] Jacobs DG, Deutsch NL, Brewer M. Suicide, depression, and isotretinoin: is there a causal link? J Am Acad Dermatol 2001;45:S168–75.
[33] Ng CH, Schweitzer I. The association between depression and isotretinoin use in acne. Aust N Z J Psychiatry 2003;37:78–84.
[34] O'Donnell J. Overview of existing research and information linking isotretinoin (Accutane), depression, psychosis, and suicide. Am J Ther 2003;10:148–59.
[35] Cotterill JA. Dermatological non-disease: a common and potentially fatal disturbance of cutaneous body image. Br J Dermatol 1981;104:611–9.
[36] Hazen PG, Carney JF, Walker AE, et al. Depression: a side effect of 13-cis-retinoic acid therapy. J Am Acad Dermatol 1983;9:278–9.
[37] Lindemayr H. Isotretinoin intoxication in attempted suicide. Acta Derm Venereol 1986;66:452–3.
[38] Burket JM, Storrs FJ. Nodulocystic infantile acne occurring in a kindred of steatocystoma. Arch Dermatol 1987;123:432–3.
[39] Scheinman PL, Peck GL, Rubinow DR, et al. Acute depression from isotretinoin. J Am Acad Dermatol 1990;22:1112–4.
[40] Hepburn NC. Deliberate self-poisoning with isotretinoin. Br J Dermatol 1990;122:840–1.
[41] Gatti S, Serri F. Acute depression from isotretinoin. [letter] J Am Acad Dermatol 1991;25:132.
[42] Duke EE, Guenther L. Psychiatric reactions to the retinoids. Canadian Journal of Dermatology 1992;5:467.
[43] Bravard P, Krug M. RJC. Isotretinoin and depression: care is needed. [letter] Nouv Dermatol 1993;12:215.
[44] Byrne A, Hnatko G. Depression associated with isotretinoin therapy. Can J Psychiatry 1995;40:567.
[45] Aubin S, Lorette G, Muller C, et al. Massive isotretinoin intoxication. Clin Exp Dermatol 1995;20: 348–50.
[46] Hull PR, Demkiw-Bartel C. Isotretinoin use in acne: prospective evaluation of adverse events. J Cutan Med Surg 2000;4:66–70.
[47] Robusto O. Depression caused by an anti-acne agent. Acta Med Port 2002;15:325–6.
[48] van Broekhoven F, Verkes RJ, Janzing JG. Psychiatric symptoms during isotretinoin therapy. Ned Tijdschr Geneeskd 2003;147:2341–3.
[49] Millard LG. Adverse mood and behaviour change in young patients on systemic isotretinoin. Br J Dermatol 1999;141(Suppl 55):16.
[50] Ng CH, Tam MM, Hook SJ. Acne, isotretinoin treatment and acute depression. World J Biol Psychiatry 2001;2:159–61.
[51] Shehi GM, Bryson WJ. Hypersomnia associated with isotretinoin in a patient with recurrent major depressive disorder and acne vulgaris. Sleep 2004;27:821.
[52] Barak Y, Wohl Y, Greenberg Y, et al. Affective psychosis following Accutane (isotretinoin) treatment. Int Clin Psychopharmacol 2005;20:39–41.
[53] Wray CM. Accutane and depression. Canadian Adverse Drug Reaction Newsletter 1999;9:1. Available at: http://www.hc-sc.gc.ca/hpfb-dgpsa/tpd-dpt/adrv9n1_e.html. Accessed January 31, 2005.
[54] Depression with isotretinoin. Australian Adverse Drug Reactions Bulletin 1998;17:3. Available at: http://www.tga.gov.au/docs/html/aadrbltn/aadr9808.htm#isot. Accessed January 30, 2005.
[55] Irish Medicines Board. Roaccutane. Drug Safety Newsletter. 7th Edition 1998. Available at: http://www.imb.ie/uploads/publications/7077996_Issue%208.pdf. Accessed January 30, 2005.
[56] The Danish Medicines Agency. Psychic adverse

[57] Lammy. House of Commons Hansard Written Answers for 27th January 2003. Available at: http://www.publications.parliament.uk/cgi-bin/ukparl_hl?DB=ukparl&STEMMER=en&WORDS=isotretinoin+&COLOUR=Red&STYLE=s&URL=/pa/cm200203/cmhansrd/vo030127/text/30127w46.htm#30127w46.html_spnew0. Accessed January 30, 2005.

reactions to the use of the acne medicine isotretinoin (trade name Roaccutan, Accutin, Isotretinoin, Isotrex). Danish Medicines Agency. Available at: http://www.dkma.dk/1024/visUKLSArtikel.asp?artikelID=2302. Accessed January 30, 2005.

[58] Ng CH, Tam MM, Celi E, et al. Prospective study of depressive symptoms and quality of life in acne vulgaris patients treated with isotretinoin compared to antibiotic and topical therapy. Australas J Dermatol 2002;43:262–8.

[59] Jick SS, Kremers HM, Vasilakis-Scaramozza C. Isotretinoin use and risk of depression, psychotic symptoms, suicide, and attempted suicide. Arch Dermatol 2000;136:1231–6.

[60] Wysowski DK. Methodological limitations of the study "isotretinoin use and risk of depression, psychotic symptoms, suicide, and attempted suicide [letter]. Arch Dermatol 2001;137:1102.

[61] Hersom K, Neary MP, Levaux HP, et al. Isotretinoin and antidepressant pharmacotherapy: a prescription sequence symmetry analysis. J Am Acad Dermatol 2003;49:424–32.

[62] Lewinsohn PM, Rohde P, Seeley JR. Treatment of adolescent depression: frequency of services and impact on functioning in young adulthood. Depress Anxiety 1998;7:47–52.

[63] Kovacs M, Feinberg TL, Crouse-Novak M, et al. Depressive disorders in childhood. II. A longitudinal study of the risk for a subsequent major depression. Arch Gen Psychiatry 1984;41:643–9.

[64] Keller MB, Lavori PW, Beardslee WR, et al. Depression in children and adolescents: new data on undertreatment and a literature review on the efficacy of available treatments. J Affect Disord 1991;21:163–71.

[65] Neary MP, Klaskala W, McLane J, et al. Epidemiological study of adverse events in Accutane users and matched non-users: retrospective analysis of major US health plan claims database [abstract]. Pharmacoepidemiol Drug Saf 2001;10(Suppl 1):S141.

[66] Bendich A, Langseth L. Safety of vitamin A. Am J Clin Nutr 1989;49:358–71.

[67] Restak RM. Pseudotumor cerebri, psychosis, and hypervitaminosis A. J Nerv Ment Dis 1972;155:72–5.

[68] McCance-Katz EF, Price LH. Depression associated with vitamin A intoxication. Psychosomatics 1992;33:117–8.

[69] Stuttgen G. Oral vitamin A acid therapy. Acta Derm Venereol Suppl (Stockh) 1975;74:174–9.

[70] Henderson CA, Highet AS. Depression induced by etretinate. [letter] BMJ 1989;298:964.

[71] Borbujo MJM, Casado JM, Garijo LMB, et al. An unusual secondary effect of etretinate. Med Clin (Barc) 1987;89:577.

[72] Mey J, McCaffery P. Retinoic acid signaling in the nervous system of adult vertebrates. Neuroscientist 2004;10:409–21.

[73] Campbell S, Macqueen G. The role of the hippocampus in the pathophysiology of major depression. J Psychiatry Neurosci 2004;29:417–26.

[74] Sheline YI, Mittler BL, Mintun MA. The hippocampus and depression. Eur Psychiatry 2002;17(Suppl 3):300–5.

[75] Sheline YI. Hippocampal atrophy in major depression: a result of depression-induced neurotoxicity? Mol Psychiatry 1996;1:298–9.

[76] Sheline YI, Wang PW, Gado MH, et al. Hippocampal atrophy in recurrent major depression. Proc Natl Acad Sci U S A 1996;93:3908–13.

[77] Sheline YI, Gado MH, Kraemer HC. Untreated depression and hippocampal volume loss. Am J Psychiatry 2003;160:1516–8.

[78] Sakai Y, Crandall JE, Brodsky J, et al. 13-cis Retinoic acid (Accutane) suppresses hippocampal cell survival in mice. Ann N Y Acad Sci 2004;1021:436–40.

[79] Bremner JD, Fani N, Ashraf N, et al. Functional brain imaging alterations in acne patients treated with isotretinoin [abstract]. Program No. 114.2. 2004 Abstract Viewer/Itinerary Planner. Washington: Society for Neuroscience; 2004.

[80] McCoy K. Drugmaker rebuffed call to monitor users. December 12, 2004. Available at: http://www.usatoday.com/money/industries/health/drugs/2004-12-06-accutanecover_x.htm. Accessed June 21, 2005.

[81] World Health Organization. Available at: http://who.int/mental_health/prevention/suicide/country_reports/en/index.html. Accessed June 22, 2005.

[82] US Food and Drug Administration. Dermatologic and Ophthalmic Advisory Committee. Hoffmann-La Roche. Briefing information. September 2000. Available at: http://www.fda.gov/ohrms/dockets/ac/00/backgrd/3639b1c_05.pdf. Accessed June 22, 2005.

[83] Statistics Canada. Depression. In: Health indicators, May 2002 [cat. no. 82-221-XIE]. Available at: http://www.statcan.ca:80/english/freepub/82-221-XIE/00502/hlthstatus/conditions2.htm#depression. Accessed June 22, 2005.

# Obsessive-Compulsive Disorders and Dermatologic Disease

## Bavanisha Vythilingum, FCPsych[a],*, Dan J. Stein, MD, PhD[a,b,c]

[a]MRC Research Unit on Anxiety and Stress Disorders, Department of Psychiatry, University of Stellenbosch, PO Box 19063, Tygerberg 7505, South Africa
[b]University of Cape Town, Cape Town, South Africa
[c]Department of Psychiatry, University of Florida, Gainesville, FL, USA

Obsessive-compulsive disorder (OCD) is a disorder characterized by obsessions, which are repeated intrusive thoughts, and compulsions, which are repetitive acts performed to neutralize the obsessions. There are data that patients with OCD often present to dermatologists. Fortunately, there have been substantial advances in understanding and treating OCD in recent years. This article addresses some of these developments.

The term "obsessive-compulsive spectrum disorder" has been used to describe a number of disorders with similar phenomenology (eg, unwanted repetitive behaviors) and psychobiology (eg, selective response to serotonin reuptake inhibitors). Patients with a number of these disorders (eg, trichotillomania [TTM], body dysmorphic disorder [BDD], pathologic skin picking, and onychophagia) also frequently present to dermatologists. Important advances have been made in the understanding and treatment of these disorders.

It is important for the dermatologist to be able recognize these disorders and to refer appropriately. It is also important to realize that most patients are extremely ashamed and embarrassed about their symptoms, and may hide or minimize their behavior to not seem "crazy." Patients should be approached tactfully and supportively. This article also discusses the evaluation and treatment of OCD and obsessive-compulsive spectrum disorder.

### Case 1: Obsessive-compulsive disorder

The patient is a 30-year-old man who presented to a dermatologist complaining of a rash on his hands. Examination revealed dermatitis. Further history indicated that since adolescence the patient had the repetitive thought that he would be contaminated if he were not careful, and that he spent at least an hour repetitively washing and scrubbing his hands. At times, these concerns would diminish, or be replaced by other symptoms, such as compulsively checking doors and switches. In the previous few months his washing behaviors had reappeared and worsened, resulting in his hand lesions.

OCD is characterized by the presence of obsessions, or compulsions [1]. Obsessions are defined as recurrent thoughts or images that are experienced as intrusive or senseless. Compulsions are repetitive and intentional behaviors performed to diminish present discomfort or future harm, and are also experienced as unreasonable or excessive. Both obsessions and compulsions are often resisted by the patient. The disorder affects up to 1% to 2% of the general population [2,3] and is associated with significant morbidity [4].

The prevalence in dermatology clinics has been reported to be high. For example, in a recent study of dermatology outpatients Fineberg and coworkers [5] screened 92 consecutive referrals. A total of 18 patients (20%) had OCD, of which 17 were undiagnosed. Most patients had moderate severity of OCD symptoms.

Contamination obsessions and cleaning compulsions are common, occurring in up to 16% of patients with OCD. These often take the form of repetitive

---

Drs. Vythilingum and Stein are supported by grants from the Medical Research Council of South Africa.
* Corresponding author.
E-mail address: bv@sun.ac.za (B. Vythilingum).

hand washing, bathing, or showering. This often results in excoriation and hence dermatologic presentation. The previous case report is typical of such patients with OCD, who often have onset of the disorder in childhood or adolescence [6].

Obsessions and compulsions in OCD should be differentiated from delusions in the psychotic disorders and from obsessive-compulsive personality traits in obsessive-compulsive personality disorder, symptoms that may also be seen by dermatologists. A delusion is a false personal belief based on incorrect inference about external reality and firmly sustained despite what almost everyone else believes and despite what constitutes incontrovertible and obvious proof or evidence to the contrary [1]. Dermatologists are familiar, for example, with delusions of parasitosis [7], which are seen in both functional and organic psychiatric disorders.

Obsessive-compulsive personality disorder is characterized by a pervasive pattern of perfectionism and inflexibility that causes significant impairment in social or occupational functioning, or subjective distress [1]. Patients may be excessively devoted to work and productivity, may have trouble expressing warm or tender affect or being generous, and may suffer from indecision. These symptoms have been thought common in patients with dermatologic illness [8].

Some authors have also suggested that symptoms in OCD have animal analogs [9,10]. In certain species, for example, repetitive licking and scratching of the extremities leads to localized alopecia and granulomatous lesions, or acral lick dermatitis. It is notable that canine acral lick dermatitis responds to clomipramine and the selective serotonin reuptake inhibitors (SSRIs) [11,12]. Rodent models also provide interesting insights into the neurobiology of OCD. Self-grooming in rats may be viewed as an analog to hand washing.

Patients who present to the dermatologist with chronic dermatitis from compulsive hand washing should ideally be treated in consultation with a psychiatrist. Some patients may resist referral, however, because of poor insight, embarrassment, or the stigma associated with mental illness. The dermatologist can play a key role in educating the patient about OCD and motivating them to start treatment. Patients with OCD are often extremely embarrassed about their behavior. Despite knowing that their behavior is unreasonable, they may be unable to control compulsions. Telling patients that "it's all in their head" or "they must just stop" is counterproductive. Patients should rather be approached in as supportive and sympathetic a manner as possible. In patients who resist psychiatric referral, a helpful approach is to acknowledge their concerns, but also to acknowledge the distress they are experiencing and to suggest that a psychiatrist may help them in finding ways to cope with this distress.

In patients who refuse psychiatric consultation, the dermatologist may be required to begin treatment of the OCD. Enquiry about comorbid conditions, in particular other obsessive-compulsive spectrum disorders, other anxiety disorders, depression, and substance use, should be made. The Yale Brown Obsessive Compulsive Scale is a measure of severity and is useful in monitoring treatment response.

Both pharmacotherapy and cognitive behavioral therapy are effective. The first-line drugs of choice in OCD are the SSRIs. It should be noted that relatively long treatment periods (up to 10–12 weeks) and high doses (eg, 40–60 mg fluoxetine) may be required before a response is seen. Current recommendations are to continue medication in responders for at least a year. If treatment is initiated by the dermatologist, it is advisable to start on a low dose of medication (eg, 20 mg fluoxetine) and gradually increase until a response is seen (eg, increase fluoxetine by 20 mg every 2–4 weeks). The aim is that with medication and continuing psychoeducation, the patient develops enough insight to agree to a psychiatric consultation.

Cognitive behavior therapy aims to modify the underlying irrational cognitions and modify unwanted behavior. Exposure and response prevention is the most commonly used technique. Here, the patient is exposed to the feared stimulus (eg, dirt) and then prevented from carrying out the compulsion (eg, hand washing) until the patient's anxiety decreases. Relaxation techniques are used together with this to aid the patient in managing anxiety.

Referral to an OCD support group can help the patient in coming to terms with their disorder and decrease their sense of shame and isolation. The OCD Foundation [13] is an excellent resource with links to many local support groups.

### Case 2: Trichotillomania

The patient is a 28-year-old woman who has had the symptom of hair-pulling of scalp and eyebrow hairs since adolescence. She presented to a dermatologist asking for help with her extensive alopecia. The patient stated that she now has to wear a wig. Apart from her family, nobody knew about her hair-pulling, because she was embarrassed by her behavior and was secretive about it. As a result she had few friends, and avoided intimate relationships. Her pulling tended to worsen during times of stress. She admitted to some depressed mood, stemming from the feeling that her hair-pulling would never improve, but had no other psychiatric problems.

TTM is characterized by the recurrent impulse to pull out one's hair [14]. Patients may pull out clumps of hair from their head, or may pull out individual hairs from their eyebrows, eyelashes, abdomen, or pubic hair. The extracted hair may be chewed or swallowed. Patients may also pull out hair from others, pets, or (in children) toys [15,16].

The disorder is currently classified as an impulse control disorder [1], and usually there are no associated obsessions, nor are the behaviors intended to ward off future harm. Nevertheless, the resistance to the behavior, and the relief associated with its completion are reminiscent of OCD. TTM differs from OCD in that it is seen predominantly in females (~10:1) [17]; however, this may be because women are more likely to present for treatment. TTM also differs from OCD in that some patients may report being in a "trancelike" or dissociated state while pulling, often unaware that they are pulling until after the episode [12], which is very unlike the focused compulsions of OCD. Furthermore imaging studies show differences in morphology between patients with TTM and OCD [18].

Consequences of TTM include avoidance of social situations and intimate relationships, alopecia, and less commonly medical complications, such as carpal tunnel syndrome (from repetitive pulling or manipulation of hair) and intestinal obstruction (after hair swallowing) [17].

With the recent awareness of TTM as a mental health disorder, many patients acknowledge their pulling. In patients who deny pulling, however, covering of the scalp with a bandage to observe regrowth may be helpful [17], and scalp biopsy shows characteristic findings: catagen hairs, pigment casts, traumatized hair bulbs, and trichomalacia.

Recent work has put forward two animal models for TTM. Greer and Capecchi [19] have shown that mice with disruption of the Hoxb8 gene show excessive grooming leading to hair removal and also excessively groom cagemates. Interestingly, Hoxb8 is expressed in the striatum and orbitofrontal cortex areas known as "the OCD circuit." In another study of mice Garner and coworkers [20] identified a subpopulation that engaged in abnormal fur and whisker trimming. These "barber" mice resembled patients with TTM in that they plucked focused areas of hair and engaged in postplucking manipulatory and oral behaviors.

Serotonin and dopamine have been postulated to be involved in the neurobiology of TTM. Swedo and coworkers [21] demonstrated in a double-blind crossover study that TTM responds preferentially to clomipramine compared with desipramine (a norepinephrine reuptake blocker). Trials of the SSRIs, however, have shown mixed results. Dopamine blockers have been shown to have a role in the augmentation of SSRIs, and opioid and hormonal systems have also been implicated [22].

The evaluation of TTM involves determining the extent and consequences of pulling (both physical and emotional). The Massachusetts General Hospital Hair Pulling Scale is the usual measure to quantify this and aids in evaluating treatment efficacy. Psychoeducation plays an important role in the management of the disorder. Many patients experience considerable shame over their behavior, and knowing that that they have a recognized disorder often provides a measure of relief. Online resources, such as the Trichotillomania Learning Center [23], are useful for providing information and connecting the patient with support groups.

The evaluation of TTM should also include a search for comorbid conditions. OCD and other obsessive-compulsive spectrum disorders often coexist, and depression and substance use are particularly important to rule out.

The treatment of TTM involves both pharmacotherapeutic and psychotherapeutic approaches. Cognitive behavior therapy, in particular the technique of habit reversal, has proved effective [24] and remains the first-line treatment, particularly in children and patients without comorbid psychopathology. The place of pharmacotherapy in the treatment of TTM is less clear. Clomipramine has been shown to be effective, but trials of SSRIs show conflicting results and response is not always maintained. In patients with comorbid psychopathology or severe TTM, however, a trial of medication is warranted in conjunction with cognitive behavioral therapy.

### Case 3: Compulsive skin picking

This patient is a 24-year-old woman with an 18-month history of compulsive picking. The picking began after she started a new job, which she found very stressful. She reported that her picking had continued since then, but became worse when she was more stressed at work. The patient had multiple excoriations on her face, chest, back, arms, and legs. Tension rose as she tried to resist picking, and removal of scabs led to a feeling of relief. She presented to a dermatologist, requesting a topical cream to help prevent the picking.

Compulsive skin picking is a self-injurious behavior produced by ritualistic picking, usually of skin lesions, but also of normal skin, that may cause severe tissue damage [25]. It has been described under various names including dermatotillomania, neurotic excoriation, and acne excoriée. There is no formal *Diagnostic and Statistical Manual-IV* diagnostic category for compulsive skin picking. It is perhaps best classified as a stereotypic movement disorder not otherwise specified. he incidence in dermatology clinics has been estimated to be about 2% [25].

Other kinds of lesions that may be related to pathologic skin picking include onychodystrophy with paronychia hypertrophy secondary to rubbing the nail folds, circumscribed areas of lichen simplex chronicus, and prurigo nodularis [1]. The disorder has been noted to be exacerbated by stress.

Neurobiologically, stereotyped behaviors are thought to be mediated by dopamine (among other neurotransmitters) and it is postulated that stress causes release of β-endorphin and cortisol in the brain, stimulating dopamine release in the striatum and activating basal ganglia motor programs [26]. This fits in findings that fur-biting chinchilla's (a putative animal model for skin picking) show Cushingoid changes [27].

The phenomenology of pathologic skin picking is once again reminiscent of stereotypic movement disorder more than OCD. Picking is repetitive and ritualistic, and leads to tension reduction, as do compulsions. Patients do not invariably report that the behavior is designed to prevent or neutralize future harm, but they do often admit that the urge to scratch themselves is senseless and intrusive, in the same way that obsessive-compulsive symptoms are often ego-dystonic.

Compulsive picking, unlike OCD, may have an early or late onset, and is more common in females [1]. Comorbidity with other psychiatric disorders is high, notably with OCD, mood disorders, substance use disorders, TTM, BDD, and eating disorders [28]. In a comparison of patients with TTM, patients with skin picking were found to be similar with regard to demographics, high comorbidity of mood and anxiety disorders, and personality dimensions [29], suggesting an overlap between these disorders.

It is important to differentiate compulsive skin picking from other self-injurious behaviors, particularly those associated with borderline personality disorder. Here, self-injury is usually associated with suicidal ideation, dissociation, impulsivity, and aggression [30], in contrast to skin picking, which is often a compulsive act and usually relieves tension.

There is growing evidence on the treatment of compulsive skin picking. Open and controlled trials have documented efficacy of the SSRIs and clomipramine [29,31,32], and case studies have documented success with naltrexone and dopamine antagonists. No controlled trial of psychotherapeutic interventions exists, however, given the considerable overlap between skin picking and TTM [29]. Cognitive behavioral therapy seems to be a logical option, and case studies of habit reversal suggest that it is a promising treatment [23].

## Case 4: Body dysmorphic disorder

This patient is a 32-year-old woman who presented on multiple occasions to dermatologists and plastic surgeons complaining that prominent veins on her face made her unattractive. Reassurance that the defect was imagined did not help. The patient insisted on using cosmetics to cover the imagined defect, and carefully avoided mirrors.

BDD is characterized by preoccupation with some imagined defect in appearance in a normal-appearing person [33]. Any area of the body may be a focus of concern but concerns most often involve the nose, skin, and hair [34]. Patients with this disorder frequently present to dermatologists with rates of between 10% and 14% being found [35]. In fact, dermatologists may be the health care provider most often consulted by patients with BDD.

The disorder is currently classified as a somatoform disorder [6], implying that these preoccupations differ from obsessions in not being intrusive and senseless. By definition they also are not of delusional intensity. Nevertheless, the resistance to and the fixity of the preoccupation vary greatly, and may change in the individual patient over time, a phenomena seen also in OCD [36]. Patients with BDD often engage in compulsive behaviors, such as mirror checking and camouflage, and may seek repeated reassurance. Compulsive skin picking may also be a feature [34].

The authors have also noted that body dysmorphic patients may have other obsessions and compulsions, and that OCD patients may have concerns about body defects or disease. A number of validators, such as course, prevalence, age of onset, comorbid illnesses, level of impairment, age of onset, and sex ratio seem to be similar in BDD and OCD [37]. At times there may be a family history of OCD in patients with BDD [38].

BDD symptoms have been reported to be exacerbated with marijuana [38], and has been reported secondary to cyproheptadine [39] suggesting possible serotonergic involvement. Furthermore, clomipramine (a serotonergic agent) was shown to be more effective than desipramine (a noradrenergic agent) [33]. Imaging studies have shown anomalies in the caudate nucleus [40] and parietal areas [41], which is consistent with the theory that patients have altered processing of their body perception.

Patients with BDD respond to SSRIs, which should be used as the first-line of treatment. As with OCD, BDD requires high doses and long duration of treatment and treatment should be maintained for at least 1 year [34]. Antipsychotics may be needed as augmentation in the delusional patient.

Cognitive behavior therapy is also an effective modality. It can be used alone in mild cases, but with more severe BDD should be used in combination with medication [34].

Getting the patient to accept psychiatric treatment may be difficult. As in TTM, many patients, experience shame over their behavior and insist that theirs is a purely physical problem. Here, the dermatologist can play a crucial role in educating the patient, and informing them about the potential benefit of psychiatric treatment in improving their mood and functioning. In those who are reluctant to consult a psychiatrist, starting an SSRI may improve symptoms and insight enough for the patient to consent to psychiatric treatment.

## Summary

OCD, TTM, pathologic skin picking, and BDD may share aspects of phenomenologic presentation, neurobiologic underpinning, or pharmacotherapeutic response. Recent epidemiologic studies have demonstrated that OCD, which was once thought a rare disorder, is in fact a relatively common psychiatric disorder [42].

Although the prevalence of many of the OCD-related disorders has not yet been established, it seems clear that many of these disorders are frequently seen by dermatologists. One reason for this frequent presentation may be that that these disorders represent grooming action repertoires that have been aberrantly triggered. Graybiel [43,44] posits that basal ganglia recodes cortically derived information into action "chunks" to facilitate storage and easy retrieval, with different striatal circuits coding for different "chunks." Disturbances in these circuits lead to emergence of unwanted behaviors, and also help explain the symptom overlap between the various disorders.

These theoretical considerations also seem to have important practical applications. The notion of an OCD-related spectrum reminds physicians to enquire about important comorbid symptoms in the patient and family, avoids unnecessary procedures, and suggests particular avenues of treatment including antiobsessional medication. It is important for the dermatologist to be aware of these conditions; to look for them in patients; and once diagnosed to provide support, education, and appropriate referral.

## References

[1] American Psychiatric Association. Diagnostic and statistical manual of mental disorders-revised. 4th edition. Washington: American Psychiatric Association; 2000.

[2] Stein MB, Forde DR, Anderson G, et al. Obsessive-compulsive disorder in the community: an epidemiologic survey with clinical reappraisal. Am J Psychiatry 1997;154:1120–6.

[3] Bebbington PE. Epidemiology of obsessive-compulsive disorder. Br J Psychiatry Suppl 1998;35:2–6.

[4] Murray CJ, Lopez AD. Alternative projections of mortality and disability by cause 1990–2020: Global Burden of Disease Study. Lancet 1997;349:1498–504.

[5] Fineberg NA, O'Doherty C, Rajagopal S, et al. How common is obsessive-compulsive disorder in a dermatology outpatient clinic? J Clin Psychiatry 2003;64: 152–5.

[6] Stein DJ. Obsessive-compulsive disorder. Lancet 2002;360:397–405.

[7] Berrios GE. Delusional parasitosis and physical disease. Compr Psychiatry 1985;26:395–403.

[8] Hall Smith SP, Norton A. Psychiatric survey of a random sample of skin outpatients. BMJ 1952;2(4781): 417–21.

[9] Holland HC. Displacement activity as a form of abnormal behavior in animals. In: Beech HR, editor. Obsessional states. London: Methuen; 1974.

[10] Stein DJ, Shoulberg N, Helton K, et al. The neuroethological approach to obsessive-compulsive disorder. Compr Psych 1992;33(4):274–81.

[11] Stein DJ, Mendelsohn I, Potocnik F, et al. Use of the selective serotonin reuptake inhibitor citalopram in a possible animal analogue of obsessive-compulsive disorder. Depress Anxiety 1998;8:39–42.

[12] Rapoport JL, Ryland DH, Kriete M. Drug treatment of canine acral lick: an animal model of obsessive-compulsive disorder. Arch Gen Psychiatry 1992;49: 517–21.

[13] The Obsessive-Compulsive Disorder Foundation. Available at: http://www.ocfoundation.org.

[14] Krishnan KR, Davidson JR, Guajardo C. Trichotillomania: a review. Compr Psychiatry 1985;26:123–8.

[15] Buxbaum E. Hair pulling and fetishism. Psychoanal Study Child 1960;15:243–60.
[16] Galski T. Hair pulling (trichotillomania). Psychoanal Rev 1983;70:331–46.
[17] Stein DJ, Simeon D, Cohen LJ, et al. Trichotillomania and obsessive-compulsive disorder. J Clin Psychiatry 1995;56(Suppl 4):28–34.
[18] Stein DJ, Coetzer R, Lee M, et al. Magnetic resonance brain imaging in women with obsessive-compulsive disorder and trichotillomania. Psychiatry Res 1997;74:177–82.
[19] Greer JM, Capecchi MR. Hoxb8 is required for normal grooming behavior in mice. Neuron 2002;33:23–34.
[20] Garner JP, Weisker SM, Dufour B, et al. Barbering (fur and whisker trimming) by laboratory mice as a model of human trichotillomania and obsessive-compulsive spectrum disorders. Comp Med 2004;54:216–24.
[21] Swedo SE, Leonard HL, Rapoport JL. A double-blind comparison of clomipramine and desipramine in the treatment of trichotillomania (hair-pulling). N Engl J Med 1989;321:497–500.
[22] Keuthen NJ, O'Sullivan RL, Sprich-Buckminster S. Trichotillomania: current issues in conceptualization and treatment. Psychother Psychosom 1998;67:202–13.
[23] Trichotillomania Learning Center. Available at: http://www.trich.org.
[24] Deckersbach T, Wilhelm S, Keuthen NJ, et al. Cognitive-behavior therapy for self-injurious skin picking: a case series. Behav Modif 2002;26:361–77.
[25] Gupta MA, Gupta AK, Haberman HF. Neurotic excoriations: a review and some new perspectives. Compr Psychiatry 1986;27:381–6.
[26] Dodman NH, Shuster L, Court MH, et al. Investigation into the use of narcotic antagonists in the treatment of a stereotypic behavior pattern (crib-biting) in the horse. Am J Vet Res 1987;48:311–9.
[27] Tisljar M, Janic D, Grabarevic Z, et al. Stress-induced Cushing's syndrome in fur-chewing chinchillas. Acta Vet Hung 2002;50:133–42.
[28] Arnold LM, Auchenbach MB, McElroy SL. Psychogenic excoriation: clinical features, proposed diagnostic criteria, epidemiology and approaches to treatment. CNS Drugs 2001;15:351–9.
[29] Lochner C, Simeon D, Niehaus DJ, et al. Trichotillomania and skin-picking: a phenomenological comparison. Depress Anxiety 2002;15:83–6.
[30] Winchel RM, Stanley M. Self-injurious behavior: a review of the behavior and biology of self-mutilation. Am J Psychiatry 1991;148:306–17.
[31] Bloch MR, Elliott M, Thompson H, et al. Fluoxetine in pathologic skin-picking: open-label and double-blind results. Psychosomatics 2001;42:314–9.
[32] Simeon D, Stein DJ, Gross S, et al. A double-blind trial of fluoxetine in pathologic skin picking. J Clin Psychiatry 1997;58:341–7.
[33] Hollander E, Allen A, Kwon J, et al. Clomipramine vs desipramine crossover trial in body dysmorphic disorder: selective efficacy of a serotonin reuptake inhibitor in imagined ugliness. Arch Gen Psychiatry 1999;56:1033–9.
[34] Phillips KA. Body dysmorphic disorder: diagnostic controversies and treatment challenges. Bull Menninger Clin 2000;64:18–35.
[35] Phillips KA, Dufresne Jr RG, Wilkel CS, et al. Rate of body dysmorphic disorder in dermatology patients. J Am Acad Dermatol 2000;42:436–41.
[36] Insel TR, Akiskal HS. Obsessive compulsive disorder with psychotic features: a phenomenological analysis. Am J Psychiatry 1986;143:1527–33.
[37] Hollander E, Cohen L, Simeon D, et al. Fluvoxamine treatment of body dysmorphic disorder. J Clin Psychopharmacol 1994;14:75–7.
[38] Allen A, Hollander E. Body dysmorphic disorder. Psychiatr Clin North Am 2000;23(3):617–28.
[39] Craven JL, Rodin GM. Cyproheptadine dependence associated with atypical somatoform disorder. Can J Psychiatry 1987;32:143–5.
[40] Rauch SL, Phillips KA, Segal E, et al. A preliminary morphometric magnetic resonance imaging study of regional brain volumes in body dysmorphic disorder. Psychiatry Res 2003;122:13–9.
[41] Carey P, Seedat S, Warwick J, et al. SPECT imaging of body dysmorphic disorder. J Neuropsychiatry Clin Neurosci 2004;16:357–9.
[42] Karno M, Golding JM, Sorenson SB, et al. The epidemiology of obsessive-compulsive disorder in five US communities. Arch Gen Psychiatry 1988;45:1094–9.
[43] Graybiel AM. The basal ganglia and chunking of action repertoires. Neurobiol Learn Mem 1998;70:119–36.
[44] Graybiel AM. Network-level neuroplasticity in cortico-basal ganglia pathways. Parkinsonism Relat Disord 2004;10:293–6.

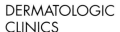

# Psychologic Factors in Psoriasis: Consequences, Mechanisms, and Interventions

Dónal G. Fortune, ClinPsyD, PhD[a],*, Helen L. Richards, ClinPsyD, PhD[b,c], Christopher E.M. Griffiths, MD[b]

[a]*Department of Behavioral Medicine, Clinical Sciences Building, Hope Hospital, Salford Royal Hospitals NHS Trust, Manchester, UK*
[b]*Dermatology Center, University of Manchester School of Medicine, Hope Hospital, Salford Royal Hospitals NHS Trust, Manchester, UK*
[c]*Academic Department of Clinical Psychology, Wythenshawe Hospital, University of Manchester, Manchester, UK*

A comprehensive review by Ginsburg [1] addressed psychologic and psychophysiologic aspects of psoriasis. Psoriasis does not have to be visible to other people for the patient to fear and anticipate their censure, and it does not need to be objectively severe to warrant significant disability and distress. A substantial proportion of patients with psoriasis live with the condition as a source of significant psychologic stress. In addition, the belief that such psychologic stress affects the course of the condition tends to have common currency in the experience of patients [2–7]. Although clinical researchers have addressed the first statement with perhaps a keener focus than the latter, researchers have made some increasingly comprehensive attempts to provide at least the beginnings of a focus of investigation into the effects of elements of stress or distress on the expression of psoriasis and on the nature of psychologically informed interventions to combat such negative outcomes. This article reviews the research evidence from 1995 to January 2005 about psychologic factors in psoriasis. The English-language research literature concerning psychologic aspects of psoriasis published since 1995 was identified through searches of Medline, Psychlit, and Cinahl and through hand searching relevant medical and psychologic journals. To be included in this review, articles had to be empirical investigations addressing psychosocial issues in patients with psoriasis. Articles were not included if they were reviews or case studies or if the object of the study was the development of a measure without additional data. This process yielded 121 empirical articles in three broad areas. These three areas are reviewed, followed by an examination of the impact of the condition on patients' psychologic functioning and quality of life. Next this article addresses the link between stress and psoriasis and examines proposed mechanisms. Studies of psychologic interventions for psoriasis are reviewed. Finally, future directions for research that have potential for informing clinical practice are examined.

## Consequences

Generally accepted estimates of the prevalence of psoriasis are 2% to 3% of the population [8]. Research has shown that psoriasis has the potential for significant psychologic and social morbidity [1,9–12]; although estimates vary, generally about one in four patients experiences significant psychologic distress [11]. Dermatologists' ability to identify clinically relevant distress in their patients has been shown to be unsatisfactory [10]. Richards and colleagues [13] reported that only 39% of patients

* Corresponding author.
  *E-mail address:* donal.fortune@manchester.ac.uk (D.G. Fortune).

who had psoriasis with clinically relevant distress were identified correctly by dermatologists. When physicians did identify patients as clinically distressed (anxiety or depression), further action to address such difficulties through referral to appropriate specialists was taken in only one third of cases [13], despite the potential effects of distress on adherence to treatment [14,15] and the effectiveness of treatment [16]. This study is commensurate with the suggestion [17] that for many skin conditions dermatologists may not have an accurate perception of the extent of psychiatric morbidity.

A range of deleterious phenomena has been reported in research studies charting the psychology of the psoriasis patient. In the main, researchers have tended to investigate the impact of this condition in terms of diminution in quality of life and magnification of disability. Such psychologic and social sequelae are complex phenomena, however, and studies reviewed here suggest that the psychologic impact may not be simply reducible to the severity, extent, or duration of disease.

## Psychologic impact on patients

### Disability and quality of life

The consequences of psoriasis on patients' quality of life have been well documented, and there is general consensus among research studies that objective clinical severity is insufficient as an assessment of the burden of disease [8,18–29]. One study suggests that simply being diagnosed with the condition can carry significant emotional consequences for patients [30], whereas another found psoriasis patients to have better health status than a comparison group of patients with atopic dermatitis [31]. Generally the impact of psoriasis appears comparable with other major diseases, however, and patients with psoriasis have been shown to experience decrements in their quality of life comparable to that found in patients with chronic diseases such as cancer and heart disease [32], to score significantly lower on quality of life measures and disability than healthy controls [33–36], and to be willing to incur significant costs for a cure [9,37,38].

Most studies undertaken in relation to disability have considered hospital-based rather than community-based patients with psoriasis. Community-based studies have shown, however, a high extent of disability in patients [39]. In one of relatively few community-based studies [40], the level of disability in the community sample was only slightly lower than that in hospital-based studies. This finding suggests that the use of hospital-based samples may not overinflate the level of disability experienced by individuals with psoriasis.

### Predictors of disability and quality of life.
Clinical variables have been shown to have a direct impact on disability. de Jong and colleagues [41] reported that nail involvement contributed to restrictions in daily activities in almost two thirds of individuals. Patients with palmoplantar pustulosis reported significantly greater disability and physical discomfort, but not more psychologic distress, than patients without palmoplantar involvement [42]. Patients with an additional diagnosis of arthritis show greater impairment in quality of life than patients without arthritis [43], although the relationship between clinical severity of psoriasis and health status tends to be greater for younger patients [44]. Older patients [29,45] and patients in a stable relationship [29,46] tend to report less impairment in quality of life. The effects of gender are less clear, with some studies reporting that women experience greater impairment than men [47,48], and other studies reporting no significant differences [25,46].

Studies have suggested that disability or quality of life improves as a result of treatment for psoriasis [48–51]. Although statistically significant, the improvements tend to be modest and, in general, physical clearance of psoriasis by more than 50% needs to occur before meaningful change in quality of life is reported [52]. The results of these studies suggest no clear relationship between quality of life and clinical features of the disease. One study indicated that after successful treatment of psoriasis by psoralen and ultraviolet A radiation photochemotherapy (PUVA), levels of psoriasis-specific disability and life stress improved, but more general levels of distress (anxiety and depression) did not change significantly from baseline [53]. Gupta and colleagues [54] suggested that almost one fifth of patients' disability scores remain stable or worsen despite improvement or clearance of psoriasis.

Two studies [34,55] found that perception of stigmatization was the principal predictor of disability in patients with psoriasis. Similar results of the effects of patients' responses to stigma were reported by Hill and Kennedy [56], who found that anticipatory and avoidance coping behaviors used by patients to deal with the stigma of psoriasis and venting emotions were associated significantly with disability. This study is concordant with the finding of Fortune and colleagues [20,57] that disability is best accounted for by anticipatory and avoidant coping behavior and experiences of rejection. These results illustrate that what patients do and think as they attempt to make sense of their condition [36,58,59] is important in disability or quality of life. Many illness beliefs have been illustrated to be important in accounting for disability in psoriasis. Beliefs that psoriasis has greater consequences, stronger beliefs that the condition could be controlled, and coping through marshaling support from others have been shown to be important contributors to the variance in patients' functioning [60]. At 1 year of follow-up, passive coping and beliefs about symptoms accounted for small but significant proportions of the variance in physical functioning [61]. Patients who have more severe psoriasis report more disability, but do not differ from patients with relatively mild psoriasis in their use of particular strategies to cope with their condition [62]. It seems that patients with more severe disease may not recognize the gap between the demands of their condition and the utility of particular coping strategies in mediating subjective disability. The protective effects on quality of life of particular coping strategies, such as disclosing disease status to others, is unclear [63], and the effect of coping strategies on disability in cross-sectional studies tends to be modest. Beliefs about the condition and the reactions of others seem to be the most important factors accounting for self-reported disability in psoriasis.

*Depression*

Studies investigating the prevalence of depression in patients with psoriasis have reported a range from 10% [55] to 58% [64]. Differences in estimates are likely to be due to differences in the choice of samples (outpatients versus inpatients) and in the methods and measures used to assess depression. Patients with psoriasis have been reported to be more depressed than controls on the Beck Depression Inventory [64,65] and to have generally higher rates of depression or psychopathology than patients with lichen planus [64], leprosy [66], and vitiligo [67,68], but rates of psychopathology tend to be significantly lower than in Behçet's disease [69]. Studies [70,71] suggest that inpatients with psoriasis express more suicidal ideation than outpatients with rates in psoriasis higher than that seen in patients with acne, alopecia areata, atopic dermatitis, or general medical conditions [70].

*Predictors of depression.* There is general agreement that the clinical severity of psoriasis is not the principal predictor of depression in psoriasis. Although many studies have shown a correlation between depression and psoriasis severity [61,65,70] or visibility of plaques [72], one study suggested this may be more prevalent in women than in men [12]. The magnitude of the association with severity tends to be modest, however. Other studies have reported the absence of an association that suggests that any effect of disease severity on depression is mediated by other factors [53,55,73].

Symptoms of psoriasis, especially pruritus, are related to depression in patients with psoriasis [74], with the implication that the depressed state decreases the threshold for itch perception via an increase in central nervous system opiate levels. Similarly, there is evidence [75] that patients who report high levels of stress experience pruritus more frequently than patients with lower stress levels. The effects of other symptoms are less clear. In a survey of 225 hospital outpatients with psoriasis, Fortune and colleagues [73] reported that depression was best predicted by gender, reporting more symptoms, a stronger belief in the severity of the consequences of psoriasis, and less use of coping strategies that help the patient to reappraise the impact of the condition on his or her life. Regardless of the clinical severity of patients' psoriasis, depression also has been associated with feelings of stigma that arise from deprivation of social touch [76]. Attempts to cope through venting emotions and the use of alcohol and nonprescription drugs also have been associated with depression in psoriasis outpatients [56]. Although the noneffectiveness of treatment has been shown to be associated with higher levels of distress [77], Schmid-Ott and colleagues [78] showed that patients whose psoriasis was rated as worse after 1 year were significantly more likely to engage in coping strategies such as the use of religion and rumination. Although rumination may be considered unhelpful, the palliative effects of coping through the use of religion/spirituality require further investigation.

*Anxiety*

Studies of anxiety in psoriasis also have tended to employ different methods of assessment and to report on different aspects of the experience. The proportion of patients meeting criteria for an anxiety disorder is notably higher than that for depression in patients with psoriasis. Richards and colleagues [55] found 43% of attendees at a tertiary clinic for psoriasis were cases for anxiety as defined by the Hospital Anxiety and Depression Scale. This level of caseness was much higher than figures of 20% reported in other major chronic medical conditions such as cancer [79]. Some studies have not found that patients with psoriasis have elevated levels of anxiety. Devrimci-Ozguven and colleagues [65] reported no significant differences between patients with psoriasis and controls on levels of anxiety as assessed by the Speilberg State-Trait Anxiety Scale. The sample size was small ($n = 50$), and the authors emphasize that the concentration of low psoriasis severity scores may have influenced results. Fear of negative evaluation [80] gives a particular social component to the anxiety experienced by patients with psoriasis, and social anxiety/avoidance has been reported to be higher in patients with psoriasis than in patients with atopic or contact dermatitis, acne, and vitiligo [81].

*Predictors of anxiety.* Anatomic location of psoriasis has not been assessed adequately in terms of its relation to distress in patients. Some studies have suggested a relationship between anxiety and presence of psoriasis on the face and hands [82]. Williamson and colleagues [83] reported results from patients with nail involvement and found that greater nail involvement was associated with anxiety. Patients with more severe nail involvement by psoriasis also tended to have more severe arthritis and psoriatic arthropathy, however, which makes inferences about the specificity of the findings solely to anatomic location of psoriasis problematic.

Greater use of two coping strategies, avoidance of anxiety-provoking situations and emotion-focused coping, tend to be associated significantly with greater levels of anxiety [56,73]. It is suggested that reliance on the use of anticipation and avoidance as a coping strategy serves to maintain the patient's anxiety [7,84]. Similarly, excessive worrying—the cognitive component of anxiety—tends to be best predicted by social evaluative concerns and patients' beliefs about their state of mind being responsible for their psoriasis [2]. The belief in emotional causes of psoriasis tends to be associated with a wide array of measures of psychologic well-being [6].

Questionnaire studies in psoriasis suggest that one of the major ways that anxiety is experienced and maintained is in terms of vigilance by patients toward the potential for social evaluation coupled with subsequent avoidance of such social evaluative threat. Fortune and colleagues [85] conducted an experimental test of this hypothesis by presenting lists of disease-specific, social-evaluative, self-evaluative, and neutral words to patients and controls via computer. Patients with psoriasis responded significantly more slowly than controls to social evaluative, self-evaluative, and disease-related words. Results suggested that patients show an attentional bias toward stimuli relating to these areas of concern, and such material is processed differently by patients (involving initial hypervigilance and subsequent avoidance processes), slowing their ability to name particular types of words and maintaining their anxiety.

Anxiety is an important feature associated with psoriasis. Inevitably the cognitive processes that accompany anxiety, in particular, fears relating to interpersonal processes such as perceived stigma experiences and worrying, also seem to be important in terms of its impact and in terms of informing patients' understanding of the condition.

One research group has begun to examine the effects of excessive worrying in psoriasis [2,16,53,73, 86–89]. Some initial work has suggested that 40% of patients attending a tertiary referral clinic for psoriasis meet criteria for pathologic levels of worry [2]; 25% of patients have worry scores similar to scores found in patients with a diagnosis of generalized anxiety disorder [2]. Further work has illustrated this finding to be consistent [16,87]. Pathologic worry in patients with psoriasis seems to be associated with social evaluative concerns and beliefs about the cause of psoriasis being due to the patient's state of mind, rather than more disease-oriented variables [2,73]. A role for pathologic worrying in slowing the response of psoriasis to photochemotherapy has been reported [16].

*Interpersonal concerns and stigma*

Patients with psoriasis often report numerous interpersonal concerns related to their condition. In a survey of the National Psoriasis Foundation, Krueger and colleagues [4] reported that 27% of individuals cited difficulties with sexual activities, 81% were embarrassed if psoriasis was visible, and 88% expressed concerns about the disease worsening. Gupta and Gupta [90] reported that more than 40% of their sample of psoriasis patients were affected sexually by their condition. This group had slightly more psoriasis affecting the perineal region, greater joint pain, and higher levels of depression, but the severity of psoriasis was no different from the nonsexually affected group.

*Stigmatization*

The concept of stigma underpins many difficulties experienced by patients. Although the literature in relation to anxiety or stress has shown the importance of "felt" stigma—the perception and anticipation of the reaction of others to a person's psoriasis—patients also may have to contend with enacted stigma—that which arises from uninformed public attitudes to the condition and discriminatory behaviors by others toward the patient. There have been many more recent investigations in relation to stigma and psoriasis [25,34,55,76,80,91–93]. As previously outlined, perceptions of stigmatization have been shown to be significantly related to psychologic distress and disability in patients with psoriasis and to account for a significant proportion of the variance in disability over and above general psychologic distress. Vardy and colleagues [34] showed that experiences of stigmatization mediated the impact of severity of psoriasis on quality of life. Gupta and colleagues [76] reported that perception of stigmatization was the most significant factor in predicting depression in psoriasis. According to Schmid-Ott and colleagues [92], stigmatization in their sample of patients was predicted by age, sex, and age at onset. These variables together predicted only 7% of the variance, however, suggesting the importance of other unmeasured factors. Perceived helplessness has been shown in one study to be the most important factor predicting stigmatization in psoriasis and atopic dermatitis [94], whereas fear of negative evaluation has been shown to be associated with stigma. Stigmatized individuals have been shown to be more distressed about symptoms and reported greater interpersonal impact and lower quality of life than their nonstigmatized counterparts [80].

*Personality and psoriasis*

The suggestion that patients with psoriasis have an underlying personality style is contentious, and to date research has not addressed adequately the role of normal and abnormal personality features in adjustment to the condition and in terms of interacting with the disease process in psoriasis. Rubino and colleagues [95] assessed patients using the Millon Clinical Multiaxial Inventory and found that psoriasis patients reported higher scores and frequencies on all scales on the inventory than a comparison group of dental and surgical patients. Using a cluster analysis from the Delusions-Symptom-States Inventory, they reported that only 18.2% of patients had no personality disorder. This finding has been challenged [96] on the basis of inappropriate control groups and poor appreciation that the psychologic stress of living with a medical condition can bring about a short-term change in one's personality traits [97]. One study has suggested that onset of psoriasis before age 40—a time when personality is being established—may lead to poorer emotional regulation with concomitant effects on patients' ability to deal with stress [98].

One area of enduring self-characteristics, alexithymia, has been investigated more comprehensively in psoriasis. It is suggested that individuals with alexithymia have difficulties identifying feelings, difficulty describing individual feelings, impoverishment of fantasy life, and excessive preoccupation with physical symptoms and external events [73,99,100]. It is suggested that this poor emotional regulation may lead to undifferentiated affect and eventual physical pathology.

One study [99] found a nonsignificant trend for psoriasis patients with recent exacerbations to have higher scores on a standardized measure of alexithymia (Twenty-Item Toronto Alexithymia Scale) than patients with other skin conditions. Patients with psoriasis also were more likely to score above the cutoff for borderline alexithymia than controls. Using the more conservative cutoff score, studies in outpatient samples have suggested that between one quarter [99] and one third of psoriasis outpatients [73,100] and 42% of psoriasis patients in a trial of cognitive-behavioral psychotherapy [84] have scores indicating the presence of alexithymia. There is some debate as to whether the close concordance between alexithymia and anxiety sensitivity may imply that alexithymia may be more important in accounting for poor psychologic adjustment in patients with psoriasis than in the expression of disease [73]. In cross-sectional studies, alexithymia tends not to correlate with clinical severity, duration, or onset of disease [73,100], and the overlap or shared variance with anxiety and depression tends to be high [73].

Regardless of any effect of alexithymia on the disease process in psoriasis, one study has shown that alexithymia has negative effects on the ability of patients with psoriasis to construe benefits from living with the disease [101]. The idea that patients may experience psychologic growth as a result of dealing with ongoing adversity has important clinical implications for psoriasis. In this study, patients who were able to find meaning in the experience of living with a chronic skin disease tended to have fewer alexithymic characteristics, a younger age at onset of psoriasis, and a stronger belief about chronicity or recurrence of the condition than patients who did not achieve clinically significant psychologic growth. Such a lack of psychologic mindedness may bring about difficulties in the self-regulation of emotion and an inability to develop alternative viewpoints and perspectives on the condition and its impact.

*Impact on family members*

To date, only one peer-reviewed quantitative study has addressed the effects of psoriasis on family members. Richards and colleagues [89] examined the nature of beliefs held by patients and their spouses and reported that divergence in patient/spouse beliefs about the emotional impact of psoriasis and beliefs about how long the condition would last were the main predictors of depression in partners and worry in patients. Lack of consensus between the beliefs of patients and family members regarding the sequelae of psoriasis has important implications for mental health of patients and family members.

*Conclusions*

The literature reviewed indicates that psoriasis is a condition that provides patients and their families with frequent and disabling physical, psychologic, and social effects. There is compelling evidence that patients with psoriasis experience a range of psychosocial difficulties, such as elevated levels of disability, diminution in quality of life, anxiety, depression, worry, stigmatization, and avoidance of social activities. It also is clear that such effects are not simply reducible to the extent or severity of the condition. Difficulty in the self-regulation of emotion seems pertinent in a subgroup of patients with psoriasis; however, there is inconclusive evidence as to whether these characteristics occur as a result of living with psoriasis or whether they predispose the individual to the condition. Beliefs and to a lesser extent coping strategies seem important in adjustment to the condition. It seems plausible that the obvious psychologic distress encountered in living with a condition such as psoriasis may constitute a low-grade chronic stressor, which may have an impact on the skin condition itself. Mechanisms by which psychologic factors may affect psoriasis are addressed next.

## Mechanisms

Evidence for a potential role of psychologic factors in the etiology and pathogenesis of psoriasis is growing; however, the question of whether stress or psychologic distress directly contributes to exacerbation or maintenance of psoriasis is not particularly well established [99]. Despite the recognition by Ginsburg [1] in 1995 of the absence of well-controlled, longitudinal studies examining the relationship between stress and psoriasis, this deficiency has yet to be adequately addressed. Consequently the relationship between stress and the mechanisms involved in exacerbations of psoriasis is unclear. Numerous areas of investigation have gained increasing acceptance, however, in consideration of this relationship. In reviewing the literature in this area, first investigations of the relationship between stress and psoriasis are examined before considering potential mechanisms of action.

*Stress and psoriasis*

Some of the most persuasive indications of a link between stress and psoriasis come from patients themselves, with studies illustrating that 37% to 88% of patients [3,5–7,102,103] believe stress or psychologic distress is a factor in the manifestations of their condition. In recent years, the conceptualization of stress in the context of psoriasis has developed to embrace the assertion that stress not only concerns significant life events, which have been shown to be important [104], but also may entail chronic, recurrent, low-grade stresses or daily hassles that occur largely as a result of living with a chronic disfiguring disease [105]. In one of the largest surveys involving approximately 6000 patients in Norway, Zachariae and colleagues [7,43] examined reports of stress as associated with disease onset and activity from patients and members of numerous national psoriasis associations; 71% of members of psoriasis associations and 66% of patients examined recalled exacerbations of psoriasis at times of stress. Self-reported psoriasis "stress reactors" were more likely to be female and to have a family history of psoriasis, greater disease severity, higher levels of psoriasis-related stress, and greater impairment in psoriasis-related quality of life.

In a smaller uncontrolled study ($n = 38$), Harvima and colleagues [106] divided patients into high-stress and low-stress groups on the basis of responses to psychometric questionnaires. No differences were identified between the groups on the basis of Psoriasis Area and Severity Index (PASI) scores, although patients in the high-stress group were reported to have significantly more active psoriasis and joint symptoms. In addition, activity of psoriasis was significantly associated with depression, psychosomatic reactivity, and life events. Pacan and colleagues [107] found no relationship, however, between intensity of depression and the PASI score or between intensity of stress and severity of depression. One case-controlled study [108] investigated 73 patients with acute guttate psoriasis. Stressful life events in the 6 months before diagnosis were found to be significant risk factors for the onset of psoriasis. Although the study did not take into account more chronic psychologic stressors, it did attempt to control for the potential phenomenon that stress is purely related to the chronic course of psoriasis. Kupfer and colleagues [109] used a dispositional construct called "sense of coherence," which relates to an individual's positive appraisal that demands are challenges that are generally predictable and that can be met with appropriate psychologic resources. There were 72 patients assessed at three time points (before, immediately after, and 15–18 months after treatment), and results suggested that patients with low sense of coherence experienced their first relapse 3.5 months after therapy, whereas patients with high sense of coherence experienced their first relapse after 10 months.

Several attempts have been made to identify the timeline associated with the experience of psychologic distress and expression of psoriasis. One study illustrated that psoriasis patients compared with controls experienced more stress 3 months before onset [65]. Picardi and colleagues [99], in a comparison of psoriasis patients with a recent onset or exacerbation of psoriasis ($n = 40$) and patients experiencing other skin conditions in which psychosomatic factors usually are considered insignificant ($n = 116$), found no significant differences in terms of either the number of stressful life events or the nature of events experienced between the groups. Commensurate with the study by Naldi and colleagues [108], there was a nonsignificant trend for patients with guttate psoriasis to have experienced more stressful events than controls. Although suggestive, on the basis of only a few studies in the 1990s, it is difficult to draw conclusions about the timing of stressful events and disease exacerbations. Further research is warranted, examining daily stressors and life events to clarify this relationship.

One of a few prospective studies examining the influence of psychologic distress on disease manifestations and treatment efficacy has suggested that psychologic distress in the form of pathologic worry may be implicated in the response of psoriasis to standard pharmacologic care [16]. In this study, patients attending centers in the United Kingdom and Republic of Ireland underwent a standard photochemotherapy treatment protocol (PUVA). Results suggested that patients who were classified as high worriers were 1.8 times less likely to achieve clearance of psoriasis at the same time point as their low worry counterparts (median difference 19 days). This result held constant even when disease severity, skin type, sex, anxiety, depression, age of the patient, and duration with active disease were controlled. Such a finding provides compelling evidence of the deleterious impact of psychologic distress on the response of psoriasis to treatment and further highlights the importance of examining potential psychophysiologic mechanisms in psoriasis.

*Brain-skin axis*

Numerous studies have attempted to clarify pathways between psychologic factors and biologic events pertinent to the disease process in psoriasis. Among them, the action of the hypothalamic-pituitary-adrenal (HPA) axis, physiologic reactivity, endocrine factors, and immunologic changes have been examined.

The HPA axis is discussed frequently as one of the major pathways through which the central nervous system exerts control over the immune system under stressful conditions. There is increasing evidence to support the notion that an inappropriate reactivity of the HPA axis in its response to a stimulus may have an impact on an individual's defense against physical disease and severe and enduring psychologic states [101,110]. There have been some limited examinations of HPA axis function in patients with psoriasis. A pilot study by Schmid-Ott and colleagues [111] examined cardiovascular, endocrine, and immunologic responses after a public speaking and mental arithmetic task in psoriasis patients and healthy controls. The data suggested that psoriasis patients showed more marked increases in heart rate, blood pressure, and adrenaline, but lower plasma cortisol and dehydroepiandrosterone plasma concentrations compared with control subjects after the stress task. The group suggested that these findings may offer some evidence of a hypocortisolic response. In a further investigation of HPA axis function, Thaller and colleagues [112] compared psoriasis patients, patients with posttraumatic stress disorder, and normal controls. Psoriasis and posttraumatic stress disorder patients had lower 24-hour urinary cortisol levels compared with healthy controls, and psoriasis patients had significantly lower 8 AM plasma cortisol levels. This study adds weight to the assertion that in chronic stress-related diseases there may be altered HPA axis function, which is incompetent to realize its immunoregulatory function so that consequently clinical signs persist. The study was underpowered (19 psoriasis patients), there were no assessments of psychologic status undertaken, factors known to affect cortisol response (eg, menstrual status) were not controlled for, and responses to HPA axis stimulation were not measured. In a more recent study that attempted to control for such factors, Richards and colleagues [110] reported that patients with psoriasis who believed that their disease was stress responsive exhibited altered HPA responses to acute social stress. Psoriasis patients had significantly lower salivary cortisol levels after completion of an acute social performance stressor than patients who believed stress had no impact. In contrast, there was no difference between the groups for change in pulse rate after stressor.

Schmidt-Ott and colleagues [111] found that natural killer lymphocyte ($CD16^+$, $CD56^+$) numbers were significantly less in patients treated with PUVA ($n = 4$) compared with healthy control subjects ($n = 7$) and untreated psoriasis patients with stable chronic plaque psoriasis ($n = 7$) after an acute laboratory stressor. The untreated psoriasis patients showed natural killer cell responses similar to healthy controls. The same group built on this work [113] and compared patients with psoriasis ($n = 15$), atopic dermatitis ($n = 15$), and healthy controls ($n = 15$). Participants completed the same stressful task. Results suggested poststressor increases in the number of circulating T lymphocytes ($CD8^+/CD11b^+/CD16^-$) in psoriasis patients compared with healthy controls and increases in $CD16^+$ natural killer cells. These findings suggest that stress induces changes in the number of cytotoxic T lymphocytes, and this may be associated with exacerbation of psoriasis.

*Conclusions*

The literature implies that for some patients there is the possibility of a link between psychologic distress and various physical manifestations of psoriasis. The possible routes connecting psychologic factors with the appearance, worsening, or resistance of psoriatic lesions to treatment, although suggestive, remain uncertain. The question as to how stress modulates the physiologic homeostasis is complex and is likely to involve multifaceted interactions between many cardiovascular, endocrine, and immunologic parameters. Further well-designed, adequately powered, and hypothesis-driven research is required to investigate further potential psychophysiologic mechanisms in individuals with psoriasis.

## Interventions

In the absence of clear psychophysiologic data, one further source of evidence for the link between stress and psoriasis is the improvement in clinical parameters as a result of psychologic intervention. Although psychologic interventions in psoriasis are few, the most compelling tend to favor an approach to treatment that derives from cognitive and behavioral principles.

Cognitive behavioral therapy (CBT) specifically targets patterns of unhelpful thoughts and beliefs held by patients and the effects of such cognitions on mood and behavior. Zachariae and colleagues [114] reported results from 21 patients in a CBT group and 23 patients receiving standard care. CBT consisted of seven individual sessions over 12 weeks. Results showed slight but significant reductions in severity of a randomly chosen psoriatic reference lesion and a nonsignificant trend for a greater overall reduction in severity of psoriasis as assessed by dermatologists in the intervention group, but not in the control group. A more recent study [86] reported results from 91 patients that showed patients who opted for a group CBT intervention in addition to their standard treatment showed significantly greater reductions in anxiety and depression, in self-reported disability and stress, and in objective clinical severity of psoriasis compared with patients receiving standard care only. Only 23% of patients on standard treatment achieved greater than 75% clearance of psoriasis over the 6 weeks of the study, whereas 64% of patients in the CBT group achieved the same degree of clearance. One study [84] looked more specifically at the mechanisms underlying change as a result of psychologic intervention and showed that changes in patients' beliefs about symptoms, their beliefs about the severity of the consequences of psoriasis in everyday life, and strength of beliefs in emotional causes are the cognitions most likely to be altered by CBT intervention. Not all patients who might benefit from such adjunctive interventions participate, however, because elevated worry, anxiety, and feelings of stigmatization can impede patients from attending such programs [88]. Although statistically and clinically effective, CBT interventions are complex and expensive to deliver.

Kabat-Zinn and colleagues [115] examined a less involved treatment modality and investigated the utility of patients being guided in stress management via audiotape in a mindfulness-meditation–based stress reduction as they underwent treatment with phototherapy (PUVA or UVB). Patients who listened to the audiotape showed a median difference in the time taken to achieve clearance of psoriasis of 49.5 days compared with patients receiving standard PUVA without the relaxation tape. The effects were not significant for UVB-treated patients, and the subject numbers for the PUVA group were small ($n = 8$). Changes in psychologic measures did not reach statistical significance. The clear potential for being able to reduce the number of treatments required as a result of such an intervention would seem to hold important benefits for patients with psoriasis, but may have limited relevance to patients who are experiencing greater psychologic difficulties.

Education and stress management procedures also have been shown to be helpful in children and adolescents. Scheewe and colleagues [116] found that a 10-session program resulted in a significant improvement in self-estimated skin condition, self-estimated attractiveness, self-efficacy, and specific social impairment in the intervention group ($n = 34$) relative to the control group ($n = 21$). Anxiety was not affected significantly by participation, suggesting that more severe psychologic difficulties require a more comprehensive therapeutic intervention.

Support alone has been reported to be helpful for patients [117], but methodologic issues, such as lack of control groups or the use of single case design, mean that conclusions that reliably could inform clinical practice are uncertain. Other approaches that have shown early promise include music therapy, which has been shown to bring about a reduction in blood pressure and heart rate and a reduction in urge to scratch in psoriasis patients who received three sessions of 30-minute music intervention [118], and respondent techniques such as hypnosis. Tausk and Whitmore [119] performed a small ($n = 11$), randomized, double-blind controlled trial of hypnosis and reported significant improvement in individuals who were highly susceptible to hypnosis ($n = 5$).

The quality of these studies varies widely, and there is a lack of consensus on the use of outcome measures, which is unhelpful in deciding on whether variation in outcome between studies constitutes clinically meaningful differences or results simply from methodologic diversity. Psychologic interventions and methods require further refining and consensus to elucidate the active ingredients of particular therapeutic approaches.

## Future directions

### Brain-skin axis

A key area for future research in psoriasis is the interface between the brain and skin. There is presently insufficient evidence to state categorically that what happens in the skin is a reflection of an individual's psychologic state. The burgeoning evidence of a brain-skin axis is suggestive, however, and many research avenues seem promising, including investigations of factors contributing to hypocortisolism, patient self-monitoring of everyday stressors and the link with the onset, amplitude and timing of relapse, and experimental studies investigating the endocrine and immunologic aspects of induced and chronic low-grade stress or daily hassles.

### Refining clinical interventions

Therapeutic approaches specifically for patients with psoriasis must derive from a compelling empirical and theoretical base. These interventions need not be targeted solely at the individual patient; rather the knowledge that psoriasis has a crucial social component warrants a broader view to psychologic intervention. Antistigma interventions targeted at changing public attitudes toward disfiguring diseases require further investigation. Work with the families or partners of patients with psoriasis also is a critical area that is significantly underrepresented in the research literature and warrants further attention.

### Toward a positive psychology

There is probably a case for agreeing on a moratorium on unidimensional studies highlighting that living with psoriasis leads to decrements in quality of life because such studies do little now to advance knowledge in this area. It seems timely to move away from research that is simply descriptive toward research that recognizes and adequately appraises the complexity and multivariate features of this biopsychosocial condition. Although living with psoriasis can be a source of significant stress and distress [120,121], it also is important to recognize that psoriasis can leave the individual transformed in ways that may not be universally negative. Dealing with everyday adversity arising from psoriasis can bring about substantial growth experiences for patients [101]. An overreliance on research into deficits in functioning may mean that evidence of human thriving or adversarial growth in the context of suffering can be overlooked, and an opportunity for a truly collaborative clinical relationship can be missed. Future research would be well placed examining the patterns and predictors of adversarial growth in patients and their families.

## Summary

This article has examined the literature pertinent to psychologic aspects of psoriasis published since 1995. The studies reviewed have suggested that the consequences of this condition for patients and their families can be significant. Numerous factors seem to mediate the impact of the condition, chiefly beliefs about the consequences, causes, and emotional impact of the condition. Cognitive and behavioral strategies engaged in by patients also seem to have risk and protective properties depending on the outcome being studied and seem more helpful for anxiety, disability, and quality of life rather than depression. Alexithymia—a deficit in the self-regulation of emotion—also seems to function as a risk factor for the emergence and maintenance of distress, and excessive worry may have significant implications for resistance of disease to treatment. Although inconclusive, studies investigating HPA axis function suggest that hypocortisolism may be an important feature of stress-responsive psoriasis. Given the high levels of distress and the proposed interaction between psychologic factors and disease process, structured psychologic interventions that are integrated into standard care packages are likely to be of most benefit to patients with this complex disease. The next decade will reveal findings from studies currently being undertaken by research teams worldwide that will further understanding of the interplay between different, yet related facets of this condition. These facets include, but are not restricted to, the use of brain imaging in the context of acute stress in psoriasis, the role of early adversity as a risk factor in chronicity, family perspectives and stigma, in-depth examinations of the interplay between stress and the HPA system, interventions targeting specific psychologic processes and outcomes, and the use of longitudinal designs to address adequately the putative stress-psoriasis link. A truly collaborative research and clinical impetus that may facilitate meaningful changes for patients may be closer than is realized.

## References

[1] Ginsburg IH. Psychological and psychophysiological aspects of psoriasis. Dermatol Clin North Am 1995;13:793–804.

[2] Fortune DG, Richards HL, Main CJ, et al. Pathological worrying, illness perceptions, and disease severity in patients with psoriasis. Br J Heal Psychol 2000;5:71–82.

[3] Fortune DG, Richards HL, Main CJ, et al. What patients with psoriasis believe about their condition. J Am Acad Dermatol 1998;39:197–201.

[4] Krueger G, Koo J, Lebwohl M, et al. The impact of psoriasis on quality of life: results of a 1998 National Psoriasis Foundation patient membership survey. Arch Dermatol 2001;137:280–4.

[5] Nevitt GJ, Hutchinson PE. Psoriasis in the community: prevalence, severity and patients' beliefs and attitudes towards the disease. Br J Dermatol 1996; 135:533–7.

[6] O'Leary CJ, Creamer D, Higgins E, et al. Perceived stress attributions and psychological stress in psoriasis. J Psychosom Res 2004;57:465–71.

[7] Zachariae R, Zachariae H, Blomqvist K, et al. Self-reported stress reactivity and psoriasis-related stress of Nordic psoriasis sufferers. J Eur Acad Dermatol Venereol 2004;18:27–36.

[8] Kirby B, Richards HL, Woo P, et al. Physical and psychologic measures are necessary to assess overall psoriasis severity. J Am Acad Dermatol 2001;45: 72–6.

[9] Finlay AY, Coles EC. The effect of severe psoriasis on the quality of life of 369 patients. Br J Dermatol 1995;132:236–44.

[10] Picardi A, Amerio P, Baliva G, et al. Recognition of depressive and anxiety disorders in dermatological outpatients. Acta Derm Venereol 2004;84:213–7.

[11] Picardi A, Abeni D, Melchi CF, et al. Psychiatric morbidity in dermatological outpatients: an issue to be recognised. Br J Dermatol 2000;143:983–91.

[12] Picardi A, Abeni D, Renzi C, et al. Increased psychiatric morbidity in female outpatients with skin lesions on visible parts of the body. Acta Derm Venereol 2001;81:410–4.

[13] Richards HL, Fortune DG, Weidman A, et al. Detection of psychological distress in patients with psoriasis—low consensus between doctor and patient. Br J Dermatol 2004;151:1227–33.

[14] Renzi C, Picardi A, Abeni D, et al. Association of dissatisfaction with care and psychiatric morbidity with poor treatment compliance. Arch Dermatol 2002;138:337–42.

[15] Richards HL, Fortune DG, O'Sullivan TM, et al. Patients with psoriasis and their compliance with medication. J Am Acad Dermatol 1999;41:581–3.

[16] Fortune DG, Richards HL, Kirby B, et al. Psychological distress impairs clearance of psoriasis in patients treated with photochemotherapy (PUVA). Arch Dermatol 2003;139:752–6.

[17] Sampogna F, Picardi A, Melchi CF, et al. The impact of skin diseases on patients: comparing dermatologists' opinions with research data collected on their patients. Br J Dermatol 2003;148:989–95.

[18] Feldman SR, Fleischer AB, Reboussin DM, et al. The self-administered psoriasis area and severity index is valid and reliable. J Invest Dermatol 1996;106: 183–6.

[19] Fleischer AB, Feldman SR, Rapp SR, et al. Disease severity measures in a population of psoriasis patients: the symptoms of psoriasis correlate with self administered Psoriasis Area and Severity Index Scores. J Invest Dermatol 1996;107:26–9.

[20] Fortune DG, Main CJ, O'Sullivan TM, et al. Quality of life in psoriasis: the contribution of clinical variables and psoriasis-specific stress. Br J Dermatol 1997;137:755–60.

[21] Jenner N, Campbell J, Plunkett A, et al. Cost of psoriasis: a study on the morbidity and financial effects of having psoriasis in Australia. Austral J Dermatol 2002;43:255–61.

[22] Kirby B, Fortune DG, Bhushan M, et al. The Salford Psoriasis Index: an holistic measure of psoriasis severity. Br J Dermatol 2000;142:728–32.

[23] Main CJ, Richards HL, Fortune DG. Why put new wine in old bottles: the need for a biopsychosocial approach to the assessment, treatment, and understanding of unexplained and explained symptoms in medicine. J Psychosom Res 2000;48:511–4.

[24] Nichol MB, Margolies JE, Lippa E, et al. The application of multiple quality-of-life instruments in individuals with mild-to-moderate psoriasis. Pharmacoeconom 1996;10:644–53.

[25] Perrott SB, Murray AH, Lowe J, et al. The psychosocial impact of psoriasis: physical severity, quality of life, and stigmatization. Physiol Behav 2000;70:567–71.

[26] Sampogna F, Picardi A, Chren MM, et al. Association between poorer quality of life and psychiatric morbidity in patients with different dermatological conditions. Psychosom Med 2004;66:620–4.

[27] Sampogna F, Sera F, Abeni D. IDI Multipurpose Psoriasis Research on Vital Experiences (IMPROVE) investigators: measures of clinical severity, quality of life, and psychological distress in patients with psoriasis: a cluster analysis. J Invest Dermatol 2004;122:602–7.

[28] Wahl A, Moum T, Hanestad BR, et al. The relationship between demographic and clinical variables, and quality of life aspects in patients with psoriasis. Qual Life Res 1999;8:319–26.

[29] Zachariae R, Zachariae H, Blomqvist K, et al. Quality of life in 6497 Nordic patients with psoriasis. Br J Dermatol 2002;146:1006–16.

[30] Fried RG, Friedman S, Paradis C, et al. Trivial or terrible? The psychosocial impact of psoriasis. Int J Dermatol 1995;34:101–5.

[31] Kiebert G, Sorensen SV, Revicki D, et al. Atopic dermatitis is associated with a decrement in health-related quality of life. Int J Dermatol 2002;41:151–8.

[32] Rapp SR, Feldman SR, Exum ML, et al. Psoriasis causes as much disability as other major medical diseases. J Am Acad Dermatol 1999;41:401–7.

[33] O'Neill P, Kelly P. Postal questionnaire study of disability in the community associated with psoriasis. BMJ 1996;313:919–21.

[34] Vardy D, Besser A, Amir M, et al. Experiences of stigmatization play a role in mediating the impact of disease severity on quality of life in psoriasis patients. Br J Dermatol 2002;147:736–42.

[35] Wahl A, Loge JH, Wiklund I, et al. The burden of psoriasis: a study concerning health-related quality of life among Norwegian adult patients with psoriasis compared with general population norms. J Am Acad Dermatol 2000;43:803–8.

[36] Wahl AK, Gjengedal E, Hanestad BR. The bodily suffering of living with severe psoriasis: In-depth interviews with 22 hospitalized patients with psoriasis. Qual Health Res 2002;12:250–61.

[37] Clark CM, McKay RA, Fortune DG, et al. Use of alternative treatments by patients with psoriasis. Br J Gen Pract 1998;48(437):1873–4.

[38] Lundberg L, Johannesson M, Silverdahl M, et al. Quality of life, health-state utilities and willingness to pay in patients with psoriasis and atopic eczema. Br J Dermatol 1999;141:1067–75.

[39] Poyner TE, Fell PJ. A survey of patients with plaque psoriasis who had not consulted their doctor in the past year. Br J Clin Res 1995;6:201–7.

[40] Harlow D, Poyner T, Finlay AY, et al. Impaired quality of life of adults with skin disease in primary care. Br J Dermatol 2000;143:979–82.

[41] de Jong EM, Seegers BA, Gulinck MK, et al. Psoriasis of the nails associated with disability in a large number of patients: results of a recent interview with 1,728 patients. Dermatology 1996;193:300–3.

[42] Pettey AA, Balkrishnan R, Rapp SR, et al. Patients with palmoplantar psoriasis have more physical disability and discomfort than patients with other forms of psoriasis: implications for clinical practice. J Am Acad Dermatol 2003;49:271–5.

[43] Zachariae H, Zachariae R, Blomqvist K, et al. Quality of life and prevalence of arthritis reported by 5,795 members of the Nordic Psoriasis Associations: data from the Nordic Quality of Life Study. Acta Derm Venereol 2002;82:108–13.

[44] Husted JA, Gladman DD, Farewell VT, et al. Validating the SF-36 health survey questionnaire in patients with psoriatic arthritis. J Rheumatol 1997;24:511–7.

[45] McKenna KE, Stern RS. The impact of psoriasis on the quality of life of patients from the 16-center PUVA follow-up cohort. J Am Acad Dermatol 1997;36:388–94.

[46] Gupta MA, Gupta AK. Age and gender differences in the impact of psoriasis on quality of life. Int J Dermatol 1995;34:700–3.

[47] Gelfand JM, Feldman SR, Stern RS, et al. Patients with more extensive psoriasis have greater reductions in quality of life: female patients and young patients are affected to a greater extent. J Invest Dermatol 2004;122:60.

[48] Mazzotti E, Picardi A, Sampogna F, et al. Sensitivity of the Dermatology Life Quality Index to clinical change in patients with psoriasis. Br J Dermatol 2003;149:318–22.

[49] Lebwohl M, Christophers E, Langley R, et al. An international, randomized, double-blind, placebo-controlled phase 3 trial of intramuscular Alefacept in patients with chronic plaque psoriasis. Arch Dermatol 2003;139:719–27.

[50] Salek MS, Finlay AY, Lewis JJ, et al. Quality of life improvement in treatment of psoriasis with intermittent short course cyclosporin (Neoral). Qual Life Res 2004;13:91–5.

[51] Touw CR, Hakkaart-Van Roijen L, Verboom P, et al. Quality of life and clinical outcome in psoriasis patients using intermittent cyclosporin. Br J Dermatol 2001;144:967–72.

[52] Ellis CN, Mordin MM, Adler EY. Randomized, placebo-controlled phase II trial: effects of alefacept on health-related quality of life in patients with psoriasis: results from a randomized, placebo-controlled phase II trial. Am J Clin Dermatol 2003;4:131–9.

[53] Fortune DG, Richards HL, McElhone K, et al. Successful treatment of psoriasis improves psoriasis-specific but not more general aspects of patients' well-being. Br J Dermatol 2004;151:1219–26.

[54] Gupta G, Long J, Tillman DM. The efficacy of narrowband ultraviolet B phototherapy in psoriasis using objective and subjective outcome measures. Br J Dermatol 1999;140:887–90.

[55] Richards HL, Fortune DG, Griffiths CEM, et al. The contribution of perceptions of stigmatisation to disability in patients with psoriasis. J Psychosom Res 2001;50:11–5.

[56] Hill L, Kennedy P. The role of coping strategies in mediating subjective disability in people who have psoriasis. Psychol Health Med 2002;7:261–9.

[57] Fortune DG, Main CJ, O'Sullivan TM, et al. Assessing illness-related stress in psoriasis: the psychometric properties of the Psoriasis Life Stress Inventory. J Psychosom Res 1997;42:467–76.

[58] Metz D, Jemec GBE. Coping and psoriasis—a framework for targeted interventions. J Eur Acad Dermatol Venereol 1996;6:27–31.

[59] Wahl A, Hanestad BR, Wiklund I, et al. Coping and quality of life in patients with psoriasis. Qual Life Res 1999;8:427–33.

[60] Scharloo M, Kaptein AA, Weinman J, et al. Illness perceptions, coping and functioning in patients with rheumatoid arthritis, chronic obstructive pulmonary disease and psoriasis. J Psychosom Res 1998;44:573–85.

[61] Scharloo M, Kaptein AA, Weinman J, et al. Patients' illness perceptions and coping as predictors of functional status in psoriasis: a 1-year follow-up. Br J Dermatol 2000;142:899–907.

[62] Fortune DG, Richards HL, Main CJ, et al. Patients' strategies for coping with psoriasis. Clin Exp Dermatol 2002;127:177–85.

[63] Rapp SR, Cottrell CA, Leary MR. Social coping strategies associated with quality of life decrements among psoriasis patients. Br J Dermatol 2001;145:610–6.

[64] Akay A, Pekcanlar A, Bozdag KE, et al. Assessment of depression in subjects with psoriasis vulgaris and lichen planus. J Eur Acad Dermatol Venereol 2002;16:347–52.

[65] Devrimci-Ozguven H, Kundakci TN, Kumbasar H, et al. The depression, anxiety, life satisfaction and affective expression levels in psoriasis patients. J Eur Acad Dermatol Venereol 2000;14:267–71.

[66] Bharath S, Shamasundar C, Raghuram R, et al. Psychiatric morbidity in leprosy and psoriasis—a comparative study. Ind J Leprosy 1997;69:341–6.

[67] Mattoo SK, Handa S, Kaur I, et al. Psychiatric morbidity in vitiligo and psoriasis: a comparative study from India. J Dermatol 2001;28:424–32.

[68] Sharma N, Koranne RV, Singh RK. Psychiatric morbidity in psoriasis and vitiligo: a comparative study. J Dermatol 2001;28:419–23.

[69] Calikoglu E, Onder M, Cosar B, et al. Depression, anxiety levels and general psychological profile in Behcet's disease. Dermatology 2001;203:238–40.

[70] Gupta MA, Gupta AK. Depression and suicidal ideation in dermatology patients with acne, alopecia areata, atopic dermatitis and psoriasis. Br J Dermatol 1998;139:846–50.

[71] Zachariae R, Zachariae C, Ibsen HH, et al. Psychological symptoms and quality of life of dermatology outpatients and hospitalized dermatology patients. Acta Derm Venereol 2004;84:205–12.

[72] Niemeier V, Nippesen M, Kupfer J, et al. Psychological factors associated with hand dermatoses: which subgroup needs additional psychological care? Br J Dermatol 2002;146:1031–7.

[73] Fortune DG, Richards HL, Griffiths CEM, et al. Psychological stress, distress and disability in patients with psoriasis: consensus and variation in the contribution of illness perceptions, coping and alexithymia. Br J Clin Psychol 2002;41:157–74.

[74] Gupta MA, Gupta AK. Depression modulates pruritus perception: a study of pruritus in psoriasis, atopic dermatitis and chronic idiopathic urticaria. Ann N Y Acad Sci 1999;885:394–5.

[75] Reich A, Szepietowski JC, Wisnicka B, Pacan P. Does stress influence itching in psoriatic patients? Dermatol Psychosom 2003;4:151–5.

[76] Gupta MA, Gupta AK, Watteel GN. Perceived deprivation of social touch in psoriasis is associated with greater psychologic morbidity: an index of the stigma experience in dermatologic disorders. Cutis 1998;61:339–42.

[77] Picardi A, Abeni D, Renzi C, et al. Treatment outcome and incidence of psychiatric disorders in dermatological out-patients. J Eur Acad Dermatol Venereol 2003;17:155–9.

[78] Schmid-Ott G, Hofste N, Niederauer H-H, et al. Illness severity and coping in psoriasis patients: a 1-year follow-up. Dermatol Psychosom 2004;5:178–83.

[79] Hammerlid E, Ahlner-Elmqvist M, Bjordal K, et al. A prospective multicentre study in Sweden and Norway of mental distress and psychiatric morbidity in head and neck cancer patients. Br J Cancer 1999;80:766–74.

[80] Leary MR, Rapp SR, Herbst KC, et al. Interpersonal concerns and psychological difficulties of psoriasis patients: effects of disease severity and fear of negative evaluation. Health Psychol 1998;17:530–6.

[81] Stangier U, Ehlers A, Gieler U. Measuring adjustment to chronic skin disorders: validation of a self-report measure. Psychol Assess 2003;15:532–49.

[82] Kent G, Keohane S. Social anxiety and disfigurement: the moderating effects of fear of negative

evaluation and past experience. Br J Clin Psychol 2001;40:23–34.

[83] Williamson L, Dalbeth N, Dockerty JL, et al. Nail disease in psoriatic arthritis—clinically important, potentially treatable and often overlooked. Rheumatol 2004;43:790–4.

[84] Fortune DG, Richards HL, Griffiths CEM, et al. Targeting cognitive-behaviour therapy to patients' implicit model of psoriasis: results from a patient preference controlled trial. Br J Clin Psychol 2004; 43:65–82.

[85] Fortune DG, Richards HL, Corrin A, et al. Attentional bias for psoriasis-specific and psychosocial threat in patients with psoriasis. J Behav Med 2003;26: 211–24.

[86] Fortune DG, Richards HL, Kirby B, et al. A cognitive-behavioural symptom management programme as an adjunct in psoriasis therapy. Br J Dermatol 2002;146:458–65.

[87] Fortune DG, Richards HL, Griffiths CEM, et al. Worry and pathological worry in patients with psoriasis: cross sectional and longitudinal analyses of the Penn State Worry Questionnaire (PSWQ) in four samples of patients. J Clin Psychol Med Settings 2005;12:143–52.

[88] Fortune DG, Richards HL, Main CJ, et al. Developing clinical psychology services in an outpatient dermatology speciality clinic: what factors are associated with non-uptake of the service? Clin Psychol Forum 1998;115:34–6.

[89] Richards HL, Fortune DG, Chong SLP, et al. Divergent beliefs about psoriasis are associated with increased psychological distress for patients and their partners. J Invest Dermatol 2004;123:49–56.

[90] Gupta MA, Gupta AK. Psoriasis and sex: a study of moderately to severely affected patients. Int J Dermatol 1997;36:259–62.

[91] Richards HL, Fortune DG, Main CJ, et al. Stigmatization and psoriasis. Br J Dermatol 2003;149:209–11.

[92] Schmid-Ott G, Jaeger B, Kuensebeck HW, et al. Dimensions of stigmatization in patients with psoriasis in a "Questionnaire on Experience with Skin Complaints." Dermatologyg 1996;193:304–10.

[93] Schmid-Ott G, Kuensebeck HW, Jaeger B, et al. Validity study for the stigmatization experience in atopic dermatitis and psoriatic patients. Acta Derm Venereol 1999;79:443–7.

[94] Lu Y, Duller P, van der Valk PGM, et al. Helplessness as predictor of perceived stigmatization in patients with psoriasis and atopic dermatitis. Dermatol Psychosom 2003;4:146–50.

[95] Rubino IA, Sonnino A, Pezzarossa B, et al. Personality disorders and psychiatric symptoms in psoriasis. Psychol Rep 1995;77:547–53.

[96] Fukunishi I, Berger D. Personality disorders and psychiatric symptoms in psoriasis: a critical analysis. Psychol Rep 1996;79:1248–50.

[97] Berger D, Fukunishi I. Personality disorders in psoriasis. Psych Rep 1997;80:877–8.

[98] Gupta MA, Gupta AK, Watteel GN. Early onset (<40 years age) psoriasis is comorbid with greater psychopathology than late onset psoriasis: a study of 137 patients. Acta Derm Venereol 1996;76:464–6.

[99] Picardi A, Pasquinnni P, Cattaruzza MS, et al. Only limited support for a role of psychosomatic factors in psoriasis: results from a case control study. J Psychosom Res 2003;55:189–96.

[100] Richards HL, Fortune DG, Griffiths CEM, et al. Alexithymia in patients with psoriasis: clinical correlates and psychometric properties of the Toronto Alexithymia Scale-20. J Psychosom Res 2005;58: 89–96.

[101] Fortune DG, Richards HL, Griffiths CEM, et al. Adversarial growth in patients undergoing treatment for psoriasis: a prospective study of the ability of patients to construe benefits from negative events. Psychol Health Med 2005;10:44–56.

[102] Blok S, Vissers WH, van Duijnhoven M, et al. Aggravation of psoriasis by infections: a constitutional trait or a variable expression? Eur J Dermatol 2004;14:259–61.

[103] Park BS, Youn JI. Factors influencing psoriasis: an analysis based upon the extent of involvement and clinical type. J Dermatol 1998;25:97–102.

[104] Suljagic E, Sinanovic O, Tupkovic E, et al. Stressful life events and psoriasis during the war in Bosnia. Dermatol Psychosom 2000;1:56–60.

[105] Gupta MA, Gupta AK. The psoriasis life stress inventory: a preliminary index of psoriasis related stress. Acta Derm Venereol 1995;75:240–3.

[106] Harvima RJ, Viinamaki H, Harvima IT, et al. Association of psychic stress with clinical severity and symptoms of psoriatic patients. Acta Derm Venereol 1996;76:467–71.

[107] Pacan P, Szepietowski JC, Kiejna A. Stressful life events and depression in patients suffering from psoriasis vulgaris. Dermatol Psychosom 2003;4:142–5.

[108] Naldi L, Peli L, Parazzini F, et al. Family history of psoriasis, stressful life events, and recent infectious disease are risk factors for a first episode of acute guttate psoriasis: results of a case-control study. J Am Acad Dermatol 2001;44:433–8.

[109] Kupfer J, Niemeier V, Brosig B, et al. Sense of coherence among psoriatics as a predictor of symptom-free time following dermatological inpatient therapy. Dermatol Psychosom 2003;4:200–6.

[110] Richards HL, Ray DW, Kirby B, et al. The HPA response to psychological stress in patients with psoriasis. Br J Dermatol, in press.

[111] Schmid-Ott G, Jacobs R, Jäger B, et al. Stress-induced endocrine and immunological changes in psoriasis patients and healthy controls. Psychother Psychosom 1998;67:37–42.

[112] Thaller V, Vrkljan M, Hotujac L, et al. The potential role of hypocortisolism in the pathophysiology of PTSD and psoriasis. Colleg Antropol 1999;23: 611–9.

[113] Schmid-Ott G, Jaeger B, Adamek C, et al. Acute

psychosocial stress and T-cell response in patients with atopic dermatitis psoriasis, and healthy controls. J Psychosom Res 2000;48:249–50.

[114] Zachariae R, Oster H, Bjerring P, et al. Effects of psychologic intervention on psoriasis: a preliminary report. J Am Acad Dermatol 1996;34:1008–15.

[115] Kabat-Zinn J, Wheeler E, Light T, et al. Influence of a mindfulness meditation-based stress reduction intervention on rates of skin clearing in patients with moderate to severe psoriasis undergoing phototherapy (UVB) and photochemotherapy (PUVA). Psychosom Med 1998;60:625–32.

[116] Scheewe S, Schmidt S, Petermann F, et al. Long-term efficacy of an inpatient rehabilitation with integrated patient education program for children and adolescents with psoriasis. Dermatol Psychosom 2001;2:16–21.

[117] Kang Seng T, Siew Nee T. Group therapy: a useful and supportive treatment for psoriasis patients. Int J Dermatol 1997;36:110–2.

[118] Lazaroff I, Shismshoni R. Effects of medical resonance therapy music on patients with psoriasis and neurodermatitis—a pilot study. Integrat Physiol Behav Sci 2000;35:189–98.

[119] Tausk F, Whitmore SE. A pilot study of hypnosis in the treatment of patients with psoriasis. Psychother Psychosom 1999;68:221–5.

[120] Weiss SC, Kimball AB, Liewehr DJ, et al. Quantifying the harmful effect of psoriasis on health-related quality of life. J Am Acad Dermatol 2002;47:512–8.

[121] Koo J. Population-based epidemiologic study of psoriasis with emphasis on quality of life assessment. Dermatol Clin North Am 1996;14:485–96.

# Psychoneuroimmunodermatology of Atopic Dermatitis: From Empiric Data to the Evolutionary Hypothesis

Stefano Pallanti, MD[a,b,*], Torello Lotti, MD[c,d], Mauro Urpe, PhD[c,d]

[a]Institute of Neuroscience, University of Florence, Florence, Italy
[b]Mount Sinai School of Medicine, New York, NY, USA
[c]Centro Interuniversitario di Dermatologia Biologica e Psicosomatica, University of Florence, Florence, Italy
[d]University Unit of Physical Therapy and Dermatology, University of Florence, Florence, Italy

Atopic dermatitis (AD) is a chronically relapsing inflammatory skin disease characterized by dry and eczematous skin lesions, erythematosus papules, and intense pruritus. AD appears in early childhood, in approximately 90% of cases before age 5. Epidemiologic data indicate that the prevalence of AD has been increasing steadily since World War II and now affects more than 12% of children in the Western world [1,2]. AD symptomatology often results in significant morbidity associated with frequent hospitalization, school absenteeism, difficulties in attaining educational qualifications, and missed work days. Endogenous and environmental factors, such as genetic disposition, climate, allergens, and microbial organisms (eg, *Staphylococcus aureus*) are critical in determining the disease [3]. Research conducted over the past decade strongly suggests, however, an underlying immunoregulatory abnormality in patients who have AD. Although there is general agreement that stress is a factor in AD, the underlying mechanism of how this may have an impact on the pathophysiology of AD has yet to be defined.

In aInitial exposure to environmental allergens leads, in patients who have AD, to an activation of B cells, with hypersecretion of the allergen-specific immunoglobulin E (IgE). Subsequent cross-binding of IgE molecules located on basophils and mast cells by the allergen leads to the release of vasoactive and proinflammatory mediators, inducing a hypersensitivity reaction of the skin and initiating an IgE-dependent, late-phase (inflammatory) allergic response [4,5].

It is reported that surface-bound IgE enables Langerhans' cells and monocytes to process and present allergens in the skin, resulting in recruitment of T helper cells (Th). Furthermore, allergen-specific $T_H$ cells cloned from AD skin lesions secrete large amounts of interleukin (IL) 4, IL-5, and IL-13, but not interferon-$\gamma$ (IFN-$\gamma$), reflecting the establishment of a predominantly Th-2 cytokine-secreting profile. According to recent reports, the dominance of Th-2–like cytokines plays a major role in the pathogenesis of AD.

IL-4 and IL-13 stimulate IgE synthesis and induce B cells to switch from other Ig isotypes to IgE. They further stimulate the expression of vascular cell adhesion molecule–1 that is involved in the recruitment of eosinophils into sites of allergic tissue inflammation [6]. Eosinophils are inflammatory cells commonly associated with tissue damage in atopy. IL-5 further augments eosinophil production and stimulates eosinophils to secrete toxic proteins (eg, major basic protein and eosinophilic cationic protein), which are known to contribute to

---

* Corresponding author. Institute of Neuroscience, University of Florence, Viale Ugo Bassi 1, 50100 Florence, Italy.
E-mail address: s.pallanti@agora.it (S. Pallanti).

tissue injury because of their cytotoxic properties and their ability to stimulate basophil and mast cell degranulation [7].

Besides profound immunoregulatory abnormalities, an increasing number of studies argue that psychologic factors, such as stress, contribute significantly to the continuation and chronification of AD symptoms [8–12]. Early studies suggest that in a majority of cases (50%–70%), severe shock, worry, or upsetting emotional events precede the onset or aggravation of AD [11,12]. These observations are in line with more recent findings demonstrating a significant positive relationship between interpersonal life stress on a given day and skin condition in the succeeding 24 hours. Indirect confirmation of the importance of psychosocial factors in the maintenance and exacerbation of AD is provided by several studies reporting the effectiveness of psychotherapeutic interventions, including stress management and relaxation techniques. These resulted in a significant improvement of AD symptomatology [13].

The issue is how psychologic processes and stressful experiences may influence the endocrine and the immune system, leading to the immunopathogenesis of AD [14]. Is there any specificity? The hypothalamus-pituitary-adrenal (HPA) axis is pointed to most frequently as one of the major pathways through which the central nervous system exerts control over the immune system under stressful conditions. An appropriate reactivity of the HPA axis to stressful stimuli may be necessary to control immunologic processes and to prevent an immune response, for example an inflammatory response, from reaching a level that may be damaging for the host [15,16]. More recently, on the basis of animal data, it is argued that the HPA axis plays a protective role regarding chronic allergic inflammation [17–19].

The assumption that reduced HPA axis (re)activity may be involved in the maintenance and exacerbation of atopy is supported by the observation that diurnal plasma cortisol variations in patients who have AD are associated closely with the diurnal variation of atopy-relevant inflammatory parameters, such as basophils or eosinophils, and the severity of allergic symptomatology [20,21].

The pathogenic significance of a dysfunctional HPA axis in skin atopy is underlined further by an incidental observation by Laue and coworkers [22]. They report that after treatment with the glucocorticoid receptor antagonist, RU 486, healthy volunteers who had no prior history of atopy showed AD-like symptoms, such as erythema and eczematous skin. Animal data showing that blunted responsiveness of the HPA axis to stress is linked closely to increased susceptibility to inflammatory disease lend support to this model [23,24]. A recent report investigated HPA axis responsiveness in children who had allergic asthma, a chronic disorder of the airways characterized by airway inflammation and airflow obstruction. The immunopathology of allergic asthma and AD involve similar processes: IgE-mediated inflammation, Th-2–cell-predominant immune responses, and eosinophilia [25].

Allergic asthma often is considered a chronic bronchial inflammatory condition of the "atopic triad" [26]. Children who had allergic asthma and were exposed to psychosocial stress showed significantly blunted cortisol responses compared to those of a nonatopic control group, but no differences in heart rate responses or in psychologic variables, such as subjective stress experience or subjective well-being after the stressor [27].

These data support the concept that reduced HPA axis reactivity in patients who have AD probably does not reflect a specific phenomenon linked to skin atopy, rather a nonspecific phenomenon associated with allergic inflammation regardless of the target organ. Patients who have AD are reported to worsen as a consequence of various acute stressful situations, such as watching stressful film sequences [28] or being confronted with stressful interactions [29]. Investigation of this model highlights that HPA axis responsiveness is reduced significantly in patients who have AD, as indicated by a blunted cortisol level, a blunted ACTH response to the stressor, aberrant immune responses, and further worsening of atopic symptoms [30]. The latter observation supports the idea that dysfunction of the HPA axis may be located on the suprapituitary side. This is in line with animal data suggesting deficient paraventricular nucleus corticotrophin-releasing hormone–mRNA levels in Lewis (LEW/N) rats, which are characterized by hyporesponsiveness of the HPA axis and high vulnerability to inflammatory disease [31].

Distinct immunologic alterations, such as a significant increase in the number of eosinophils and in IgE levels, were found in subjects who had AD under stress but not in control subjects [32]. Recruitment and activation of eosinophils are assumed to precede exacerbation of AD [33]. When activated, eosinophils can secrete cytotoxic mediators that are correlated positively with disease severity and that are described as contributing to tissue injury [34]. IgE is a key molecule in AD and enables immediate hypersensitivity reactions by stimulating mast cells and basophils. It further propagates the recruitment and activation of atopy-relevant Th-2 cells, initiating the late phase response and chronicity of the disease [35,36].

As a result of this mechanism, AD is supposed to share the same pathophysiology as other severe conditions. As reported by Caligaris-Cappio and colleagues and Romagnani and colleagues [37,38], pathophysiologic conditions associated with prevalent Th-2 cells responses are numerous, including systemic lupus eryhtematosus, vernal conjunctivitis [39], successful pregnancy [40], and so forth. The finding of increased eosinophil numbers and IgE levels in response to stress in patients who have AD is consistent with an attenuated HPA axis response, leading to reduced ACTH and cortisol release. This hyporesponsiveness of the HPA axis is associated with a shift towards an immune response characteristic of chronic allergic inflammation. The potential pathologic relevance of these immune changes is underlined by the observation that 24 hours after the stress test, significant worsening of the skin condition in the subjects who had AD could be determined [32]. It remains to be determined if attenuated reactivity of the HPA axis in patients who have AD represents a (genetically determined) vulnerability trait or a consequence of long-term, chronic inflammation. Activation of the HPA axis by proinflammatory cytokines with later downregulation of the system is reported typically in chronic inflammatory conditions [41].

The cord blood of newborns who have an atopic predisposition (defined as having a positive family history of atopy where at least one parent was atopic) and elevated IgE levels (IgE > kU/L) has been studied to verify whether a hyporeactive HPA axis can be observed early in life and before the onset of any potential allergic inflammation. Results showed elevated cortisol responses to venipuncture stress when compared to newborns who did not have an AD predisposition [42].

The hyporeactivity of the HPA axis in individuals who have long-term AD, associated with the observation of hyperreactivity of the system in newborns who have atopic predisposition, makes it possible to propose a model wherein there is a progressive adjustment from the onset of the disease to when it becomes chronic, with the HPA axis switching from a hyper- to a hyporeactive state. Even though there are reports suggesting that the long-term release of pro-inflammatory cytokines (as observed after the onset of allergic inflammation) can diminish HPA axis responsiveness as a result of increased negative feedback produced by persistently increased endogenous cortisol concentrations [41], it is worth collecting further data with a view to validating this model.

## Other behavioral dimensions

### Maternal caring behavior

In animals, licking and grooming are implicated in regulating blunted HPA axis responsiveness to chronic stress [43]. Maternal care is activated as a relevant and influential behavioral factor in AD. Licking and grooming increase everyday stress levels, which parallels altered mother-child interactions characterized by overprotection as described by atopic patients [44]. Further studies should considered to establish a correlation between attachment style in humans and AD.

### Infant response to stress

Adverse, short-term physiologic and behavioral responses in infants to intense stress are well documented [44–46]. Physiologic response to stress invokes the sympathetic-adrenomedullary, HPA, and endogenous opiate systems. Independently, and through their interaction, these systems have widespread effects on target organs and the functioning of the immune system, including suppression of T-lymphocyte function and decreased mitogen responses [46]. Most short-term physiologic responses are the result of cortical and subcortical stimulation of centers in the hypothalamus that activate the HPA system to produce glucocorticoids (primarily cortisol) and the sympathetic-adrenomedullary system to release catecholamines (primarily epinephrine and norepinephrine) [47,48]. Measures of physiologic arousal include heart and respiratory rates, vagal tone, blood pressure, and metabolic markers (catecholamines, glucagon, insulin, and cortisol) [49]. Of these markers, cortisol and vagal tone are the most useful in studies of children.

### Temperament and stress

Temperament is defined as "individual differences in emotionality, attention, and self-regulation" [50]. Temperament is distinguished from personality because the prior is defined as a behavioral trait more genetically closely related, precognitive, and elementary less influenced from previous even precocious experiences. Temperament modulates children's behavioral and physiologic responses to stress. It also plays an important role in organizing children's responses to adverse and ordinary environmental stresses [51]; in particular, temperament is believed to influence children's behavioral expressions of activity, emotionality, sociability, and reactivity.

Response to stress has an autonomic nervous system component that includes threshold (length of time to respond to a stimulus), magnitude, and dampening or self-regulation (length of time to subdue the response). Physiologic responses may be the biologic analogue of behavioral response [52]. Behavioral manifestations of reactivity (threshold and magnitude) and self-regulation, however, are not simply reflections of physiologic response. A mounting body of evidence in the psychobiology of temperament points to the influence behavior and physiology have on each other and the relationships between behavior and genetics, development, environment, and experience [53]. In infants, initial behavioral responses to stress (reactivity) and behavioral quieting after a stressor (self-regulation) probably are relatively independent components of the stress response [54].

*The hygiene hypothesis in an evolutionary framework*

Several epidemiologic studies suggest that the increase in the prevalence of atopic disorders that has occurred over the past few decades is attributable to a reduced microbial burden during childhood, as a consequence of a Westernized lifestyle (the so-called "hygiene hypothesis"). Is the hygiene hypothesis better explained by missing immune deviation or by reduced immune suppression?

The hygiene hypothesis as the most reasonable explanation of the allergy outbreaks is strengthened by reports of pregnant mothers or their sons, in their sons' first year of life, to be expoxed to microbial products released by farm animals, which is typical of the rural lifestyle, exerts an important protective role against the development of an allergy as a consequence of the chronic stimulation of the Toll-like receptors (TLRs) expressed by cells of the innate immunity. The critical point is to identify the immunologic mechanism(s) by which the reduced microbial stimulation of TLRs on cells of the innate immunity in early life can result in easier and stronger Th-2 responses to allergens. For several years, the most likely explanation has been that a reduction in the microbial burden impairs the occurrence of immune deviation from Th-2 to Th-1, which takes place usually with increasing age. This means that reduced stimulation of TLRs on dendritic cells and natural killer cells results in decreased production of cytokines, such as IL-12 and IFN-$\gamma$, which not only promotes the development of $T_H1$ cells but also antagonizes the development of Th-2 cells [38].

Recently, however, an alternative view has emerged, suggesting the importance of reduced immune suppression rather than missing immune deviation. According to this alternative view, the lower microbial burden does not act by inducing a lower production of Th-1 polarizing cytokines but by decreasing the activity of T regulatory cells [55,56]. The mechanisms by which the reduced exposure of children to pathogenic and nonpathogenic microbes results in enhanced responses of Th-2 cells have yet to be ascertained conclusively. Initially it was argued that there is a missing immune deviation of allergen-specific responses from a Th-2 to a Th-1 profile, as a result of the reduced production of IL-12 and interferons by natural immunity cells, which are stimulated by bacterial products via their TLRs. TLRs play a critical role in early innate immunity to invading pathogens by sensing microorganisms. More recently, the role of the reduced activity of T regulatory cells has been emphasized. The epidemiologic findings and the experimental evidence available so far suggest that both mechanisms may be involved [57].

*False contamination, atopic dermatitis, and obsessive-compulsive disorder: a Darwinian view*

According to the literature summarized in this article, the psychoimmunologic pathway contributes to the origins of AD, but some issues remain. One hypothesis is that the actual models used in psychiatry (categoric diagnosis) and in other branches of medicine might not be adequate to build up a heuristic view and modeling of this complex phenomenon.

Evolutionary theory distinguishes between two different causations: proximate levels, which refer to all the possible physical factors that directly produce the given trait (biochemical, genetic, and so forth [discussed previously]); and ultimate causation, which, it is argued, refers to the adaptive function of an organism within the ancestral environment. Darwinian medicine considers that biologic systems, including psychologic functions, have evolved through natural selection because of their contribution to inclusive fitness [58]. Darwinian theorists suggest that some idiopathic psychiatric symptoms and syndromes may represent misplaced adaptive strategies or accentuated versions of original strategies that may be caused by a number of proximate factors [59–61]. The most suggestive psychiatric condition that seems to mirror allergic phenomena at the psychic level is represented by obsessive-compulsive disorder (OCD).

OCD can be interpreted as an accentuated version of an adaptive strategy that enhanced the reproductive fitness of those humans who possessed this trait over those who did not within their ancestral environment. Patients who have OCD experience obsessive thoughts as a form of "psychic parasitism" associated with internal feelings of disgust and repulsion [62]. Until now, research of AD has not considered and investigated OCD symptomatology, although this disorder is reported as the most prevalent psychiatric condition in a dermatologic setting [63]. The correlation between OCD and atopic phenomena is even more intriguing. The authors refer to the model of the mental module according to the formulation of a modular configuration for the human mind/brain [64].

*The importance of the mental scenario: a hypothesis*

Modularity suggests that the human mind consists of many domain-specific, highly tuned systems that have evolved to carry out circumscribed tasks. Rapoport and Fiske propose a modular configuration of the brain system that addresses obsessional phenomena [65].

It is contended that obsessional phenomena are archaic, involuntary, repetitive thought processes that stimulate strong aversive emotional states (eg, fear and disgust) and lead to risk-avoidance behavior. It is hypothesized that the neurobiologic system that generates these phenomena has the function of generating risk scenarios without conscious intervention and thus functions as an involuntary risk scenario generating system (IRSGS) [66]. Compulsive rituals, the other component of OCD, are conceptualized as primitive harm avoidance behavioral routines that are under semivoluntary control [67,68]. It is suggested that the IRSGS operates primarily as a self-generated conditioning system whereby individuals can develop harm-avoidance behavioral strategies without experiencing the risks involved in real-life dangers.

The adaptive function of this system is that it saves individual organisms from having to experience physical and social dangers in vivo, instead producing the same learning response in total physical safety. Therefore, the ability of some organisms to learn to avoid common dangers without the need to experience them in real life confers a clear advantage on the individuals who possess this trait over those who do not. This would have ensured the spreading of the obsessional traits within the population, but, as with most traits, extreme variants may prove harmful and can reduce reproductive fitness.

It is claimed that obsessional processes may be akin to the generation of antibodies by the immune system. Whether or not an antibody increases in concentration depends on the subsequent feedback.

Although antibodies have the function of protecting the body from invisible dangers within the body, obsessional thoughts are designed to protect individuals primarily from external dangers within the environment. It is suggested that both operate through a selectionist process, that is, the better-fit antibody or thought survives. Some investigators suggest that a similar process, involving the selection of random and spontaneously generated thoughts, lies at the heart of all human thinking [69,70].

It already is suggested that the neurobiologic system responsible for generating obsessional thoughts is the mental or psychologic analogue to the immune system. Rather than being responsible for the production of protective proteins (antibodies) that neutralize physical danger from potential invaders, it is argued that the IRSGS is charged with the production of risk scenario packages that use elements of the physical and social environment to predict certain dangers. The accompanying negative emotions of anxiety, disgust, or fear should result in avoidance behavior and a process of learning in imagery that usually renders the individual immunized. At this point, the random danger scenarios should cease or become simply dormant. Thus, if the present hypothesis is correct, OCD is analogous to a mental autoimmune disease (ie, a protective response that goes beyond the point of usefulness and becomes self-destructive) [71–73]. The heuristic value of these highly speculative hypotheses might represent a theoretic background for further empiric validations through the adoption of a new modeling in medicine.

## References

[1] Boguniewicz M. Advances in the understanding and treatment of atopic dermatitis. Curr Opin Pediatr 1997;9:577–81.
[2] Nimmagadda SR, Evans R. Allergy and epidemiology. Pediatr Rev 1999;20:111–5.
[3] Werfel M. Environmental and other major factors in atopic dermatitis. Allergy 1998;53:731–9.
[4] Leung DYM. Pathogenesis of atopic dermatitis. J Allergy Clin Immunol 1999;104:S99–108.
[5] Eedy DJ. What's new in atopic dermatitis? Br J Dermatol 2001;145:380–4.
[6] Leung DY, Soter NA. Cellular and immunologic mechanisms in atopic dermatitis. J Am Acad Dermatol 2001;44:S1–12.
[7] Martin LB, Kita H, Leiferman KM, et al. Eosinophils in allergy: role in disease, degranulation, and cytokines. Int Arch Allergy Immunol 1996;109:207–15.
[8] Buske-Kirschbaum A, Geiben A, Hellhammer D. Psychobiological aspects of atopic dermatitis: an overview. Psychother Psychosom 2001;70:6–16.

[9] Wright RJ, Cohen RT, Cohen S. The impact of stress on the development and expression of atopy. Curr Opin Allergy Clin Immunol 2005;5:23–9.

[10] Lonne-Rahm S, Berg M, Marin P, et al. Atopic dermatitis, stinging, and effects of chronic stress: a pathocausal study. J Am Acad Dermatol 2004;51:899–905.

[11] Wittkower E, Russel B. Emotional factors in skin disease. London: Cassell; 1953.

[12] Brown DG. Stress as a precipitant factor of eczema. J Psychosom Res 1972;16:321–7.

[13] Melin L, Frederiksen T, Noren P, et al. Behavioral treatment of scratching in patients with atopic dermatitis. Br J Dermatol 1986;115:467–74.

[14] Ader R. Psychoneuroimmunology. San Diego (CA): Academic Press; 2000.

[15] Chroussos GP. The hypothalamus-pituitary-adrenal axis and immune mediated inflammation. N Engl J Med 1995;332:1351–62.

[16] Sternberg EM, Hill JM, Chrousos GP, et al. Inflammatory mediator-induced hypothalamic-pituitary-adrenal axis activation is defective in streptococcal cell wall arthritis-susceptible Lewis rats. Proc Natl Acad Sci USA 1989;86:2374–8.

[17] Goujon E, Parnet P, Laye S, et al. Adrenalectomy enhances pro-inflammatory cytokines gene expression in the spleen, pituitary and brain of mice in response to lipopolysaccharide. Brain Res Mol Brain Res 1996;36:53–62.

[18] Farsky SP, Sannomiya P, Garcia-Leme J. Secreted glucocorticoids regulate leukocyte-endothelial interactions in inflammation: a direct vital microscopic study. J Leukoc Biol 1995;57:379–86.

[19] Fornhem C, Peterson CG, Scheynius A, et al. Influence of endogenous cortisol on eosinophil function in sensitized pigs: direct measurements of eosinophil peroxidase. Clin Exp Allergy 1996;26:469–78.

[20] Herrscher RF, Kasper C, Sullivan TJ. Endogenous cortisol regulates immunoglobulin-E dependent late phase reactions. J Clin Invest 1992;90:596–603.

[21] Buhles N, Holzel C, Spiteller G, et al. Disorders of steroid metabolism in inflammatory dermatoses. Z Hautk 1987;62:1356–63.

[22] Laue L, Lotze MT, Chrousos GP, et al. Effect of chronic treatment with the glucocorticoid antagonist RU 486 in man. Toxicity, immunological and hormonal aspects. J Clin Endocrinol Metab 1990;71: 1474–80.

[23] Sternberg EM, Hill JM, Chrousos GP, et al. Inflammatory mediator-induced hypothalamic-pituitary-adrenal axis activation is defective in streptococcal cell wall arthritis-susceptible Lewis rats. Proc Natl Acad Sci USA 1989;86:2374–8.

[24] Tonelli L, Webster JI, Rapp KL, et al. Neuroendocrine responses regulating susceptibility and resistance to autoimmune/inflammatory disease in inbred rat strains. Immunol Rev 2001;184:203–11.

[25] Maddox L, Schwartz DA. The pathophysiology of asthma. Annu Rev Med 2002;53:477–98.

[26] Oettgen HC, Geha RS. IgE in asthma and atopy: cellular and molecular connections. J Clin Invest 1999;104:829–35.

[27] Buske-Kirschbaum A, von Auer K, Krieger S, et al. Blunted cortisol responses to psychosocial stress in asthmatic children: a general feature of atopic disease? Psychosom Med 2003;65(5):806–10.

[28] Ritz T, Steptoe A, DeWilde S, et al. Emotions and stress increase respiratory resistance in asthma. Psychosom Med 2000;62:401–12.

[29] Kolbe J, Garrett J, Vamos M, et al. Influences on trends in asthma morbidity and mortality: the New Zealand experience. Chest 1994;106:S211–5.

[30] Buske-Kirschbaum A, Geiben A, Hollig H, et al. Altered responsiveness of the hypothalamus-pituitary-adrenal axis and the sympathetic adrenomedullary system to stress in patients with atopic dermatitis. J Clin Endocrinol Metab 2002;87:4245–51.

[31] Calogero AE, Sternberg EM, Bagdy G, et al. Neurotransmitter-induced hypothalamus-pituitary-adrenal axis responsiveness is defective in inflammatory disease-susceptible Lewis rats: in vivo and in vitro studies suggesting globally defective hypothalamic secretion of corticotropin-releasing hormone. Neuroendocrinology 1992;55:600–8.

[32] Buske-Kirschbaum A, Gierens A, Hollig H, et al. Stress-induced immunomodulation is altered in patients with atopic dermatitis. J Neuroimmunol 2002; 129:161–7.

[33] Boguniewicz M. Advances in the understanding and treatment of atopic dermatitis. Curr Opin Pediatr 1997;9:577–81.

[34] Eedy DJ. What's new in atopic dermatitis? Br J Dermatol 2001;145:380–4.

[35] Martin LB, Kita H, Leiferman KM, et al. Eosinophils in allergy: role in disease, degranulation, and cytokines. Int Arch Allergy Immunol 1996;109:207–15.

[36] Turnbull AV, Rivier CL. Regulation of the hypothalamus-pituitary-adrenal axis by cytokines: actions and mechanisms of action. Physiol Rev 1999;79:1–71.

[37] Caligaris-Cappio F, Bertero MT, Converso M, et al. Circulating levels of soluble CD30, a marker of cells producing Th2-type cytokines, are increased in patients with systemic lupus eryhtematosus and correlate with disease activity. Clin Esp Rheum 1995;13: 339–43.

[38] Romagnani S. Lymphokine production by human T cells in disease states. Annu Rev Immunol 1994; 12:227–57.

[39] Maggi E, Biswas P, Del Prete G, et al. Accumulation of Th2-like helper T cells in the conjunctiva of patients with vernal conjunctivitis. J Immunol 1991;146: 1169–74.

[40] Wegmann Th. Bidirectional cytokine interactions in the maternal-fatal relationship: is successful pregnancy a Th2 phenomenon? Immunol Today 1993;14:353–6.

[41] Nickerson P, Steurer W, Steiger J, et al. Cytokines and the Th1/Th2 paradigm in trasplantation. Curr Opin Immunol 1994;6:757–64.

[42] Buske-Kirschbaum A, Fischbach S, Rauh W, et al.

Increased responsiveness of the hypothalamus-pituitary-adrenal (HPA) axis to stress in newborns with atopic disposition. Psychoneuroendocrinology 2004; 29(6):705–11.
[43] Francis DD, Champagne FA, Liu D, et al. Maternal care and the development of stress responses. Curr Opin Neurobiol 1999;9:128–34.
[44] Anand KS. Relationships between stress responses and clinical outcome in newborns, infants, and children. Crit Care Med 1993;21:S358–9.
[45] Boyce WT, Jemerin JM. Psychobiological differences in childhood stress response. I. Patterns of illness and susceptibility. J Dev Behav Pediatr 1990;11: 86–94.
[46] Gunnar MR. Psychobiological studies of stress and coping: An introduction. Child Dev 1987;58:1403–7.
[47] Gunnar MR. Reactivity of the hypothalamic-pituitary-adrenocortical system to stressors in normal infants and children. Pediatrics 1992;90(3 Pt 2):491–7.
[48] Ramsay DS, Lewis M. Developmental change in infant cortisol and behavioral response to inoculation. Child Dev 1994;65:1491–502.
[49] Lewis M, Thomas D. Cortisol release in infants in response to inoculation. Child Dev 1990;61:50–9.
[50] Rothbart MK. Temperament and development. In: Kohnstamm GA, Bates JE, Rothbart MK, editors. Temperament in childhood. New York: Wiley; 1989. p. 187–247.
[51] Boyce WT. Temperament and the psychobiology of childhood stress. Pediatrics 1992;90:483–6.
[52] Jemerin JM, Boyce WT. Psychobiological differences in childhood stress response. II. Cardiovascular markers of vulnerability. J Dev Behav Pediatr 1990; 11:140–50.
[53] Gunnar MR. The psychobiology of infant temperament. In: Colombo J, Fagen J, editors. Individual differences in infancy: reliability, stability, prediction. Hillsdale (NJ): Lawrence Erlbaum; 1990. p. 387–409.
[54] Worobey J. Individual differences in the reactivity of young infants. Dev Psychol 1989;25:663–7.
[55] Yazdanbakhah M. Allergy, parasites, and the hygiene hypothesis. Science 2002;296:490–4.
[56] Wills-Karp M, Santeliz J, Karp CL. The germless allergic disease: revisiting the hygiene hypothesis. Nature Rev Immunol 2001;1:69–75.
[57] Romagnani S. The increased prevalence of allergy and the hygiene hypothesis: missing immune deviation, reduced immune suppression, or both? Immunology 2004;112:352–63.
[58] Hamilton WD. The genetical evolution of social behaviour I & II. J Theoret Biol 1964;7:1–52.
[59] Buss DM. Evolutionary psychology: the new science of the mind. Boston: Allyn & Bacon; 1999.
[60] McGuire A. Darwinian psychiatry. London: Oxford University Press; 1998.
[61] Stevens A. Evolutionary psychiatry: a new beginning. London: Routledge; 1996.
[62] Stein DJ. The psychobiology of obsessive-compulsive disorder: how important is the role of disgust? Curr Psychiatry Rep 2001;3:281–7.
[63] Fineberg NA, O'Doherty C, Rajagopal S, et al. How common is obsessive-compulsive disorder in a dermatology outpatient clinic? J Clin Psychiatry 2003;64: 152–5.
[64] Fodor JL. The modularity of mind. Cambridge (MA): MIT Press; 1983.
[65] Rapoport J, Fiske A. The new biology of obsessive-compulsive disorder: implications for evolutionary psychology. Perspect Biol Med 1998;41:159–79.
[66] Abed RT, DePauw KW. An evolutionary hypothesis for obsessive compulsive disorder: a psychological immune system? Behav Neurol 1998;11:245–50.
[67] Cosmides L. Cognitive adaptations for social exchange. In: Barkow JH, Cosmides L, Tooby J, editors. The adapted mind: evolutionary psychology and the generation of culture. London: Oxford University Press; 1992. p. 163–228.
[68] Bradshaw JL. Human evolution: a neuropsychological perspective. Hove: Psychology Press/Taylor & Francis; 1997.
[69] Gazzaniga MS. The mind's past. Berkley (CA): University of California Press; 1998.
[70] Plotkin H. Darwin machines and the nature of knowledge. Harmondsworth: Allen Lane; 1994.
[71] Denys D, Fluitman S, Kavelaars A, et al. Decreased TNF-alpha and NK activity in obsessive-compulsive disorder. Psychoneuroendocrinology 2004;29:945–52.
[72] Dinn WM, Harris CL, McGonigal KM, et al. Obsessive-compulsive disorder and immunocompetence. Int J Psychiatry Med 2001;31:311–20.
[73] Stein DJ. Advances in the neurobiology of obsessive-compulsive disorder. Implication for conceptualizing putative obsessive-compulsive and spectrum disorders. Psychiatr Clin North Am 2000;23:545–62.

# Evaluating Clinical Rating Scales for Evidence-Based Dermatology: Some Basic Concepts

Madhulika A. Gupta, MD, FRCPC[a,b,*], Andrew M. Johnson, PhD[c], Mary-Margaret Chren, MD[d,e]

[a]*Department of Psychiatry, University of Western Ontario, London, ON, Canada*
[b]*Mediprobe Research Inc, London, ON, Canada*
[c]*Faculty of Health Sciences, University of Western Ontario, London, ON, Canada*
[d]*University of California at San Francisco, San Francisco, CA, USA*
[e]*Health Services Research Enhancement Award Program, San Francisco Veterans Affairs Medical Center, San Francisco, CA, USA*

A greater emphasis on evidence-based medicine has contributed to the increased interest in the development of standardized clinical rating scales for dermatology [1]. Greater availability of computing technology has made statistical analysis accessible to most practitioners, making it easier to implement these measurement tools. Finally, the desire to measure variables that lie outside the range of traditional biologic outcome measures (eg, the impact of skin disorders on an individual's quality of life) has led to an increased demand for psychometric measures of health.

Because quality of life is a complex and multidimensional construct, most of the measurement tools consist of multidimensional rating scales. Although this ever-increasing choice of assessment instruments makes it more likely that a tool exists for most practitioners' decision-making needs, it makes it all the more important for practitioners to have some guidelines to evaluate instruments for clinical or research uses. This article outlines some of the basic psychometric concepts that need to be considered when evaluating a clinical rating scale.

\* Corresponding author. 645 Windermere Road, London, ON N5X 2P1, Canada.
 *E-mail address:* magupta@uwo.ca (M.A. Gupta).

## Measurement of a construct

Measurement is a fundamental activity of science. Within the behavioral sciences, psychometrics has evolved as the specialty that is concerned with the measurement of psychologic and social phenomena, and the instrument typically used is the questionnaire [2–5]. Theory plays a key role in how the variables of the measurement instrument are conceptualized. A concept is an abstraction of an empirical observation, and provides the labels used to describe the environment. Of greater relevance to clinical research, however, is the construct: a concept that is essentially unobservable without some form of systematic definition. For example, the construct quality of life, which addresses the impact of a skin disorder on the physical, social, emotional, and vocational functioning of the patient, has no physical meaning, and no clear unidimensional symptomatic presentation. Despite this fact, however, it can be described in terms of its typical manifestation, and its relationship to other (sometimes similarly unobservable) concepts. This systematic definition is called an operational definition, and it is the first step in translating a construct into a variable (ie, a measurable quantity). It is the development and testing of these definitions that forms the basis of measurement.

## Basic measurement properties of psychometric instruments

Some of the basic indicators to be considered when evaluating the accuracy of any assay, including psychometric rating scales, are precision, reliability, validity, and standardization [2–5]. A high level of reliability is a prerequisite for validity.

### Precision

The ability of an instrument to produce a particular type of measurement is of paramount importance. The precision of an instrument, its capacity to detect small differences, is constrained by its level of measurement. Four levels of measurement are generally used in describing the precision of a variable: (1) nominal, (2) ordinal, (3) interval, and (4) ratio. Categorical data may be either nominal or ordinal, depending on whether an order is imposed on the categories. Nominal data simply classifies subjects (eg, male-female is a nominal scaling classification). In ordinal data, the subjects are ranked but it is not possible to assume any consistent distance between the ranks. For example, if one were to divide the spectrum of symptom severity into three stages (mild, moderate, and severe), the distance between mild and moderate may not be equivalent to the distance between moderate and severe. The use of interval and ratio measurements, however, introduces the concept of continuous measurement, a level of precision at which one may assume that adjacent points on the measurement scale are equidistant. The primary difference between interval and ratio measurements is the presence of a meaningful zero, which indicates a complete absence of the construct. Most psychometric instruments rely on interval-level measurement (eg, when assessing the psychosocial burden of psoriasis, a patient may be asked to rate the degree to which the cosmetic impact of the psoriasis bothers them, using a five-point scale, ranging from "very little" to "all the time"). Because the lowest measure on the scale is not truly indicative of a complete absence of the construct, this is an interval measure. Clinical measures related to duration (eg, "how long have you had the disorder?") or size (eg, "what is the size of the lesion?") are ratio-level measures, because a zero represents a complete absence of the construct.

The precision of a variable provided in a questionnaire is an important consideration, because of the fact that it determines the types of statistics that may be done on the measure. Nominal data may only be described by frequencies, because any ordering of categories is wholly arbitrary. Ordinal data may be described by frequencies or by a median. Both interval-level and ratio-level measurements may be described using means, medians, modes, and standard deviations, but only ratio-level measurements may be expressed multiplicatively. This means that it is not appropriate to express one interval-level measurement as a multiple of another [4]. For example, if the pretreatment score on an interval-level quality of life scale is 6 out of 10 and the posttreatment score is 9 out of 10, one cannot infer that the 3 point or 50% improvement in scores indicates a 50% improvement in the quality of life.

### Reliability

Reliability refers to the extent to which a variable may be demonstrated to be measured in a reproducible fashion, or the extent to which the results measuring a stable variable may be relied on to be the same on each subsequent administration. Unfortunately, there is no gold standard for reliability that is appropriate for all testing situations; the measure of reliability on which a good instrument selection decision is based varies according to the purpose for which the instrument is intended. Reliability is generally assessed using one of four methods: (1) test-retest reliability, (2) parallel forms reliability, (3) internal consistency reliability, and (4) interrater reliability.

For the demonstration of temporal reliability (ie, stability across time, provided the subjects have not changed), one needs to look for the test-retest reliability of a measure, a statistic that assesses the extent to which two separate administrations of the same measure are significantly correlated. Test-retest reliability may be raised artifactually if the time between testing periods is too short and there is a carryover effect because the subject remembers the responses from the original testing session. For situations in which this carryover effect is likely, it is often preferable to use parallel forms reliability, where equivalent or parallel forms of items are constructed and subjects take an entirely separate test for the retest.

Another common form of reliability analysis is internal consistency, usually measured with Cronbach's alpha (sometimes called coefficient alpha). The desirability of internal consistency reliability is based on the proposition that if one item is measuring a variable, then the other items must be consistent with this measurement if they are to be considered to be measuring the same variable. Conversely, some psychometricians have argued that if all items are highly intercorrelated (ie, highly consistent), that provides no new information, arguing that the ideal test should have items that do not correlate strongly with each other but correlate strongly with the criterion under study. In practice, the truth probably lies somewhere between these two extremes. For measures that have a single, unitary construct, a measure of internal consistency is useful. For measures that are multidimensional, or for measures that use single-item measurements of content domains within the general construct, measures of internal consistency are inappropriate, unless used to demonstrate the homogeneity of the measure's subscales [5,6]. It has been suggested [5,6] that a coefficient alpha of greater than 0.70 is necessary to demonstrate that a measure is assessing a single construct.

To increase the discriminating power of a test, it may be desirable to have several items that address a wide range of concepts within the construct. This usually reduces the item intercorrelations, and thereby the internal consistency of the scale. For example, when assessing the impact of a skin disorder on socialization, a scale with five items that address the impact of the disorder on social interactions with (1) the spouse or partner, (2) friends, (3) family, (4) strangers, and (5) the workplace is likely to have greater discriminating power but less internal consistency that a scale with two items that address the impact of the disorder on social interactions in the home and outside the home. What this implies is that when a test is constructed, one has to decide the degree to which its discriminating power is important, because this is usually achieved at the cost of internal consistency. This is one area that needs to be addressed carefully in dermatology, because a scale with a reduced discriminating power may be insensitive to important improvements following treatment.

For evaluations that involve the use of subjective measures administered by multiple raters, it is advisable to assess the extent to which all raters are measuring the same thing, through the measurement of interrater reliability. This is an important consideration for most clinical settings. There are a variety of statistical methods for assessing this form of reliability, but the most common methods are Pearson's correlation coefficient (for continuous, interval-level measurements) and Cohen's kappa (for categorical, nominal-level measurements).

*Validity*

A test is valid if it measures what it purports to measure. There are a variety of ways of demonstrating the validity of a test. In general, one is most concerned with construct validity, which assesses the extent to which a measurement tool manages accurately to capture all relevant aspects of a particular construct. Unfortunately, there is no construct validity coefficient; estimates of construct validity are arrived at through the careful application of psychometric methodology and by comparing empirical evidence with expectations derived from the theory underlying the construct.

In identifying the construct validity of a measure one is primarily concerned with the concordance between the theoretical underpinnings of the questionnaire, and the items in that measure. The most direct testing of construct validity is accomplished through the known-groups method, or through the calculation of convergent and discriminant validity coefficients. With the known-groups method, one is primarily interested in demonstrating that there are systematic differences between groups of individuals with known levels of a construct. For example, in a clinical study of the impact of treatment on the quality of life of the psoriasis patient, one might create two distinct groups: one in which the psoriasis patients are receiving the treatment, and one in which they are not. The demonstration of construct validity is accomplished by showing that the treatment group has more favorable quality of life scores (assuming, of course, that one expects treatment to improve the quality of life) than the control group. Convergent and discriminant validity rely on more specific predictions. For convergent validity, one demonstrates a correlation (positive or negative) between variables that one expects to be correlated, based on theory. For example, one might expect a positive correlation between a quality of life measure, and a measure of earned income. For discriminant validity, one demonstrates a null correlation between variables that should not be correlated (eg, one might expect a null correlation between overall quality of life score, and whether or not the patient uses corrective lenses).

Other tests of validity that are frequently encountered include face validity and content validity. Face validity is concerned with clinical sensibility of the test items [7,8], specifically if the items of the test seem to be measuring the variables they are supposed to be measuring. Typically, face validity is considered to be the weakest form of validity, because it does not explicitly speak to the actual accuracy of a measure, but rather its apparent utility. Under some circumstances, however, face validity can become important in clinical evaluation, particularly for the purpose of reassuring participants that the questions being asked as part of a survey are not frivolous, but rather are reflective of bona fide areas of concern within the disorder. Content validity is often evaluated in a manner similar to that of face validity investigations, but the goal is subtly different. With content validity, one is most concerned with the extent to which all facets of a construct are represented within an instrument. In practice, content validity is ensured by having experts in the field evaluate an item pool, to determine whether it represents an accurate and comprehensive coverage of the construct.

*Standardization*

If the purpose for using a psychometric instrument is to eliminate some of the subjectivity involved in a clinical evaluation, the instrument should demonstrate some evidence of standardization. Through standardization, it is possible to compare a patient's score with that of the general population, or other relevant patient groups. One crucial aspect of standardization is sampling (ie, the sample that is used to generate the normative scores should be representative of the target population, and should be sufficiently large to produce a reasonable standard error of the normative data). A second important component of standardization involves a description of the experimenter-participant interaction. This should be evident through the presentation of standard testing protocols within the scoring manual that specifically outline the instructions given to participants, and the procedures that one is required to follow throughout the administration of the test.

## Power analysis considerations and choice of instrument

The power of a study is the probability that it demonstrates a difference between groups when the null hypothesis is, in fact, false [9]. The two most important considerations in maximizing power are sample size (ie, the number of participants that one is testing) and effect size. Effect size refers to the degree to which the phenomenon is present in the population (eg, the size of relationship, or the magnitude of the difference between groups). The larger the effect size, the greater the power of the test (alpha value or significance criterion and sample size being equal). Similarly, the larger the effect size (significance criterion and desired power being equal), the smaller the sample necessary to detect it. This is particularly relevant to one's choice of clinical instrument when considering a very specific area of a clinical construct as one must choose the instrument that produces the largest effect size. This is usually accomplished by selecting an instrument that is sufficiently reliable to produce consistent results, and sufficiently precise to make fine distinctions within a construct.

## Summary

The need for evidence-based medicine has necessitated the use of standardized rating scales and assessment of abstract and multidimensional constructs, such as the quality of life. This has resulted, in the past decade, in the publication of large numbers of rating scales that assess the psychosocial burden of dermatologic disorders. It is important for the clinician to consider some of the basic psychometric properties of these rating scales, such as reliability, validity, standardization, and discriminatory ability, before choosing a particular scale. Careful attention to these parameters increases the statistical power (ie, the probability of rejecting the null hypothesis when it is false) of the studies that use these tests to evaluate treatment outcomes.

## References

[1] Chren M, Weinstock MA. Conceptual issues in measuring the burden of skin diseases. J Investig Dermatol Symp Proc 2004;9:97–100.
[2] DeVellis RF. Scale development: theory and applications. Newbury Park (CA): SAGE Publications; 1991.
[3] Kline P. A handbook of test construction: introduction to psychometric design. New York: Methuen; 1986.
[4] Portney LG, Watkins MP. Foundations of clinical research: applications to practice. 2nd edition. Upper Saddle River (NJ): Prentice Hall Health; 2000.
[5] Pedhazur EJ, Schmelkin LP. Measurement, design, and analysis: an integrated approach. Hillsdale (NJ): Lawrence Erlbaum Associates; 1991.
[6] Streiner DL. Being inconsistent about consistency: when coefficient alpha does and doesn't matter. J Pers Assess 2003;80:217–22.
[7] Gill TM, Feinstein AR. A critical appraisal of the quality of quality-of-life measurements. JAMA 1994;272: 619–26.
[8] Guyatt GH, Feeny DH, Patrick DL. Measuring health-related quality of life. Ann Intern Med 1993;118:622–9.
[9] Cohen J. Statistical power analysis for the behavioral sciences. New York: Academic Press; 1977.

# A Critical Review of Quality-of-Life Scales for Psoriasis

Victoria J. Lewis, BMedSci, MBBS, MRCP,
Andrew Y. Finlay, MBBS, FRCP*

*Department of Dermatology, Wales College of Medicine, Cardiff University, Heath Park, Cardiff CF14 4XN, UK*

Psoriasis, in addition to causing significant physical morbidity in some patients, also can have a major impact on their lives in psychologic and practical ways. A study of 17,000 patients who had psoriasis [1] demonstrated this, revealing that many patients who had psoriasis believed that their physician was not aggressive enough with therapy.

For day-to-day management of these patients, and for research into psoriasis, quality-of-life measures may be practical and useful tools. Their use may allow clinicians to make more informed choices regarding the effects of therapy and other health service research measures on their patients.

When faced with the myriad of general and disease-specific measures of quality of life currently used, it is difficult for clinicians to choose the most appropriate and most powerful measure. This article outlines all health-related quality-of-life measures that are used in psoriasis and critically evaluates their use, hoping to provide readers with a straightforward and robust guide for reference.

## An outline of quality-of-life measures

### General health-related quality-of-life measures

#### Short Form 36

The Short Form 36 (SF-36) consists of 36 items that measure 8 broad topics as listed in Box 1 [2,3]. There is an additional question on change in respondents' health in the past year. For each variable, the items are converted into a scale from 0 (worst health state) to 100 (best health state).

#### Sickness Impact Profile assessment

The Sickness Impact Profile (SIP) is a broadly based assessment of performance of daily activities [4]. One hundred thirty-six individual statements relating to daily activities can be agreed or disagreed with by patients. These are grouped into 7 main categories and 5 subcategories (Box 2).

#### General Health Questionnaire

The General Health Questionnaire (GHQ) is a self-administered screening questionnaire [5]. There are 60-, 30-, 28-, and 12-item versions. The 12- and 28-item versions are used for skin conditions. The 28-item version has 4 subscales (Box 3).

#### Nottingham Health Profile

The Nottingham Health Profile (NHP) consists of 38 statements combined to form six scales reflecting health problems, such as physical mobility and pain, and seven other statements about areas of daily life affected most often by health [6]. A weighting formula is applied to the tick-box answers.

### Dermatology-specific quality-of-life measures

#### Dermatology Life Quality Index

The Dermatology Life Quality Index (DLQI) consists of 10 questions concerning symptoms and feelings, daily activities, leisure, work and school, personal relationships, and treatment [7,8].

Each question is answered by a tick box: not at all, a little, a lot, or very much. Each answer is scored

---

Prof. Finley is joint copyright owner of PDI, DLQI, and CDLQI. His department gains income from their use.
* Corresponding author.
*E-mail address:* finlayay@cf.ac.uk (A.Y. Finlay).

> **Box 1. SF-36**
>
> 1. Physical functioning (10 items)
> 2. Social functioning (2 items)
> 3. Role limitations resulting from physical problems (4 items)
> 4. Role limitations resulting from emotional problems (3 items)
> 5. Mental health (5 items)
> 6. Energy and vitality (4 items)
> 7. Pain (2 items)
> 8. General perception of health (5 items)
>
> *Data from* Jenkinson C, Coulter A, Wright L. Short form 36 (SF-36) health survey questionnaire: normative data for adults of working age. BMJ 1993;306:1437–40; and Garratt AM, Ruta DA, Abdalla MI, et al. The SF36 health survey questionnaire: an outcome measure suitable for routine clinical use within the NHS? BMJ 1993;306:1440–4.

from 0 to 3 and the scores summed, giving a range from 0 (no impairment of life quality) to 30 (maximum impairment). All questions relate to "the last week." DLQI was designed for use in adults over age 16.

> **Box 2. SIP**
>
> 1. Physical: ambulation
>    A. Mobility
>    B. Body care and movement
> 2. Psychosocial: social interaction
>    A. Alertness behavior
>    B. Emotional behavior
>    C. Communication
> 3. Sleep and rest
> 4. Eating
> 5. Work
> 6. Home management
> 7. Recreation and pastimes
>
> *Data from* Bergner M, Bobbitt RA, Carter WB, et al. The Sickness Impact Profile: development and final revision of a health status measure. Med Care 1981;19:787–805.

> **Box 3. GHQ**
>
> 1. Somatic symptoms
> 2. Anxiety and insomnia
> 3. Social dysfunction
> 4. Severe depression
>
> *Data from* Goldberg DP, Hillier VF. A scale version of the General Health Questionnaire. Psychol Med 1979;9:139–45.

*Children's Dermatology Life Quality Index*

The Children's Dermatology Life Quality Index (CDLQI) is the children's version of the DLQI and consists of a similar format of questions and the same scoring system. Text [9] and cartoon [10] versions of this are described: the cartoon version is completed more quickly by children than the text-only version and is preferred by them.

*Skindex*

Skindex initially was described as a 61-item questionnaire, with 8 scales (Box 4), each addressing a specific effect of the respondents' skin disease [11]. Each item is scored from 0 (no effect) to 100 (maximum effect). Questions relate to "the last 4 weeks." Revision of Skindex in 1997 produced a 29-item version [12], and this was shortened again in 2001 to a 16-item one-page version [13], which proved easier for respondents to use.

*Dermatology quality-of-life scales*

The Dermatology Quality of Life Scales (DQOLS) complements the DLQI by placing greater emphasis

> **Box 4. Skindex**
>
> 1. Cognitive effects
> 2. Social effects
> 3. Depression
> 4. Fear
> 5. Embarrassment
> 6. Anger
> 7. Physical discomfort
> 8. Physical limitations
>
> *Data from* Chren MM, Lasek RJ, Quinn LM, et al. Skindex, a quality of life measure for patients with skin disease: reliability, validity and responsiveness. J Invest Dermatol 1996;107:707–13.

on the psychosocial domain [14]. Each item is scored on a 5-point scale (from *very slightly or not at all*, *a little*, *moderately*, *quite a bit*, to *extremely*). Items are grouped into 4 psychosocial and 4 activities subscales (Box 5).

*German Instrument for the Assessment of Quality of Life in Skin Diseases*

The German Instrument for the Assessment of Quality of Life in Skin Diseases (DIELH) consists of 36 quality-of-life questions in 7 domains (Box 6) [15,16]. Each question is scored on a tick-box system: 0 (not applicable), 1 (not at all), and 5 (very much). The maximum score is 180.

*Dermatology Specific Quality of Life*

The Dermatology Specific Quality of Life (DSQL) is a 52- or 53-item questionnaire (52 for atopic dermatitis, 53 for acne) [17]. It consists of five scales, reflecting the frequency of limitations from skin disease. It also consists of two scales of the SF-36 and eight global items, which focus on the intensity of limitations and the ratings of satisfaction.

*Psoriasis-specific quality-of-life measures*

*Psoriasis Disability Index*

The Psoriasis Disability Index (PDI) consists of a series of 15 questions related to daily activities, work, or school; personal relationships; leisure; and treat-

---

**Box 5. DQOLS**

*Psychosocial subscales*

1. Embarrassment
2. Despair
3. Irritableness
4. Distress

*Activities subscales*

1. Everyday
2. Summer
3. Social
4. Sexual

*Data from* Morgan M, McCreedy R, Simpson J, et al. Dermatology quality of life scales – a measure of the impact of skin disease. Br J Dermatol 1997;136:202–6.

---

**Box 6. DIELH**

1. Symptoms
2. Psychosocial
3. Daily living
4. Work/school
5. Leisure time
6. Personal relationships
7. Treatment/therapy

*Data from* Schafer T, Staudt A, Ring J. Development of the German scale for assessing quality of life in skin diseases. Hautarzt 2001;52:492–8; and Schafer T, Staudt A, Ring J. German instrument for the assessment of quality of life in skin diseases (DIELH). Internal consistency, reliability, convergent and discriminant validity and responsiveness. Hautarzt 2001;52:624–8.

---

ment [18–20]. All of the questions relate to the past 4 weeks. The PDI can be scored on a visual analog scale of 1 to 7, producing a score range of 15 to 105. If the total PDI is expressed as a percentage, the scores should be converted first to a range of 0 to 90 and the score out of 90 converted to a percentage.

The 15 questions were published in a revised version in 1995 [19], when a choice of two scoring systems (visual analog scale or tick box) was introduced. For the visual analog scale and for the tick-box scoring systems, the higher the score, the greater the disability. The tick-box system is scored from 0 to 3 per question, producing a range of 0 to 45. The standard answer choice for each question is 3 (very much), 2 (a lot), 1 (a little), and 0 (not at all). Scores using both methods should be expressed as percentages to provide equivalence for comparative purposes.

*Psoriasis Life Stress Inventory*

The Psoriasis Life Stress Inventory (PLSI) consists of 15 items, measuring the social impact of psoriasis and the effect of others' behavior toward respondents' appearance [21]. Each item is scored on a 4-point scale: 3 (a great deal); 2 (moderate degree); 1 (slight degree); and 0 (not at all). The overall score is from 0 to 45, with a higher rating indicating higher stress. A score greater than 10 is believed to indicate greater overall psoriasis severity. The questions relate to the previous month.

*Salford Psoriasis Index*

The Salford Psoriasis Index (SPI) [22] comprises 3 individually scored measures (Box 7). The 3-item signs, psychosocial disability, and interventions follow the same concept as the tumor/nodes/metastasis classification used for cancer staging.

*Psoriasis Index of Quality of Life*

The Psoriasis Index of Quality of Life (PSOR-IQol) consists of 25 negative statements intended to assess the impact of physical disability on psychologic and social problems in psoriasis [23]. Respondents score 1 point for every negative statement they agree with. The final score is between 0 and 25, a higher score indicating greater psychologic impact of the respondents' psoriasis.

*Utility measures*

These assess the hypothetic value placed by people on their health and are qualititative expressions of preference for potential health states.

*The Quality Adjusted Life Year*

The Quality Adjusted Life Year (QALY) can be used for health-care allocation [24]. One year of perfect health-life expectancy is taken as 1, but 1 year of less than perfect health-life expectancy is less than 1. Therefore, calculation of QALY can express the relative cost-effectiveness of different therapies. This concept has been applied to acne [25].

*Willingness to pay*

One example of this approach is to ask patients how much they are prepared to pay for a cure for their skin condition. When information about their disposable income is taken into account, a more meaningful measure is produced. This approach is used for acne [26], psoriasis [19,27], and atopic eczema [28].

*Time trade-off*

This can be measured in several ways, including asking the length of time that patients are prepared to spend treating their skin each day if it results in normal skin. Alternatively, patients may be asked to choose between living with their skin condition for the remainder of their lives or selecting a shorter life span in perfect health. Questions about time trade-off have been used in psoriasis [19,27,29] and atopic eczema [28].

*Others*

A comparison with other chronic conditions also is used [19] in cases where a choice between two alternatives is offered (a standard gamble) [24]. This comparison is important particularly in psoriasis, where utility measures are used to make decisions to use methotrexate, when its side effects and psoriasis severity are taken into account [29].

## A critical review of quality-of-life measures

Articles and abstracts in which all the quality-of-life measures are used are identified by searching *MEDLINE* and PubMed up to December 2004. All measures are summarized in Table 1.

*General health-related quality-of-life measures*

*Short Form 36*

The SF-36 originally was validated by being sent to a large normal population and to people who had specific illnesses [2,3]. Internal consistency was high (Cronbach's alpha 0.76–0.9). Further analysis [3] of specific illness groups use factor analysis for adjustment of age, gender, and socioeconomic status.

The SF-36 has been used in more than 200 studies of quality of life in a variety of diseases, nine of which are dermatologic. It is used in parallel with the DLQI, CDLQI, Skindex, and PDI and compared

---

**Box 7. SPI**

1. Signs: scores are converted from the Psoriasis Assessment and Severity Index (PASI) measurement to a scale of 0 to 10.
2. Psychosocial disability: a visual analog scale of 0 to 10 measuring the effect of psoriasis on the respondent's day-to-day life at the time of assessment, where 0 means not at all affected and 10 means completely affected.
3. Interventions: extra points added for historical disease severity, relating to systemic therapies, inpatient admissions, and episodes of erythroderma.

*Data from* Kirby B, Fortune DG, Bhushan M, et al. The Salford Psoriasis Index: an holistic measure of psoriasis severity. Br J Dermatol 2000;142:728–32.

Table 1
A summary of quality of life measures used in dermatology

| Quality of life measure | No. of studies (dermatology) | No. of skin diseases studied | Comparison with other relevant outcome measures | First author, year [Ref.] |
|---|---|---|---|---|
| **General health-related** | | | | |
| SF36 | >200 (29) | 9 | DLQI, CDLQI, Skindex, PDI, PASI | Jenkinson et al, 1993 [2] |
| SIP | >2000 (3) | 2 | PDI, PASI | Bergner et al, 1981 [4] |
| GHQ | >1500 (31) | 6 | PASI, DLQI, Skindex, PDI, PLSI, DQOLS | Goldberg et al, 1979 [5] |
| NHP | >600 (8) | 4 | DLQI | Hunt et al, 1989 [6] |
| **Dermatology-specific** | | | | |
| DLQI | 95 | 35 | SF-36, SIP, GHQ-28, PGI, NHP, CESD-10, APSEA, AQOLS, CADI, LAIS, PDI, PDS, PQOL | Finlay et al, 1994 [7] |
| CDLQI | 13 | 11 | SF-36, CLQI, FDI, SCORAD, EASI | Lewis-Jones et al, 1995 [9] |
| Skindex | 31 | 15 | GHQ-12, DLQI, PDI, PLSI, PASI, SCORAD | Chren et al, 1996; 1997; 2001 [11–13] |
| DQOLS | 5 | >2 | SF-36, NHP, DLQI | Morgan et al, 1997 [14] |
| DIELH | 3 | >14 | DLQI, SF-36 | Shafer et al, 2001 [15] |
| DSQL | 4 | 2 | — | Anderson et al, 1997 [17] |
| **Psoriasis-specific** | | | | |
| PDI | 31 | 1 | SF-36, GHQ-12, SIP, EQ-5D, CESD-10, HADS, PLSI, SPI, PASI | Finlay et al, 1987; 1995 [18,19] |
| PLSI | 8 | 1 | SF-36, DLQI, Skindex-29, PDI, PASI | Gupta et al, 1995 [21] |
| SPI | 3 | 1 | HADS, PDI, PASI, IPQ | Kirby et al, 2000 [22] |
| PSORIQoL | 1 | 1 | DLQI, GWBI | McKenna et al, 2003 [23] |

*Abbreviations:* APSEA, Assessment of the Psychological and Social Effects of Acne; AQOLS, Acne Quality of Life Scale; CADI, Cardiff Acne Disability Index; CESD, Center for Epidemiological Studies Depression Scale; CLQI, Children's Life Quality Index; EASI, Eczema Assessment of Severity Index; EQ, EuroQol; FDI, Family Dermatitis Index; GWBI, General Well-Being Index; HADS, Hospital Anxiety and Depression Scale; IPQ, Illness Perception Questionnaire; LAIS, Life Activity Impairment Score; PDS, Physicians Disease Severity; PGI, Patient General Index; PSORIQoL, Psoriasis Quality of Life Questionnaire.

directly with PASI scores, showing significant correlation [30]. Its use in dermatology is most appropriate for comparison of skin conditions with other systemic diseases. In conditions where a small area of affected skin can cause marked impairment of function, however, such as hand dermatitis, the SF-36 is considered a better measure of mental health than other dermatology-specific quality-of-life measures [31].

### Sickness Impact Profile

The SIP was designed to be applicable broadly across a wide range of types and severities of illness and across demographic and cultural subgroups [4]. Its initial design was validated by a high test-retest reliability ($r = 0.92$) and internal consistency ($r = 0.94$). It also was tested for its clinical validity against clinical measures in the categories of hip replacement, hyperthyroidism, and rheumatoid arthritis.

In more than 20 years, over 2000 articles have been published describing the use of the SIP in a broad range of diseases. Its validity in psoriasis is assessed by Finlay and coworkers [32], who showed that scores correlated well with PDI but not with PASI scores. Therefore, it can be considered an appropriate tool to compare the disability experienced by psoriatic patients with that of patients suffering from other systemic diseases.

### General Health Questionnaire

The GHQ is aimed at detecting diagnosable psychiatric disorders [5]. The 28- and 12-item versions are used in dermatology, the 12-item version is used in a general dermatology clinic setting [33], and the 28- item version is used in patients who have port-wine stains [34] or psoriasis [35].

### Nottingham Health Profile

The NHP originally was designed for the survey of population health problems but also is used to evaluate the outcome of medical or social intervention [6]. It has been used for patients who have leg ulcers [36] and urticaria [37]. It can be used in clinical practice, for example, as an adjunct to clinical interviews. The items of the scales represent severe problems, so is less suited to patients who have more minor health problems.

*Dermatology-specific quality-of-life measures*

*Dermatology Life Quality Index*

The DLQI was the first dermatology-specific, health-related, quality-of-life questionnaire published [7,8]. There now are more than 10 years' experience, with 95 articles describing its use. It is used in published research in more than 17 countries and translated into 21 languages. It also assesses at least 35 skin conditions.

It initially was validated by comparison with a normal population, where it shows a high specificity, and shows high repeatability and internal consistency scores (Cronbach's alpha scores 0.83–0.93). It also is used in parallel with seven other dermatology-specific measures and with seven general health measures. Its sensitivity to change is confirmed in 44 studies in 11 diseases and in seven different health service research settings [8]. An illustrated version of the DLQI is evaluated [38], but it is not possible to demonstrate exact equivalence to the text-only version.

*Children's Dermatology Life Quality Index*

The CDLQI has been used in 13 studies in 11 types of skin disease, particularly in children who had atopic eczema, and eight studies also assessed its impact on their families [9,10]. It was validated by comparing it with a normal population and also by demonstrating acceptable repeatability on test-retest analysis. Further validation included using the CDLQI across the spectrum of skin disease and demonstrating strong correlation with the Children's Life Quality Index, a generic measure of chronic illness [39].

The cartoon and text version of the CDLQI is equivalent to the previously validated text-only CDLQI version but is faster and easier to use and is preferred by children and parents [10].

*Skindex*

The design of Skindex was validated by demonstration of a high degree of internal consistency (Cronbach's alpha 0.76–0.86) and a high test-retest coefficient (Pearson's coefficient 0.68–0.9) [11–13]. The revised Skindex-29 and Skindex-16 versions also proved to have high test-retest reliability ($r = 0.8$–80.9) and internal consistency (Cronbach's alpha 0.86–0.93) [13].

Skindex is used in more than 15 skin diseases in eight countries. It is used in parallel with physical measures of skin disease, such as PASI scores and Scoring in Atopic Dermatitis (SCORAD). It also has been used alongside four other quality-of-life measures.

*Dermatology Quality of Life Scales*

The DQOLS was developed to assess the impact of skin conditions on patients' psychosocial state and everyday activities, aiming to assess "bother" from skin disease [14]. In its construction it showed high internal consistency (Cronbach's alpha–psychosocial scale, 0.92; –activity scale, 0.83) and test-retest values (range of $r = 0.66$–0.86).

Although first tested on a broad range of skin conditions, further studies have concentrated on only acne and psoriasis, with recent published trials of biologic therapies in psoriasis using this method of evaluation [40].

*German Instrument for the Assessment of Quality of Life in Skin Diseases*

The DIELH initially was validated by testing it on 110 unselected dermatology outpatients [15,16]. Internal consistency was high (Cronbach's alpha 0.71–0.91) as was test-retest reliability ($r = 0.73$–0.86). It was compared with the DLQI and SF-36. Correlation was high with the DLQI but not with the SF-36.

*Dermatology Specific Quality of Life*

The DSQL initially was tested on patients who had acne and contact dermatitis who were enrolled in clinical trials [17]. The scales were found to have high internal consistency (0.7 to >0.9) and test-retest reliability ($r = 0.81$–0.89). The DSQI showed a moderately high level of correlation with global ratings of bothersome symptoms and overall disease severity. Sensitivity to change has not been tested.

*Psoriasis-specific quality-of-life measures*

*Psoriasis Disability Index*

The PDI was constructed by analysis of a group of patients who had chronic plaque psoriasis, focusing on which specific questions, on factor analysis, correlated best with disability and symptoms [18–20]. No other validation was performed in its construction. It since has been used for almost 20 years, however, with 31 published articles describing its use. It is used in parallel with seven dermatology-specific and general health measures and also in

Table 2
Measures of validity

| Quality of life measure | Reliability | | Validity: construct |
|---|---|---|---|
| | Internal consistency | Test–retest | |
| **General health-related** | | | |
| SF-36 | Cronbach alpha 0.76–0.9 | NR | Comparison with normal population<br>Comparison with other dermatologic QoL and PASI scores |
| SIP | $r = 0.94$ | $r = 0.92$ | Comparison with 4 other conditions<br>Comparison with PDI and PASI scores |
| GHQ | NR | NR | Comparison with DLQI, Skindex, and PDI |
| NHP | NR | NR | Comparison with normal elderly population and those with chronic disease<br>Comparison with DLQI and DQOLS |
| **Dermatology-specific** | | | |
| DLQI | Cronbach alpha 0.83–0.93 | Overall $r = 0.99$ $P < 0.0001$ Individual questions $r = 0.95–0.98$ $P < 0.001$ | Comparisons with 100 normal controls and 200 general dermatology patients<br>Comparison with general and dermatology-specific quality of life measures and PASI scores, and with psychological measures<br>Demonstration of sensitivity to change with treatment and in health service research |
| CDLQI | NR | $r = 0.86$ $P < 0.0001$ | Comparison with 47 normal controls and 55 general paediatric clinic attendees, plus 233 general paediatric dermatology attenders<br>Comparison with CLQI |
| Skindex | Cronbach alpha 0.76–0.86 | $r = 0.68–0.9$ | Comparison between patients with inflammatory dermatoses and those with isolated lesions<br>Comparison with clinician: judged severity<br>Demonstration of sensitivity to change |
| DQOLS | Cronbach alpha Psychosocial: 0.92 Activity: 0.83 | $r = 0.66–0.86$ | Comparison between a range of skin diseases<br>Demonstration of sensitivity to change |
| DIELH | Cronbach alpha 0.71–0.91 | $r = 0.73–0.86$ | Comparison with general and dermatology-specific quality of life scales<br>Demonstration of sensitivity to change with treatment |
| DSQL | Cronbach alpha 0.7 to >0.9 | $r = 0.81–0.89$ | Comparison with global rating of bothersome symptoms and overall disease severity<br>Comparison of a range of skin diseases |
| **Psoriasis-specific** | | | |
| PDI | NR | NR | Comparison with general and dermatology-specific quality of life measures, PASI scores, and with psychologic measures<br>Demonstration of sensitivity to change |
| PLSI | Cronbach alpha 0.9 | NR | Comparison with other dermatology-specific and psychologic measures |
| SPI | NR | NR | Comparison with other dermatology-specific quality of life measures<br>Demonstration of sensitivity to change with treatment |
| PQOL | Cronbach alpha 0.94 | $r = 0.89$ | Comparison of different areas of the body with psoriasis |

*Abbreviations:* CDLQI, Children's Dermatology Life Quality Index; DLQI, Dermatology Life Quality Index; DQOLS, Dermatology Quality of Life Scales; NR, not recorded; PQOL, Psoriasis Quality of Life Questionnaire.

conjunction with four physical measures of psoriasis, in particular PASI scores.

It also has been used alongside psychologic measures of disability in 12 studies and in a primary and secondary care setting. It demonstrates sensitivity to change in 15 studies relating to treatment outcomes and five studies relating to health service research. It is used in published research in 20 countries and translated into 13 languages [20].

*Psoriasis Life Stress Inventory*

The PLSI was designed to obtain an index of the stress associated with having to cope with a variety of psoriasis-related events [21]. It was constructed by questioning psoriasis patients about specific events and asking them to assess the physical appearance and symptoms of their skin. A high degree of internal consistency was found within the items (Cronbach's alpha 0.9). It also was found that groups who had high PLSI (ie, $\geq 10$) also had a greater overall severity of psoriasis and greater psoriasis severity in body regions that led to the greatest cosmetic disfigurement.

The PLSI is used alongside the SF-36 and PDI, in addition to other psychologic measures. It shows comparability with PASI scores. It also is used to assess patients suffering from psoriatic arthritis [41].

*Salford Psoriasis Index*

The SPI was designed to incorporate current clinical extent of psoriasis, psychosocial disability, and past severity based on treatment history, taking a more holistic approach when determining psoriasis severity [22]. It had high reproducibility and was able to demonstrate sensitivity to change on its first construction. The Psychosocial Impact Score correlated strongly with the PDI but correlated poorly with clinical extent scores, such as the PASI.

*Psoriasis Index of Quality of Life*

Initial evaluation of the PSORIQoL demonstrated a high test-retest reliability ($r = 0.89$) and high internal consistency (Crohnbach's alpha 0.94), higher than that of the DLQI [23]. It was designed primarily for use in clinical trials in psoriasis. No publications, however, demonstrate its sensitivity to change or comparison with other psoriasis-specific quality-of-life measures.

**Which measure to use?**

In choosing which quality-of-life measure to use in psoriasis, first consider the reason for its use. This could be for clinical, research, audit, or financial purposes. If psoriasis is to be compared with other nondermatologic disease, a general health-related quality-of-life questionnaire is appropriate. If it is to be compared with other skin conditions, a dermatology-specific quality-of-life measure is likely to produce a more sensitive and meaningful comparison.

When deciding on a quality-of-life instrument to use, it is important to be aware of how reliable it is, in terms of its initial validation, and the spectrum of its subsequent use. Reliability and sensitivity to change are specific aspects of the instrument to be considered. A summary of the measures of validity for the individual instruments is contained in Table 2. Several reviews also consider this aspect [42–44].

When assessing sensitivity to change, the time context over which the questionnaire is based is fundamental. For example, a questionnaire relating to the past 4 weeks should not be readministered until a further 4 weeks has elapsed.

It also is useful to consider the setting in which the questionnaire is used. A postal survey or busy clinic gains a higher response rate when using a short, simply constructed questionnaire. If research staff are present, however, a longer, more detailed questionnaire with more complex scoring can be used. This setting allows researchers to choose the most powerful and appropriate instrument for their studies.

If the language required is different from that of the original questionnaire design and is administered in a different cultural setting, revalidation of a translated questionnaire is required. Some of the quality-of-life instruments are validated already in a number of languages.

Utility measures (discussed previously) may be most appropriate, for political and financial reasons, to represent burden of disease. They can be used alone or in combination with other health-related quality-of-life measures, and their use is increasing [45].

In conclusion, instruments designed for the measurement of quality-of-life in psoriasis are numerous and variable. This article aims to summarize these in a logical order and to guide researchers or clinicians in choosing the instrument that is most appropriate to their research.

**References**

[1] Kreuger G, Koo J, Lebwohl M, et al. The impact of psoriasis on quality of life: results of a 1998 National Psoriasis Foundation patient-membership survey. Arch Dermatol 2001;58:280–4.

[2] Jenkinson C, Coulter A, Wright L. Short form 36

(SF-36) health survey questionnaire: normative data for adults of working age. BMJ 1993;306:1437–40.
[3] Garratt AM, Ruta DA, Abdalla MI, et al. The SF36 health survey questionnaire: an outcome measure suitable for routine clinical use within the NHS? BMJ 1993;306:1440–4.
[4] Bergner M, Bobbitt RA, Carter WB, et al. The Sickness Impact Profile: development and final revision of a health status measure. Med Care 1981;19:787–805.
[5] Goldberg DP, Hillier VF. A scale version of the General Health Questionnaire. Psychol Med 1979;9:139–45.
[6] Hunt SM, McKenna SP. The Nottingham Health Profile User's Manual. Manchester: Galen Research and Consultancy; 1989.
[7] Finlay AY, Khan GK. Dermatology Life Quality Index (DLQI): a simple practical measure for routine clinical use. Clin Exp Dermatol 1994;19:210–6.
[8] Lewis VJ, Finlay AY. Ten years experience of the Dermatology Life Quality Index. J Invest Dermatol Symp Proc 2004;9:169–80.
[9] Lewis-Jones MS, Finlay AY. The Children's Dermatology Life Quality Index (CDLQI): initial validation and practical use. Br J Dermatol 1995;132:942–9.
[10] Holme SA, Man I, Sharp JL, et al. The Children's Dermatology Life Quality Index: validation of the cartoon version. Br J Dermatol 2003;148:285–90.
[11] Chren MM, Lasek RJ, Quinn LM, et al. Skindex, a quality of life measure for patients with skin disease: reliability, validity and responsiveness. J Invest Dermatol 1996;107:707–13.
[12] Chren MM, Lasek RJ, Flocke SA, et al. Improved discriminative and evaluative capability of a refined version of Skindex, a quality-of-life instrument for patients with skin disease. Arch Dermatol 1997;133:1433–40.
[13] Chren MM, Lasek RJ, Sahay AP, et al. Measurement properties of Skindex-16: a brief quality-of-life measure for patients with skin diseases. J Cutan Med Surg 2001;5:105–10.
[14] Morgan M, McCreedy R, Simpson J, et al. Dermatology quality of life scales – a measure of the impact of skin disease. Br J Dermatol 1997;136:202–6.
[15] Schafer T, Staudt A, Ring J. Development of the German scale for assessing quality of life in skin diseases. Hautarzt 2001;52:492–8.
[16] Schafer T, Staudt A, Ring J. German instrument for the assessment of quality of life in skin diseases (DIELH). Internal consistency, reliability, convergent and discriminant validity and responsiveness. Hautarzt 2001;52:624–8.
[17] Anderson RT, Rajagopalan R. Development and validation of a quality of life instrument for cutaneous diseases. J Am Acad Dermatol 1997;37:41–50.
[18] Finlay AY, Kelly SE. Psoriasis—an index of disability. Clin Exp Dermatol 1987;12:8–11.
[19] Finlay AY, Coles EC. The effect of severe psoriasis on the quality of life of 369 patients. Br J Dermatol 1995;132:236–44.
[20] Lewis VJ, Finlay AY. Two decades experience of the Psoriasis Disability Index. Dermatology 2005;210(4):261–8.
[21] Gupta MA, Gupta AK. The Psoriasis Life Stress Inventory: a preliminary index of psoriasis-related stress. Acta Derm Venereol 1995;75:240–3.
[22] Kirby B, Fortune DG, Bhushan M, et al. The Salford Psoriasis Index: an holistic measure of psoriasis severity. Br J Dermatol 2000;142:728–32.
[23] McKenna SP, Cook SA, Whalley D, et al. Development of the PSORIQoL, a psoriasis-specific measure of quality of life designed for use in clinical practice and trials. Br J Dermatol 2003;149:323–31.
[24] Torrance GW. Utility approach to measuring health-related quality of life. J Chronic Dis 1987;40:593–600.
[25] Simpson NB. Social and economic aspects of acne and the cost-effectiveness of isotretinoin. J Dermatol Treat 1993;4(Suppl. 2):S6–9.
[26] Motley RJ, Finlay AY. How much disability is caused by acne? Clin Exp Dermatol 1989;14:194–8.
[27] Schiffner R, Schiffner-Rohe J, Gerstenhaur M, et al. Willingness to pay and time trade-off: sensitive to changes of quality of life in psoriasis patients? Br J Dermatol 2003;148:1153–60.
[28] Finlay AY. Measures of the effect of adult severe atopic eczema on quality of life. J Eur Acad Dermatol Venereol 1996;7:149–54.
[29] Zug KA, Littenberg B, Baughman RD, et al. Assessing the preferences of patients with psoriasis. A quantitative utility approach. Arch Dermatol 1995;131:561–8.
[30] Heydendael VM, de Borgie CA, Spuls PI, et al. The burden of psoriasis is not determined by disease severity only. J Invest Dermatol Symp Proc 2004;9:131–5.
[31] Wallenhammar LM, Nyfjall M, Lindberg M, et al. Health-related quality of life and hand eczema- a comparison of two instruments, including factor analysis. J Invest Dermatol 2004;122:1381–9.
[32] Finlay AY, Khan GK, Luscombe DK, et al. Validation of sickness impact profile and psoriasis disability index in psoriasis. Br J Dermatol 1990;123:751–6.
[33] Wessely SC, Lewis GH. The classification of psychiatric morbidity in attenders at a dermatology clinic. Br J Psychiatry 1989;155:686–91.
[34] Lanigan SW, Cotterill JA. Psychological disabilities among patients with port wine stains. Br J Dermatol 1989;121:209–15.
[35] Root S, Kent G, Al-Abadie MSK. The relationship between disease severity, disability and psychological distress in patients undergoing PUVA treatment for psoriasis. Dermatology 1994;189:234–7.
[36] Lindholm C, Bjellerup M, Christensen OB. Quality of life in chronic leg ulcer patients. Acta Derm Venereol (Stockh) 1993;73:440–3.
[37] O'Donnell BF, Lawlor F, Simpson J, et al. Chronic urticaria—impact on quality of life. Br J Dermatol 1995;133(Suppl 45):27.

[38] Loo W-J, Diba V, Chawla M, et al. Dermatology Life Quality Index: influence of an illustrated version. Br J Dermatol 2003;148:279–84.

[39] Beattie PE, Lewis-Jones MS. Impairment of quality of life in children with skin disease: further validation studies of the Children's Dermatology Life Quality Index © and the Children's Life Quality Index ©. Br J Dermatol 2003;149(Suppl 64):77–8.

[40] Feldman SR, Menter A, Koo JY. Improved health-related quality of life following a randomized controlled trial of alefacept treatment in patients with chronic plaque psoriasis. Br J Dermatol 2004;150: 317–26.

[41] Zachariae H, Zachariae R, Blomqvist K, et al. Quality of life and prevalence of arthritis reported by 5,795 members of the Nordic Psoriasis Associations. Data from the Nordic Quality of Life Study. Acta Derm Venereol 2002;82:108–13.

[42] Ashcroft DM, Li Wan Po A, Williams H, et al. Quality of life measures in psoriasis: a critical appraisal of their quality. J Clin Pharm Ther 1998;23:391–8.

[43] de Korte J, Sprangers MAG, Mombers FMC, et al. Quality of life in patients with psoriasis: a systematic literature review. J Invest Dermatol Symp Proc 2004;9:140–7.

[44] Finlay AY. Quality of life measurement in dermatology: a practical guide. Br J Dermatol 1997;136: 305–14.

[45] Chen SC, Bayoumi AM, Soon SL, et al. A catalog of dermatology utilities: a measure of the burden of skin diseases. J Invest Dermatol Symp Proc 2004;9: 160–8.

# Massage Therapy for Skin Conditions in Young Children

Tiffany Field, PhD

*Touch Research Institutes, University of Miami School of Medicine, PO Box 016820, Miami, FL 33101, USA*

Skin conditions in young children can be painful, uncomfortable, and embarrassing. Although they are primarily treated by medications, alternative therapies, such as relaxation and massage therapy, have been noted to reduce stress associated with skin problems and improve their clinical condition. This article reviews two studies that highlight the positive effects of massage therapy on skin conditions in young children including burns and eczema (atopic dermatitis).

## Children's distress during burn treatment is reduced by massage therapy

In the United States approximately 83,000 children were hospitalized for burns during 1997 [1]. Dressing change procedures for treating severe burns can be painful and stressful for young patients. Anxiolytics have been used to reduce fear and anticipatory procedural anxiety; however, side effects of these medications can lead to respiratory dysfunction [2]. The addition of complementary treatments to standard care may lead to greater pain management and may offer a safer approach for reducing pain and procedural anxiety for burn patients.

In a controlled study, adult burn patients who received daily massage therapy reported reduced anxiety and pain and their cortisol (stress) hormone levels were also reduced [3]. Massage therapy has not been evaluated for reducing procedural anxiety or pain for burned children, although it has been shown to reduce pain, cortisol (stress) hormone levels, and anxiety in children with rheumatoid arthritis [4], and improve mood in children hospitalized for depression [5]. The present study examined if massage therapy attenuated burned children's distress to dressing change [6].

### Participants

Twenty-four children (mean age, 29.3 months) were enrolled in this study shortly after admission (mean days, 5.5) at a burn unit in a trauma center at a large university hospital. The children were randomly assigned to a massage therapy (N = 12) or standard care control group (N = 12).

### Procedures

*Standard medical care*

Approximately 30 minutes before debridement or dressing change, 23 of the 24 children were administered an oral, intravenous, or intramuscular analgesic.

*Attention control group*

To control for attention or placebo effects, the massage therapist spent 15 minutes with children assigned to the control group before dressing change. The massage therapist sat next to the child's bed and talked with the child.

*Massage therapy*

Children assigned to the massage therapy group received a 15-minute massage before the dressing change from a trained therapist. Box 1 lists the

---

This research was supported by National Institute of Mental Health grant MH46586 and Research Scientist Award grant MH00331 to Dr. Field and funding from Johnson & Johnson to the Touch Research Institutes.

E-mail address: tfield@med.miami.edu

> **Box 1. Strokes applied to the areas of the child's body with moderate pressure**
>
> *Face*
>
> > Small circles to entire scalp (as if shampooing hair)
> > Using flats of fingers, long stroking to both sides of face
> > Starting at midline of forehead, stroking with flats of fingers outward toward temples
> > Small circular stroking over the temples and jaw area
> > Using flats of fingers, stroking over the nose, cheeks, jaw, and chin
>
> *Legs*
>
> > Three long gliding strokes from the feet to the hips
> > Squeezing and twisting in wringing motion from the feet to the knees
> > Gliding thumbs across the bottom of each foot followed by squeezing and tugging of each toe
> > Stretching the Achilles tendons by flexing and extending each foot
>
> *Arms*
>
> > Stroking from hands to shoulders
> > Same procedure as for legs
>
> *Back and shoulders*
>
> > Long gliding downward stroking along the back from the neck to the hip
> > Hand-over-hand movements from the upper to the lower back
> > Starting at the top of the spine, alternating hand strokes across the back working down toward the tail bone (never pressing the spine) and reaching over to include sides
> > Rubbing and kneading shoulders
> > Small, circular rubbing along the base of the neck
> > Long, gliding stroking from the base of the neck and down the length of the back to the tail bone

strokes applied to the areas of the child's body with moderate pressure that were not burned.

*Assessments*

*Behavior observations*

Immediately following the intervention, an observer unaware of the child's group assignment (massage versus control) recorded the child's behavior before and during the dressing change. The observer distinguished between the two phases as follows: the before dressing change, or baseline observation, was the period immediately after the therapist completed the 15-minute massage or control period and up until the time the nurse approached the child to start the dressing procedure; during the dressing change the observation started when the nurse began the procedure and ended when the procedure was completed.

The Children's Hospital of Eastern Ontario Pain Scale [7] was used to code the distress behaviors during the observations before and during the dressing change. Six behaviors were recorded, as shown in Table 1.

*Results*

The massage therapy group showed only an increase in torso movements during the dressing changes. In contrast, the control group showed an increase in (1) facial grimacing, (2) torso movement, (3) crying, (4) leg movement, and (5) reaching out during the dressing change (see Table 1).

*Discussion*

During the dressing change, the children who received massage therapy showed minimal distress

Table 1
Means of Children's Hospital of Eastern Ontario Pain Scale ratings (0–3) of distress behaviors observed before and during dressing change

| Variables | Massage therapy | | Control | |
| --- | --- | --- | --- | --- |
| | Before dressing | During dressing | Before dressing | During dressing |
| Crying | $1.4_a$ | $1.7_a$ | $1.4_a$ | $2.0_b$ |
| Facial | $1.3_a$ | $1.5_a$ | $1.4_a$ | $1.6_b$ |
| Verbal | $0.9_a$ | $0.9_a$ | $1.1_a$ | $1.2_a$ |
| Torso | $1.1_a$ | $1.5_b$ | $1.3_a$ | $1.7_b$ |
| Touch | $1.2_a$ | $1.3_a$ | $1.2_a$ | $1.4_b$ |
| Legs | $1.2_a$ | $1.3_a$ | $1.1_a$ | $1.4_b$ |

Subscript denotes significant differences at $P<0.05$ for adjacent means within group.

behaviors and no increase in movement other than torso movement. Unaware of the children's group assignment, the nurses also reported less difficulty conducting the procedure on the massaged children. Future research might study the efficacy of teaching parents to massage their children before burn care procedures to reduce the anticipatory stress level of both parties. Assessing stress hormone levels (salivary cortisol) or neuropeptide pain levels (substance P) during stressful medical procedures could provide additional measures of massage therapy effects as an adjunct to standard burn dressing care.

**Atopic dermatitis symptoms decreased in children following massage therapy**

In a pediatric dermatology clinic study, Schachner and colleagues [8] reported that atopic dermatitis was the leading diagnosis for 456 out of 1578 children, exceeding the second most diagnosed disorder, impetigo, by 292 patients. Because there is evidence suggesting that eczema outbreaks and their severity are influenced by psychologic stress, some have used stress reduction as a course of treatment [9]. Although pharmacotherapies are often effective with atopic dermatitis, stress reduction therapies can be a helpful adjunct to pharmacologic therapy. The atopic dermatitis condition may improve and the need for medication may decrease (and the cost of treatment decline) following stress-reduction therapies.

Massage therapy might improve children's dermatitis because massage therapy also decreases stress, anxiety, and stress hormones (cortisol and norepinephrine) in children [5]. Patients with atopic dermatitis itch, particularly in response to stress. Massage therapy, by providing touch and relaxation, might reduce stress, leading to decreased itching and scratching and improvement of the dermatitis. In this study, the parents performed the massage therapy while applying medications, emollients, and creams [10].

*Participants*

Twenty children (7 girls) with atopic dermatitis (2–8 years old, mean 3.8 years) who received standard atopic therapy were recruited from the dermatology department. The study design called for half the group to receive standard care and the other half to receive standard care plus a 20-minute massage daily. The children were given the diagnosis of atopic dermatitis an average of 2 months previously and had experienced the current flare for an average of 12 months.

*Procedures*

*Standard care*

The children continued to receive treatment from a dermatologist consisting mainly of emollients and topical corticosteroids.

---

**Box 2. Five regions of the child's body stroked in sequence**

1. Face
   - Strokes along both sides of the face
   - Flats of fingers across the forehead
   - Circular strokes over the temples and the hinge of the jaw
   - Flat finger strokes over the nose, cheeks, jaw, and chin
2. Chest
   - Strokes on both sides of the chest with the flats of the fingers, going from midline outward
   - Cross strokes on sides of the chest going over the shoulders
   - Strokes on sides of the chest toward the shoulder
3. Stomach
   - Hand-over-hand strokes in a paddlewheel fashion, avoiding the ribs and the tip of the rib cage
   - Circular motion with fingers in a clockwise direction starting at the appendix
4. Legs
   - Strokes from hip to foot
   - Gently squeeze and twist in a wringing motion from hip to foot
   - Massage foot and toes
   - Stretch the Achilles tendon
   - Gently stroke the legs upward toward the heart
5. Arms
   - Strokes from the shoulder to the hand
   - The same procedure as for the legs

*Massage therapy*

The massage therapy group of patients was given daily 20-minute massages by their parents. During the first session the therapist gave the parents a 20-minute massage to acquaint the parents with the techniques and how the massage feels. Then the therapists demonstrated the massage techniques on the child. Finally, the parents were given a videotape and a written description of the massage to take home and review. The massage consisted of two standardized phases. During the first phase, the child was placed in a supine position and the standard medication was used as an emollient (instead of oil) to ensure smooth, stroking movements. Box 2 shows the five regions of the child's body the parents stroked in sequence. Any severely affected atopic dermatitis areas of the body that were sensitive were avoided.

*Dermatologic assessment*

The clinical status of the atopic dermatitis was defined both globally and focally on a scale of 0 to 3 for the parameters of redness, lichenification, scaling, excoriation, and pruritus. These assessments were made by the dermatologist and the dermatology fellow who were blind to the child's group assignment.

*Results*

*Presession and postsession comparisons: children's behavior and parent anxiety*

Comparisons revealed the following effects favoring the massage group (Table 2): the parents' reported anxiety levels decreased after the first massage session and by the last day of treatment; and the massaged children's affect improved and their anxiety decreased.

Table 2
Means for pre- and postsession child and parent measures on the first and last days of the study

| Measures | Massage | | Control | |
|---|---|---|---|---|
| | First day | Last day | First day | Last day |
| Parent | | | | |
| Anxiety[a] | 41.5 | 35.3* | 38.9 | 38.8 |
| Child | | | | |
| Affect | 2.6 | 3.0* | 2.8 | 2.7 |
| Anxiety | 2.7 | 3.0* | 2.3 | 3.0 |

[a] Lower score is optimal only for the State-Trait Anxiety Inventory scale measure.
* Statistically different means for pre- and postmeasures.

Table 3
Means for first day and last day children's skin assessments for the massage and control groups

| Focal area | Massage group | | Control group | |
|---|---|---|---|---|
| | First day | Last day | First day | Last day |
| Redness | 2.1 | 1.4* | 1.5 | 1.4 |
| Lichenification | 1.8 | 0.9** | 1.7 | 1.7 |
| Scaling | 1.3 | 0.6** | 1.9 | 1.4** |
| Excoriation | 1.7 | 0.6*** | 1.5 | 1.1 |
| Pruritus | 1.9 | 1.5** | 1.5 | 1.7 |

Lower score is optimal for all measures. First versus last day's means are statistically different.
* $P = .001$; ** $P = .05$; *** $P = .01$.

*First-day and last-day comparisons: children's skin assessments*

For the focal area assessment, all measures (redness, lichenification, scaling, excoriation, and pruritus) were numerically and statistically significantly improved by the last day of treatment. Scaling was the only measure on which both groups showed statistically significant improvement over the 1-month period (Table 3).

*Discussion*

The observed improvements in the children's conditions may have been mediated by massage decreasing anxiety levels in the parents and children. The children's behavior was less anxious and their affect and activity levels improved. In addition, the parents perceived their children's anxiety levels as having decreased. The parents also reported that their own anxiety levels decreased and their feelings about their children improved. Although this study did not assess the long-term effects of the massage intervention, it is hypothesized that the observed improvement in the children's condition would stabilize or continue to improve if the parents continued to administer the massage protocol. It is a very cost-effective adjunct therapy because the massage and instruction are given by the therapist one time, at a cost of $30.

**Summary**

These studies suggest that massage therapy can reduce a child's stress associated with skin conditions and improve the skin condition itself. The therapy can be cost-effective when done by parents.

## Acknowledgments

I thank the children and parents who participated in these studies and the researchers who conducted them.

## References

[1] Housing and Urban Development Report. October 1998.
[2] Latarjet J, Choinere M. Pain in burn patients. Burns 1995;21:344–8.
[3] Field T, Peck M, Krugman S, et al. Burn patients benefit from massage therapy. J Burn Care Rehabil 1998;19:241–4.
[4] Field T, Hernandez-Reif M, Seligman S, et al. Juvenile rheumatoid arthritis: benefits from massage therapy. J Pediatr Psychol 1997;22:607–17.
[5] Field T, Morrow C, Valdeon C, et al. Massage reduces anxiety in child and adolescent psychiatric patients. J Am Acad Child Adolesc Psychiatry 1992;31:123–31.
[6] Hernandez-Reif M, Field T, Largie S, et al. Children's distress during burn treatment is reduced by massage therapy. J Burn Care Rehabil 2001;22:191–5.
[7] McGrath P, Johnson G, Goodman J, et al. CHEOPS: a behavioral scale for rating postoperative pain in children. Adv Pain Res Ther 1985;9:395–402.
[8] Schachner L, Ling NS, Press S. A statistical analysis of a pediatric dermatology clinic. Pediatr Dermatol 1983;1:157–64.
[9] McMenamy C, Katz R, Gipson M. Treatment of eczema by EMG biofeedback and relaxation training: a multiple baseline analysis. J Behav Ther Exp Psychiatry 1988;19:221–7.
[10] Schachner L, Field T, Hernandez-Reif M, et al. Atopic dermatitis symptoms decreased in children following massage therapy. Pediatr Dermatol 1998;15:390–5.

# Complementary Psychocutaneous Therapies in Dermatology

Philip D. Shenefelt, MD, MS

*Division of Dermatology and Cutaneous Surgery, College of Medicine, University of South Florida, 12901 Bruce B. Downs Boulevard, MDC 79, Tampa, FL 33612, USA*

The skin and the nervous system develop side by side in the fetus as cutaneous ectoderm and neuroectoderm. They remain intimately interconnected and interactive throughout life. The skin and cutaneous nerves are the body's largest sense organ, providing touch, itch, pain, heat, cold, pressure, and vibration sensory input to the central nervous system. The central nervous system controls skin blood flow, sweating, and arrector pili erection. In addition, the central nervous system strongly influences hormonal regulation and immune responses that affect the skin. A person's behavior and environment determine the exposure of skin to ultraviolet light and other radiation, irritants, toxins, allergens, heat and cold, humidity and water, solvents, cosmetics, abrasion, friction, trauma, picking, scratching, rubbing, infectious agents, and therapeutic interventions. An individual's appearance to self and others is based partially on underlying bony and muscular structure but most directly on the visible appearance of the skin and its color, texture, hair distribution, hair color, hair texture, and nails.

Skin appearance and skin diseases affect self-image via the central nervous system, whereas autonomic, psychoneuroimmunologic, and behavioral factors interweave to affect skin appearance and skin diseases. The Griesemer index rates dermatologic disorders on a percentage scale from 100% to 0% based on emotional triggering of a condition (Table 1) [1]. It is important to keep this complex interplay of skin and nervous system in mind when considering complementary psychocutaneous therapies in dermatology.

In some areas of complementary therapies, it is difficult for science to catch up to practice. This is in part because of lack of funding for appropriate studies and in part because of the nature of some of the therapies that makes it challenging to do studies approaching the gold standard of double-blind, randomized, controlled trials with sufficient numbers of subjects and good statistical analysis. In other areas of complementary therapies, it is difficult for practice to catch up to science as new information is discovered. In general, well-conducted, randomized, controlled trials with a sufficient number of subjects provide the strongest evidence for the effectiveness of a given therapy. Nonrandomized controlled trials are next in strength, followed by case series and multiple case reports. Single case reports provide the weakest evidence for the effectiveness of a given therapy.

## Nonpharmacologic complementary psychocutaneous therapies

### Acupuncture

Focal stimulation of cutaneous nerves with needle acupuncture at specified sites is reported as helpful in the treatment of acne, atopic dermatitis, postherpetic neuralgia, psoriasis, and urticaria [2]. Generally, these are single case reports or case series in the Chinese literature. There is a risk of blood-borne pathogen infection from nonsterile acupuncture needles. Nonneedle acupuncture methods

E-mail address: pshenefe@hsc.usf.edu

Table 1
Griesemer index

| Diagnosis | Emotionally triggered (%) | Time elapsed from stressor to clinical change |
| --- | --- | --- |
| Hyperhidrosis | 100 | Seconds |
| Lichen simplex chronicus | 98 | Days to 2 weeks |
| Neurotic excoriations | 97 | Seconds |
| Alopecia areata | 96 | 2 weeks |
| Warts: multiple and spreading | 95 | Days |
| Rosacea | 94 | 2 days |
| Pruritus | 86 | Seconds |
| Lichen planus | 82 | Days to 2 weeks |
| Dyshidrotic hand dermatitis | 76 | 2 days for vesicles |
| Atopic dermatitis | 70 | Seconds for itching |
| Factitial dermatosis | 69 | Seconds |
| Urticaria | 68 | Minutes |
| Psoriasis | 62 | Days to 2 weeks |
| Traumatic dermatitis | 56 | Seconds |
| Dermatitis not otherwise specified | 56 | Days |
| Acne vulgaris | 55 | 2 days for papules |
| Telogen effluvium | 55 | 2–3 weeks |
| Nummular dermatitis | 52 | Days |
| Seborrheic dermatitis | 41 | Days to 2 weeks |
| Herpes simplex and zoster | 36 | Days |
| Vitiligo | 33 | 2–3 weeks |
| Pyoderma and bacterial infections | 29 | Days |
| Nail dystrophy | 28 | 2–3 weeks |
| Cysts | 27 | 2–3 weeks |
| Warts: single and multiple | 17 | Days |
| Contact dermatitis | 15 | 2 days |
| Fungal infections | 9 | Days to 2 weeks |
| Basal cell carcinoma | 0 | NA |
| Keratoses | 0 | NA |
| Nevi | 0 | NA |

*Abbreviation:* NA, not applicable.
*Data from* Griesemer RD. Emotionally triggered disease in a dermatological practice. Psychiatr Ann 1978;8:49–56.

include moxibustion, cupping, acupressure, and, more recently, laser acupuncture.

*Aromatherapy*

Aromatherapy, involving application of an essential oil diluted in a carrier oil, is used for atopic dermatitis, contact dermatitis, psoriasis, and seborrheic dermatitis. The essential oils may have some direct pharmacologic action on the skin disorder. For example, oil of Bergamont is reported to have antiseptic and antidepressant properties.

Lavender oil reportedly has analgesic, antiseptic, bacteriocidal, anti-inflammatory, and sedative effects. Lemon balm (melissa) is believed to be an antidepressant. Jasmine oil is purported to have antidepressant, sedative, and relaxant properties. Geranium oil is supposed to be an antiseptic, an antidepressant, and a stimulator of granulation tissue.

Sandalwood oil is believed to be an antiseptic and antidepressant. The carrier oils, such as avocado oil, wheat germ oil, sweet almond oil, evening primrose oil, and coconut oil, also may have some pharmacologic activities [3]. Again, these are based on case reports and case series. Adversely, allergic contact dermatitis is reported from aromatherapy [4]. Non-contact aromatherapy coupled with relaxation can link a specific fragrance with the relaxation response. That specific fragrance then can be used as a conditioned stimulus to induce the relaxation response.

*Biofeedback*

Biofeedback is useful in some skin disorders that have an autonomic nervous system component, such as biofeedback of galvanic skin resistance (GSR) for hyperhidrosis and biofeedback of skin temperature for Raynaud's syndrome. Using biofeedback, individuals may learn consciously how to alter the autonomic response and with enough repetition (typically 20–40 sessions) may establish new habit patterns. Hypnosis or autogenic training may enhance the effects obtained by biofeedback.

Hyperhidrosis, in a young man described by Panconese [5] who had a low initial GSR at the beginning of treatment, improved slowly over 20 sessions that combined GSR biofeedback with autogenic relaxation training, a variant of hypnosis. Follow-up at 3 and 6 months after treatment, during which the patient continued to practice the autogenic training exercises, showed persistent reduction in palmar sweating to near normal levels.

Patients who have Raynaud's as a feature of systemic sclerosis are able to increase finger skin temperature by an average of approximately 4°C using either hypnosis or autogenic training [6]. Two of six patients using autogenic training in addition to biofeedback report that they could shorten the duration of Raynaud attacks by autogenic training. In another study, measurement of finger-blood flow with venous occlusion plethysmography, finger temperature, and GSR in patients who had Raynaud's disease showed significant elevations in finger blood flow, finger temperature, and GSR conductance level in those given finger-temperature biofeedback compared with those who received autogenic training but no biofeedback [7]. A recent large study of patients who had Raynaud's disease compared learned hand-warming results using different biofeedback methods and found that attention to emotional and cognitive aspects of biofeedback training was important [8]. There was a significant correlation between degree of hypnotic ability and ability to lower finger temperature using biofeedback in 30 subjects given the Stanford Hypnotic Susceptibility Scale, Form C (SHSS-C) in a study by Piedmont [9]. In another study, biofeedback combined with hypnosis permitted voluntary control of skin temperature in some individuals who had moderate to high hypnotic ability as measured by the SHSS-C [10]. This can be used to increase local peripheral circulation in such conditions as Raynaud's disease.

Biofeedback of muscle tension via electromyogram can enhance teaching of relaxation. Relaxation can have a positive effect on inflammatory and emotionally triggered skin conditions, such as acne, atopic dermatitis, lichen planus, neurodermatitis, psoriasis, and urticaria. The mechanism is through influencing immunoreactivity [11]. Patients who have low hypnotic ability may be especially suitable for this type of relaxation training using electromyogram biofeedback.

Brainwave spectral biofeedback via filtered electroencephalogram (EEG) can, with multiple repetitions (20–40 sessions), alter pain discomfort [12], which may prove useful for chronic postherpetic neuralgia. It also has the potential to correct impulse control disorders and obsessive-compulsive disorders. In the skin, these can manifest as acne excoriée or neurodermatitis [13]. Whether or not quantitative EEG with neurofeedback will prove useful in neurogenic chronic pruritus and habit disorders, such as acne excoriée, neurodermatitis, trichotillomania, and onychotillomania, remains to be explored.

*Cognitive-behavioral methods*

Cognitive-behavioral methods deal with dysfunctional thought patterns (cognitive) or actions (behavioral) that damage the skin or interfere with dermatologic therapy. Responsive skin disorders include acne excoriée, atopic dermatitis, factitious cheilitis, hyperhidrosis, lichen simplex chronicus, needle phobia, neurodermatitis, onychotillomania, prurigo nodularis, trichotillomania, and urticaria. Addition of hypnosis to cognitive-behavioral therapy can facilitate aversive therapy and enhance desensitization and other cognitive- behavioral methods.

The first step in cognitive-behavioral therapy is to identify specific problems by listening to the patient's verbalization of thoughts and feelings, such as fear of needles, or by observing behaviors directly, such as scratching. The second step is for the dermatologist or therapist and patient to determine the goals of cognitive-behavioral therapy, such as a reduction in anxiety about needles or cessation of scratching. The third step is for the dermatologist or therapist to develop a hypothesis about the underlying beliefs or environmental events that precede (stimulate) or that maintain (reinforce) or minimize (extinguish) these thought patterns and behaviors. The fourth step is for the dermatologist or therapist to test the hypothesis of cause and effect by altering the underlying cognitions, the behavior, the environment, or all three, and to observe and document the effects on the patient's dysfunctional thoughts, feelings, and actions. The fifth step is for the dermatologist or therapist to revise the hypothesis if the desired results are not obtained or to continue the treatment if the desired results are obtained until the goals of therapy are reached (modified from Levenson and colleagues [14]).

This method draws in part on the cognitive therapies of identifying dysfunctional negative self-talk and substituting positive self-talk or reframing a thought picture by offering a new perspective. It also draws in part on alterations of behavior based on the classic conditioning described by Pavlov (with dogs) and by Watson (with people) and on the operant conditioning described by Skinner [15]. For a more detailed description of systematic desensitization, aversion therapy, operant techniques, and assertive training as applied to skin disorders, see Bär and Kuypers [16].

Picking behavior in acne excoriée responded in a young adult woman to cognitive- behavioral therapy coupled with biofeedback, minocycline, and sertraline [17]. Such a multimodal approach often is beneficial in resistant cases. In atopic dermatitis, scratching can become a conditioned response [18,19], often associated with and exacerbated by feelings of anxiety or hostility. When an itch stimulus was paired with the neutral stimulus of a sound tone (classical conditioning) and the amount of scratching and GSR changes were measured, atopic patients had a significantly higher scratching and GSR response than did a control group. Atopic patients also scored significantly higher in anxiety levels and in levels of suppressed hostility. Most atopic patients report some relief of anxiety or hostility through scratching (operant conditioning).

Substituting other activities for scratching, such as sports, music, artwork, meditating, or yoga, can, with repetition, change the conditioning. Lip licking or biting produces factitious cheilitis [20]. Topical anti-inflammatory agents combined with cognitive-behavioral counseling are effective in producing improvement or resolution.

Severe palmar hyperhidrosis in a 19-year-old woman responded after assertiveness training and systemic desensitization [16]. After 12 months, she continued to show no anxiety about social situations and was able to accept the milder hyperhidrosis that she still experienced.

Lichen simplex chronicus can arise from repetitive focal rubbing and scratching. Bär and Kuypers [16] treated a 6-year-old girl who had a 3-year history of vulvar lichen simplex chronicus by having the mother ignore all scratching but reward nonscratching behavior with a token which the girl exchanged each night for rewards. By 13 weeks, the condition resolved. They also treated a 33-year-old man who had lichen simplex chronicus by aversive therapy, with resolution of the scratching behavior after 19 days.

For needle phobia, systemic desensitization using participant modeling is effective [21]. A dermatologist or therapist first gives information about needles and interacts with them in a way that shows that the patient's fear is unrealistic or excessive. After modeling handling a needle, the dermatologist or therapist has the patient join in this performance, starting with situations that provoke relatively little anxiety and culminating in the performance of the feared activity. The patient then is instructed in self-directed practice to complete the desensitization. Approximately 10% of the population has needle phobia [22], so desensitization may be helpful in these individuals to permit performance of needed dermatologic procedures.

Ratliff and Stein report improvement of neurodermatitis in a 22-year-old man, using aversion therapy techniques [23]. Rosenbaum and Ayllon used habit reversal treatment for neurodermatitis [24]. They taught awareness of scratching, reviewed the inconveniences produced by the habit, developed a competing response practice of isometric exercise by fist clenching that was incompatible with scratching, and did symbolic rehearsal. At 1-month and 6-month follow-up, all three patents had improved and healed. Onychotillomania is damage to the nails produced by rubbing, picking, or tearing at the proximal and lateral nailfold. This differs from onychophagia, the habit of biting the free ends of the nails [25]. Onychotillomania can lead to onychodystrophy [26]. Teaching picking awareness, a competing response practice of isometric exercise gripping the hands together and pulling, and rehearsal under observation can help to reverse this habit. Trichotillomania is caused by repetitive hair twisting and pulling resulting in hair loss.

Habit reversal training involves self-monitoring of the frequency and duration of hair-pulling; habit control motivation by reviewing the inconveniences produced by the behavior; awareness training, including situational precursors or triggers; competing response training that substitutes a different motor action to prevent or interrupt hair pulling; relaxation training to reduce stress levels; and generalization training to identify and manage high-risk situations [27]. Of three patients using this process, one discontinued hair pulling and the other two decreased their hair pulling noticeably.

Psychosomatically triggered or exacerbated urticaria was reduced in a young professional woman using cognitive-behavioral therapy with specific self-talk and relaxation techniques [17]. Biofeedback also was used along with multiple-agent antihistamines in a multimodal approach to reduce the urticaria. Hypnosis may be used in cognitive-behavioral therapy with patients of medium to high hypnotic ability to produce desensitization, facilitate relaxation, or produce imagined aversive experiences [28]. It is easier and safer to have patients experience the aversive stimulus in the imagination than in real life. For patients who have low hypnotic ability, distraction or biofeedback may be more appropriate.

*Hypnosis*

Hypnosis involves guiding a patient into a trance state for a specific purpose, such as relaxation, pain or pruritus reduction, or habit modification. Hypnosis may improve or clear many skin disorders [29]. Hypnosis also can reduce anxiety and pain associated with dermatologic procedures (Box 1). Hypnosis is the intentional induction, deepening, maintenance, and termination of the trance state for a specific purpose. There are many myths about hypnosis that distort, overrate, or underrate the true capabilities of hypnosis. The purpose of medical hypnotherapy is to reduce suffering, promote healing, or help the person alter a destructive behavior.

Hypnotizability is, to a large extent, hard-wired into individual brains and tends to be consistent over time, as measured by the Hypnotic Induction Profile [30]. One biologic factor associated with degree of hypnotizability is the catechol-O-methyltransferase gene. At position 148 in this enzyme, gene coding for the amino acid valine on both alleles (homozygous) is associated with a four times more rapid degradation of dopamine and lower hypnotizability compared with gene coding for methionine on both alleles (homozygous) with slower degradation of dopamine and medium hypnotizability. Heterozygous coding for valine and methionine is associated with medium to high hypnotizability [31].

Recent evidence from EEG studies and positron emission tomography (PET) studies comparing brain activity in the same individual when alert and when in trance supports the theory that hypnosis is a describable altered state of consciousness rather than simply a social compliance with expectations. Quantitative EEG findings by Freeman and collegues [32], in a study of hypnosis versus distraction effects on cold pressor pain, show significantly greater high theta (5.5–7.5 Hz) activity for high hypnotizables (SHSS-C scores) compared with low hypnotizables at parietal and occipital sites during hypnosis and also during waking relaxation. PET subtraction studies by Faymonville and coworkers [33] demonstrate specific areas of the cerebral cortex with higher blood flow during hypnosis and other areas with lower blood flow, presumably related to cerebral activity. Pain reduction mediated by hypnosis localized to the mid anterior cingulate cortex.

How hypnosis produces improvement in symptoms and in skin lesions is not understood fully.

---

**Box 1. Dermatologic conditions responsive to hypnosis**

*Randomized controlled trials (strong evidence of effectiveness)*
    Hypnotic relaxation during procedures
    Verruca vulgaris
    Psoriasis

*Nonrandomized controlled trials*
    Atopic dermatitis

*Case series*
    Urticaria

*Single or few case reports (weak evidence of effectiveness)*
    Acne excoriée
    Alopecia areata
    Congenital ichthyosiform erythroderma
    Dyshidrotic dermatitis
    Erythromelalgia
    Furuncles
    Glossodynia
    Herpes simplex
    Hyperhidrosis
    Ichthyosis vulgaris
    Lichen planus
    Neurodermatitis
    Nummular dermatitis
    Postherpetic neuralgia
    Pruritus
    Rosacea
    Trichotillomania
    Vitiligo

---

Hypnosis can help regulate blood flow and other autonomic functions not usually under conscious control. The relaxation response that accompanies hypnosis alters the neurohormonal systems that in turn regulate many body functions [11]. Hypnosis may be used to help control harmful habits, such as scratching. It also can be used to provide immediate and long-term analgesia, reduce symptoms such as pruritus, improve recovery from surgery, and facilitate the mind-body connection to promote healing.

**Medical hypnotherapy**

Hypnosis is useful for reducing psychologic or behavioral impediments to healing. Hypnosis facilitates supportive therapies (ego strengthening), direct suggestion, symptom substitution, and hypnoanalysis (Box 2) [34–37]. Discussing the option of hypnosis with patients allows practitioners to gauge patients' receptiveness to this treatment modality. With proper selection of disease process, patients, and providers, hypnosis can decrease suffering and morbidity from skin disorders with minimal side effects. Practitioners who prefer to refer patients to hypnotherapists or who desire further information about training in hypnotherapy may obtain referrals or training information from the American Society of Clinical Hypnosis [38] or similar professional organizations. In adults, induction of the hypnotic state is achieved by methods that focus attention, soothe, or produce monotony or confusion [39,40]. In children, the hypnotic state may be induced by having them make believe that they are watching television, a movie, or a play or by using a distractive process that employs the imagination [41].

Supportive (ego-strengthening) therapies include positive suggestions and posthypnotic suggestions for self-worth and effectiveness. Reinforcement can be achieved by recording an audiocassette tape that a patient can use subsequently for repeated self-hypnosis. The strengthened ego is better able to deal with psychologic elements that inhibit healing. Direct suggestion during hypnosis can decrease skin discomfort from pain, pruritus, burning sensations, anxiety, and insomnia. Posthypnotic suggestion and repeated use of an audiocassette tape by patients for self-hypnosis help reinforce the effectiveness of direct suggestion. In highly hypnotizable individuals, direct suggestion may produce sufficiently deep anesthesia to permit cutaneous surgery. Direct suggestion also can reduce compulsive acts of skin scratching or picking, nail biting or manipulating, and hair pulling or twisting [34]. Autonomic responses in hyperhidrosis, blushing, and some forms of urticaria also can be controlled by direct suggestion. Verrucae can be induced to resolve using direct suggestion.

Symptom substitution replaces a negative habit pattern with a more constructive one [34]. Activities that can be substituted for scratching include athletics, artwork, verbal expression of feelings, or meditation.

Hypnoanalysis may help patients who have skin disorders unresponsive to other simpler approaches. Using hypnoanalysis, results also may occur more quickly than with standard psychoanalysis [34]. For hypnoanalysis, LeCron's list [42] of the seven most common factors causing emotional difficulties and illnesses is a good starting point (Box 3).

---

**Box 2. Hypnotic trance sequence for dermatologic conditions**

Trance induction
- Rapid: eyeroll
- Slow: progressive relaxation or other method

Trance deepening

Trance work (one or more)
- Ego strengthening
- Direct suggestion
- Indirect suggestion
- Hypnoanalysis
- Relaxation for procedures

Trance termination

---

**Box 3. The seven most common causes of emotional difficulties and illnesses**

1. Conflicts
2. Motivation
3. The effect of suggestion
4. Organ language
5. Identification
6. Self-punishment
7. The effect of past experiences

*Data from* LeCron LM. Self hypnotism: the technique and its use in daily living. Englewood Cliffs (NJ): Prentice-Hall; 1964. p. 77–88.

---

## Medical hypnotherapy for treating specific skin disorders

Posthypnotic suggestion was successful in reducing or stopping the picking associated with acne excoriée in two reported cases [43]. One patient was instructed to remember the word "scar" whenever she wanted to pick her face and to refrain from picking by saying "scar" instead. I have had similar success in one case [13]. Hypnosis can help reduce the picking habit aspect of acne excoriée in conjunction with standard treatments for the acne itself.

Medical hypnotherapy with five patients who had extensive alopecia areata resulted in only one patient who showed significant increase in hair growth. Although three patients had only slight increase in hair growth and one had no change, hypnosis did improve psychologic parameters in these five patients [44]. Hypnosis can be used as a supportive treatment for the psychologic impact of having alopecia areata, while not having much effect on the condition itself.

Many case reports describe improvement of atopic dermatitis in children and adults as a result of hypnotherapy [45]. In a nonrandomized controlled clinical trial, Stewart and Thomas [46] treated 18 adults who had extensive atopic dermatitis who had been resistant to conventional treatment with hypnotherapy that included relaxation, stress management, direct suggestion for nonscratching behavior, direct suggestion for skin comfort and coolness, ego strengthening, posthypnotic suggestions, and instruction in self-hypnosis. The results were statistically significant ($P<0.01$) for reduction in itch, scratching, sleep disturbance, and tension. Patient use of topical corticosteroid decreased by 40% at 4 weeks, 50% at 8 weeks, and 60% at 16 weeks. For atopic dermatitis, hypnosis can be a useful complementary therapy that can decrease the needed amount of other treatments. Remarkable clearing of congenital ichthyosiform erythroderma of Brocq in a 16-year-old boy was reported after direct suggestion for clearing under hypnosis [47]. Similar, although less spectacular, results were confirmed in two sisters, ages 8 and 6 [48], with a 20-year-old woman [49], and with a 34-year-old father and his 4-year-old son [50]. Reduction in severity of dyshidrotic dermatitis is reported with using hypnosis as a complementary treatment [51].

One case is reported of successful treatment of erythromelalgia in an 18-year-old woman using hypnosis alone followed by self-hypnosis [52]. Permanent resolution occurred.

A man who had a negative self-image and recurrent multiple Staphylococcus aureus–containing furuncles for 17 years was unresponsive to multiple treatment modalities. Hypnosis and self-hypnosis with imagined sensations of warmth, cold, tingling, and heaviness brought about dramatic improvement over 5 weeks with full resolution of the recurrent furuncles [53]. The patient also improved substantially from a mental standpoint. Conventional antibiotic therapy is the first line of treatment for furuncles, but in unusually resistant cases with significant psychosomatic overlay, complementary use of hypnosis may help end the chronic susceptibility to recurrent infection.

Oral pain, such as glossodynia, may respond well to hypnosis as a primary treatment if there is a significant psychologic component [54]. With organic disease, hypnosis may give temporary relief from pain.

Discomfort relief from herpes simplex is similar to that for postherpetic neuralgia. A reduction in the frequency of recurrences of herpes simplex after hypnosis also is reported [55].

Hypnosis or autogenic training may be useful as adjunctive therapy for hyperhidrosis [56]. A man who had ichthyosis vulgaris, which was better in summer and worse in winter, began hypnotic suggestion therapy in the summer and was able to maintain the summer improvement throughout the fall, winter, and spring [57]. Pruritus and lesions of lichen planus may be reduced in selected cases using hypnosis [34,51].

Some cases of neurodermatitis have resolved and stayed resolved with up to 4 years of follow-up using hypnosis as an alternative therapy [58–61]. Reduction of pruritus and resolution of lesions of nummular dermatitis is reported with use of hypnotic suggestion [40,56].

Pain from herpes zoster and postherpetic neuralgia can be reduced by hypnosis [34,55]. Hypnosis may be useful as a complementary therapy for postherpetic neuralgia. Hypnosis may modify and lessen the intensity of pruritus [40]. A man who had chronic myelogenous leukemia had intractable pruritus that was much improved with hypnotic suggestion [62].

Hypnosis and suggestion are demonstrated to have a positive effect on psoriasis [63–65]. In one case, a 75% clearing of psoriasis was reported using a hypnotic sensory-imagery technique [66]. In another case of extensive severe psoriasis of 20 years' duration, marked improvement occurred using sensory imagery to replicate the feelings in the patient's skin that he had experienced during sunbathing [67]. A case of severe psoriasis of 20 years' duration resolved fully with a hypnoanalytic technique [68]. Tausk and Whitmore [69] performed a small, randomized, double-blind controlled trial using hypnosis as adjunctive therapy in psoriasis with significant improvement only in the highly hypnotizable subjects and not in the moderately hypnotizable subjects. Hypnosis can be useful as a complementary therapy for resistant psoriasis, especially if there is a significant emotional factor in the triggering of the psoriasis.

The vascular blush component of rosacea is reported to improve in selected cases of resistant rosacea where hypnosis was added as complementary therapy [34,51]. Several reports of successful adjunctive treatment of trichotillomania are published [69–72].

Two cases of urticaria responded to hypnotic suggestion in one study. An 11-year-old boy had an urticarial reaction to chocolate that could be blocked by hypnotic suggestion so that hives appeared on one side of his face but not the other in response to hypnotic suggestion [73]. In a case series of 15 patients who had chronic urticaria of 7.8 years' average duration, hypnosis with relaxation therapy resulted within 14 months in 6 patients being cleared and another 8 patients improved, with decreased medication requirements reported by 80% of the subjects [74].

Many reports confirm the efficacy of hypnosis in treating warts [75–81]. One study [82], which tried to replicate the remarkable success reported by Sinclair-Gieben and Chalmers [83] of using hypnotic suggestion to cause warts to disappear from one hand but not the other in persons who had bilateral hand warts, was unsuccessful. A well-conducted, randomized controlled study resulted in 53% of the experimental group having improvement of their warts 3 months after the first of five hypnotherapy sessions, whereas none of the control group had improvement [84].

Vitiligo improved using hypnotic suggestion as complementary therapy [34,51], but it is unclear if the recovery simply was spontaneous. Hypnosis may be appropriate as a complementary supportive treatment for the psychologic impact of having vitiligo.

## Medical hypnotherapy for reducing procedure anxiety

Hypnosis can reduce anxiety, needle phobia, and pain during cutaneous procedures and reduce postoperative discomfort. Fick and colleagues [85] used self-guided imagery content during nonpharmacologic analgesia on 56 nonselected patients referred for percutaneous interventional procedures in the radiology procedure suite. They conclude that average patients can engage in imagery, but topics chosen are highly individualistic, making prerecorded tapes or provider-directed imagery likely to be less effective than self-directed imagery. I have used this technique with good success in dermatology patients [86]. A large randomized trial of adjunctive nonpharmacologic analgesia for invasive radiologic procedures conducted by Lang and coworkers [87] consisted of three groups: percutaneous vascular radiologic intraoperative standard care (control group), structured attention, and hypnotic self-guided relaxation. Pain increased linearly with time in the standard and the attention groups, but remained flat in the hypnosis group. Anxiety decreased over time in all three groups, but more so with hypnosis. Drug use was significantly higher in the standard group than in the structured attention and self-hypnosis groups. Hemodynamic stability was significantly higher in the hypnosis group than in the attention and standard groups.

Procedure times were significantly shorter in the hypnosis group than in the standard group, with the attention group intermediate. Cost analysis of this study [88] showed that the cost associated with standard conscious sedation was double the cost for sedation with adjunct hypnosis, making the latter considerably more cost effective. Findings from a meta-analysis of hypnotically induced analgesia were that hypnosis is demonstrated to relieve pain in patients who have headache, burn injury, heart disease, cancer, dental problems, eczema, and chronic back problems [33]. Pain reduction mediated by hypnosis localized to the midanterior cingulate cortex in a study [89] using PET.

To obtain good results with hypnosis, patients must be mentally intact, not psychotic or intoxicated, motivated, not resistant, and preferably medium or highly hypnotizable as rated by the Hypnotic Induction Profile [30] or SHSS and its variants. For self-guided imagery, however, a moderate or high degree of hypnotizability is not critical to success.

### Placebo

The placebo effect and the use of placebos remain controversial [90,91]. Expectations and the doctor-patient relationship can affect patients' experience of treatment, reduce pain, and influence outcome. Although positive expectations can produce positive placebo results, negative expectations can produce negative nocebo results [92]. Research on the placebo effect illustrates the extent to which the natural healing capacities of individuals can be enhanced and nurtured [93].

### Suggestion

The use of suggestion to promote healing is as old as language. Suggestion can be used to change subjective perceptions and reduce pain. Like the placebo effect, suggestion may influence outcome. Reports by Bloch [94] and Sulzberger and Wolf [95] on the efficacy of suggestion in treating verruca vulgaris have been confirmed many times to a greater or lesser degree [96–99] and failed to be confirmed in a few studies [100,101]. A recent study that showed negative results was criticized for using a negative suggestion of not feeding the warts rather than a positive suggestion about having the warts resolve [102].

## Pharmacologic complementary psychocutaneous therapies: herbs and supplements

Herbal therapy in dermatology was reviewed recently by Bedi and Shenefelt [102] and herbs and supplements in dermatology by Levin and Maibach [103]. Extensive information about individual herbs and their actions, interactions, and adverse effects is available in the *PDR for Herbal Medicines* [104] and in many textbooks and monographs. Information about nutritional supplements may be found in the *PDR for Nutritional Supplements* [105] and in many textbooks. The focus of this section is on psychoactive herbs and supplements that may have an indirect impact on skin diseases through anxiolytic, antidepressant, or soporific activities. See the *PDR for Herbal Medicines* and the *PDR for Nutritional Supplements* for details of their actions, interactions, adverse effects, and literature references.

### Anxiolytics

Lavender oil aromatherapy is demonstrated to produce a significant reduction in anxiety (see previous discussion of aromatherapy). Lemon balm is approved by the German Commission E for nervousness and insomnia. Kava Kava has moderate anxiolytic effects, but its use is not recommended because of its hepatotoxicity. Magnolia bark has moderate anxiolytic effects [106]. Passionflower is approved by the German Commission E for nervousness and insomnia.

### Antidepressants

Saint John's wort is approved by the German Commission E for depression. It is helpful in mild to moderate depression but not for severe depression. It has significant interactions with the metabolism of a number of other drugs.

### Soporifics

Melatonin is effective at producing drowsiness. Caution should be used when operating dangerous machinery. Valerian is approved by the German Commission E for insomnia caused by nervousness.

## References

[1] Griesemer RD. Emotionally triggered disease in a dermatological practice. Psychiatr Ann 1978;8: 49–56.
[2] Chen CJ. Acupuncture, electrostimulation, and reflex therapy in dermatology. Dermatol Ther 2003;16:87–92.
[3] Walsh D. Using aromatherapy in the management of psoriasis. Nurs Stand 1996;11:53–6.
[4] Weiss RR, James WD. Allergic contact dermatitis from aromatherapy. Am J Contact Dermatol 1997;8: 250–1.
[5] Panconese E, editor. Lo stress, le emozioni, la pelle. Milan (Italy): Masson; 1998. p. 94.
[6] Seikowski K, Weber B, Haustein UF. Zum einfluss der hypnose und des autogenen trainings auf die krankheitsverarbeitung bei patienten mit progressiver sklerodermie. Hautarzt 1995;46:94–101.
[7] Freedman RR. Quantitative measurements of finger blood flow during behavioral treatments for Raynaud's disease. Psychophysiology 1989;26:437–41.
[8] Middaugh SJ, Haythornthwaite JA, Thompson B, et al. The Raynaud's treatment study: biofeedback protocols and acquisition of temperature biofeedback skills. Appl Psychophysiol Biofeedback 2001; 26:251–78.
[9] Piedmont RL. Relationship between hypnotic susceptibility and thermal regulation: new directions for research. Percept Mot Skills 1983;56:627–31.
[10] Roberts AH, Kewman DG, Macdonald H. Voluntary control of skin temperature: unilateral changes using hypnosis and biofeedback. In: Wickramasekera I, editor. Biofeedback, behavior therapy and hypnosis: potentiating the verbal control of behavior for clinicians. Chicago: Nelson-Hall; 1976. p. 139–49.
[11] Tausk FA. Alternative medicine: is it all in your mind? Arch Dermatol 1998;134:1422–5.
[12] Sime A. Case study of trigeminal neuralgia using neurofeedback and peripheral biofeedback. J Neurother 2004;8:59–71.
[13] Shenefelt PD. Using hypnosis to facilitate resolution of psychogenic excoriations in acne excoriée. Am J Clin Hypn 2004;46(3):239–45.
[14] Levenson H, Persons JB, Pope KS. Behavior therapy & cognitive therapy. In: Goldman HH, editor. Review of general psychiatry. 5th edition. New York: McGraw-Hill; 2000. p. 472.
[15] Dorsett PG. Behavior and social learning psychology. In: Stoudemire A, editor. Human behavior: an introduction for medical students. 2nd edition. Philadelphia: JB Lippincott; 1994. p. 143–82.
[16] Bär LHJ, Kuypers BRM. Behaviour therapy in dermatological practice. Br J Dermatol 1973;88:591–8.

[17] Fried RG. Nonpharmacologic treatments in psychodermatology. Dermatol Clin 2002;20:177–85.
[18] Jordan JM, Whitlock FA. Emotions and the skin: the conditioning of the scratch response in cases of atopic dermatitis. Br J Dermatol 1972;86:574–85.
[19] Jordan JM, Whitlock FA. Atopic dermatitis, anxiety and conditioned scratch responses. J Psychosom Res 1974;18:297–9.
[20] Thomas JR, Greene SL, Dicken CH. Factitious cheilitis. J Am Acad Dermatol 1983;8:368–72.
[21] Ferguson JM, Taylor CB, Wermuth B. A rapid behavioral treatment for needle phobics. J Nerv Ment Dis 1978;166:294–8.
[22] Hamilton JG. Needle phobia: a neglected diagnosis. J Fam Pract 1995;41:169–75.
[23] Ratliffe R, Stein N. Treatment of neurodermatitis by behavior therapy: a case study. Behav Res Ther 1968;6:397–9.
[24] Rosenbaum MS, Ayllon T. The behavioral treatment of neurodermatitis through habit-reversal. Behav Res Ther 1981;19:313–8.
[25] Ameen Sait M, Reddy BSN, Garg BR. Onychotillomania: 2 case reports. Dermatologica 1985;171:200–2.
[26] Mortimer PS, Dawber RPR. Trauma to the nail unit including occupational sports injuries. Dermatol Clin 1985;3:415–20.
[27] Stanley MA, Mouton SG. Trichotillomania treatment manual. In: Van Hasselt VB, Hersen M, editors. sourcebook of psychological treatment manuals for adult disorders. New York: Plenum Press; 1996. p. 657–87.
[28] Dengrove E. Hypnosis. In: Dengrove E, editor. Hypnosis and behavior therapy. Springfield (IL): Charles C Thomas; 1976. p. 26–35.
[29] Shenefelt PD. Hypnosis in dermatology. Arch Dermatol 2000;136:393–9.
[30] Spiegel H, Spiegel D. Trance and treatment: clinical uses of hypnosis. 2nd edition. Washington, DC: American Psychiatric Publishing; 2004. p. 51–92.
[31] Lichtenberg P, Bachner-Melman R, Gritsenko I, et al. Exploratory association study between catechol-o-methyltransferase (COMT) high/low enzyme activity polymorphism and hypnotizability. Am J Med Genet 2000;96:771–4.
[32] Freeman R, Barabasz A, Barabasz M, et al. Hypnosis and distraction differ in their effects on cold pressor pain. Am J Clin Hypn 2000;43:137–48.
[33] Faymonville ME, Laurys S, Degueldre C, et al. Neural mechanisms of antinociceptive effects of hypnosis. Anesthesiol 2000;92:1257–67.
[34] Scott MJ. Hypnosis in skin and allergic diseases. Springfield (IL): Charles C Thomas; 1960.
[35] Scott MJ. Hypnosis in dermatology. In: Schneck JM, editor. Hypnosis in modern medicine. 3rd edition. Springfield (IL): Charles C Thomas; 1963. p. 122–42.
[36] Scott MJ. Hypnosis in dermatologic therapy. Psychosomatics 1964;5:365–8.
[37] Hartland J. Hypnosis in dermatology. Br J Clin Hypn 1969;1:2–7.
[38] American Society of Clinical Hypnosis. Available at: http://www.asch.net. Accessed June 24, 2005.
[39] Crasilneck HB, Hall JA. Clinical hypnosis. 2nd edition. Orlando (FL): Grune & Stratton; 1985.
[40] Watkins JG. Hypnotherapeutic techniques. New York: Irvington; 1987.
[41] Olness KN. Hypnotherapy in children. Postgrad Med 1986;79:95–100, 105.
[42] LeCron LM. Self hypnotism: the technique and its use in daily living. Englewood Cliffs (NJ): Prentice-Hall; 1964. p. 77–88.
[43] Hollander MB. Excoriated acne controlled by post-hypnotic suggestion. Am J Clin Hypn 1959;1:122–3.
[44] Harrison PV, Stepanek P. Hypnotherapy for alopecia areata [letter]. Br J Dermatol 1991;124:509–10.
[45] Twerski AJ, Naar R. Hypnotherapy in a case of refractory dermatitis. Am J Clin Hypn 1974;16:202–5.
[46] Stewart AC, Thomas SE. Hypnotherapy as a treatment for atopic dermatitis in adults and children. Br J Dermatol 1995;132:778–83.
[47] Mason AA. A case of congenital ichthyosiform erythroderma of Brocq treated by hypnosis. BMJ 1952;2:422–3.
[48] Wink CAS. Congenital ichthyosiform erythroderma treated by hypnosis. BMJ 1961;2:741–3.
[49] Schneck JM. Hypnotherapy for ichthyosis. Psychosomatics 1966;7:233–5.
[50] Kidd CB. Congenital ichthyosiform erythroderma treated by hypnosis. Br J Dermatol 1966;78:101–5.
[51] Tobia L. L'ipnosi in dermatologia. Minerva Med 1982;73:531–7.
[52] Chakravarty K, Pharoah PDP, Scott DGI, et al. Erythromelalgia—the role of hypnotherapy. Postgrad Med J 1992;68:44–6.
[53] Jabush M. A case of chronic recurring multiple boils treated with hypnotherapy. Psychiatr Q 1969;43:448–55.
[54] Golan HP. The use of hypnosis in the treatment of psychogenic oral pain. Am J Clin Hypn 1997;40:89–96.
[55] Bertolino R. L'ipnosi in dermatologia. Minerva Med 1983;74:2969–73.
[56] Hölzle E. Therapie der hyperhidrosis. Hautarzt 1994;35:7–15.
[57] Schneck JM. Ichthyosis treated with hypnosis. Dis Nerv Syst 1954;15:211–4.
[58] Kline M. Delimited hypnotherapy: the acceptance of resistance in the treatment of a long standing neurodermatitis with a sensory-imagery technique. Int J Clin Exp Hypn 1953;1:18–22.
[59] Sacerdote P. Hypnotherapy in neurodermatitis: a case report. Am J Clin Hypn 1965;7:249–53.
[60] Collison DR. Medical hypnotherapy. Med J Austr 1972;1:643–9.
[61] Lehman RE. Brief hypnotherapy of neurodermatitis: a case with four-year followup. Am J Clin Hypn 1978;21:48–51.
[62] Ament P, Milgram H. Effects of suggestion on

[62] pruritus with cutaneous lesions in chronic myelogenous leukemia. N Y State J Med 1967;67:833–5.
[63] Kantor SD. Stress and psoriasis. Cutis 1990;46: 321–2.
[64] Winchell SA, Watts RA. Relaxation therapies in the treatment of psoriasis and possible pathophysiologic mechanisms. J Am Acad Dermatol 1988;18: 101–4.
[65] Zachariae R, Oster H, Bjerring P, et al. Effects of psychologic intervention on psoriasis: a preliminary report. J Am Acad Dermatol 1996;34: 1008–15.
[66] Kline MV. Psoriasis and hypnotherapy: a case report. Int J Clin Exp Hypn 1954;2:318–22.
[67] Frankel FH, Misch RC. Hypnosis in a case of longstanding psoriasis in a person with character problems. Int J Clin Exp Hypn 1973;21:121–30.
[68] Waxman D. Behaviour therapy of psoriasis–a hypnoanalytic and counter-conditioning technique. Postgrad Med J 1973;49:591–5.
[69] Tausk F, Whitmore SE. A pilot study of hypnosis in the treatment of patients with psoriasis. Psychother Psychosom 1999;495:1–9.
[70] Galski TJ. The adjunctive use of hypnosis in the treatment of trichotillomania: a case report. Am J Clin Hypn 1981;23:198–201.
[71] Rowen R. Hypnotic age regression in the treatment of a self-destructive habit: trichotillomania. Am J Clin Hypn 1981;23:195–7.
[72] Barabasz M. Trichotillomania: a new treatment. Int J Clin Exp Hypn 1987;35:146–54.
[73] Perloff MM, Spiegelman J. Hypnosis in the treatment of a child's allergy to dogs. Am J Clin Hypn 1973; 15:269–72.
[74] Shertzer CL, Lookingbill DP. Effects of relaxation therapy and hypnotizability in chronic urticaria. Arch Dermatol 1987;123:913–6.
[75] Surman OS, Gottlieb SK, Hackett TP. Hypnotic treatment of a child with warts. Am J Clin Hypn 1972;15:12–4.
[76] Ewin D. Condyloma acuminatum: successful treatment of four cases by hypnosis. Am J Clin Hypn 1974;17:73–8.
[77] Johnson RFQ, Barber TX. Hypnosis, suggestions, and warts: an experimental investigation implicating the importance of "believed-in efficacy". Am J Clin Hypn 1978;20:165–74.
[78] Spanos NP, Stenstrom RJ, Johnston JC. Hypnosis, placebo, and suggestion in the treatment of warts. Psychosom Med 1988;50:245–60.
[79] Spanos NP, Williams V, Gwynn MI. Effects of hypnotic, placebo, and salicylic acid treatments on wart regression. Psychosom Med 1990;52:109–14.
[80] Ewin DM. Hypnotherapy for warts (verruca vulgaris): 41 consecutive cases with 33 cures. Am J Clin Hypn 1992;35:1–10.
[81] Noll RB. Hypnotherapy for warts in children and adolescents. J Dev Behav Pediatr 1994;15:170–3.
[82] Tenzel JH, Taylor RL. An evaluation of hypnosis and suggestion as treatment for warts. Psychosom 1969; 10:252–7.
[83] Sinclair-Gieben AHC, Chalmers D. Evaluation of treatment of warts by hypnosis. Lancet 1959;2: 480–2.
[84] Surman OS, Gottlieb SK, Hackett TP, et al. Hypnosis in the treatment of warts. Arch Gen Psychiatry 1973; 28:439–41.
[85] Fick LJ, Lang EV, Logan HL, et al. Imagery content during nonpharmacologic analgesia in the procedure suite: where your patients would rather be. Acad Radiol 1999;6:457–63.
[86] Shenefelt PD. Hypnosis-facilitated relaxation during self-guided imagery during dermatologic procedures. Am J Clin Hypn 2003;45:225–32.
[87] Lang EV, Benotsch EG, Fick LJ, et al. Adjunctive non-pharmacological analgesia for invasive medical procedures: a randomised trial. Lancet 2000;355: 1486–90.
[88] Lang EV, Rosen MP. Cost analysis of adjunct hypnosis with sedation during outpatient interventional radiologic procedures. Radiology 2002;222: 375–82.
[89] Montgomery GH, DuHamel KN, Redd WH. A meta-analysis of hypnotically induced analgesia: how effective is hypnosis? Int J Clin Exp Hypn 2000;48: 138–53.
[90] Spiegel D, Kraemer H, Carlson RW. Is the placebo powerless? [letter]. N Engl J Med 2001;345: 1276–9.
[91] Hrobjartsson A, Gotzsche PC. Is the placebo powerless? An analysis of clinical trials comparing placebo with no treatment. N Engl J Med 2001;344: 1594–602.
[92] Spiegel D. Placebos in practice [editorial]. BMJ 2004;329:927–8.
[93] Di Blasi Z, Reilly D. Placebos in medicine: medical paradoxes need disentangling [letter]. BMJ 2005; 330:45.
[94] Bloch B. Über die heilung der warzen durch suggestion. Klin Wochnschr 1927;6:2271–5; 6:2320–5
[95] Sulzberger MB, Wolf J. The treatment of warts by suggestion. Med Rec 1934;140:552–6.
[96] Obermayer ME, Greenson RR. Treatment by suggestion of verrucae planae of the face. Psychosom Med 1949;11:163–4.
[97] Ullman M. On the psyche and warts: I. Suggestion and warts: a review and comment. Psychosom Med 1959;21:473–88.
[98] Dudek SZ. Suggestion and play therapy in the cure of warts in children: a pilot study. J Nerv Ment Dis 1967;145:37–42.
[99] Sheehan DV. Influence of psychosocial factors on wart remission. Am J Clin Hypn 1978;20:160–4.
[100] Clarke GHV. The charming of warts. J Invest Dermatol 1965;45:15–21.
[101] Stankler L. A critical assessment of the cure of warts by suggestion. Practitioner 1967;198:690–4.

[102] Bedi MK, Shenefelt PD. Herbal therapy in dermatology. Arch Dermatol 2002;138:232–42.
[103] Levin C, Maibach H. Exploration of "alternative" and "natural" drugs in dermatology. Arch Dermatol 2002;138:207–11.
[104] PDR for herbal medicines. 3rd edition. Montvale (NJ): Thomson PDR; 2004.
[105] LaGow B, editor. PDR for nutritional supplements. 1st edition. Montvale (NJ): Thomson PDR; 2001.
[106] Kuribara H, Stavinoha WB, Maruyama Y. Behavioral characteristics of honkiol, an anxiolytic agent present in extracts of magnolia bark, evaluated by an elevated plus-maze test in mice. J Pharm Pharmacol 1998;50:819–26.

# Psychopharmacologic Therapies in Dermatology: An Update

Chai Sue Lee, MD[a], John Koo, MD[b],*

[a]Department of Dermatology, University of California Davis Medical Center, Sacramento, California, USA
[b]Department of Dermatology, University of California San Francisco Medical Center, San Francisco, California, USA

Many patients who have skin disorders have psychologic or psychosocial issues associated with their skin disorder. This can present in many different ways. Sometimes, the underlying psychopathology of the skin manifestation is difficult to ignore, such as delusions of parasitosis or neurotic excoriation. In other patients, psychologic factors, such as emotional stress, can exacerbate real skin disorders, such as acne or eczema. Also, some patients develop psychologic problems, such as depression, as a result of their skin disorders.

The psychotropic agents now available to physicians who are treating patients with psychiatric conditions are effective, simple to administer, have mild side effects, and generally well-tolerated. Dermatologists who wish to help their patients with psychodermatologic conditions can enhance their therapeutic armamentarium by becoming familiar with the use of a few selected psychotropic agents.

Although nonpharmacologic interventions can be effective adjunctive treatments for patients who have psychodermatologic conditions, most dermatologists have neither the training nor the time for nonpharmacologic treatments. For those interested in learning about nonpharmacologic treatments, such as biofeedback therapy, relaxation training, hypnosis, and psychotherapy, see Fried and colleagues [1].

This article reviews two clinically useful ways to classify psychodermatologic cases, which are discussed extensively in the literature [2,3]. These two classification systems can help clinicians understand what they are dealing with and with choosing the best psychotropic agent for each patient. The current status and future directions of psychopharmacology for the major types of psychopathologic conditions encountered in a dermatology practice are discussed. The intent is not to be exhaustive but to update and highlight some of the key issues that may aid clinicians in the choice of a psychotropic agent for particular patients and provide basic details on how to administer such agents.

## Classification of psychodermatologic disorders

Most psychodermatologic conditions can be classified into five categories: (1) psychophysiologic disorders, (2) primary psychiatric disorders, (3) secondary psychiatric disorders, (4) cutaneous sensory disorders, and (5) purely dermatologic (ie, nonpsychiatric) cases, for which psychotropic agents are used.

"Psychophysiologic disorders" is a term used to describe psychodermatologic cases in which real skin disorders are exacerbated by psychologic factors, such as emotional stress. There are many examples of psychophysiologic conditions in dermatology, such as acne, psoriasis, atopic dermatitis, and dyshidrosis. For each psychophysiologic condition, there are two types of patients: stress responders and stress nonresponders. Stress responders are those who experi-

* Corresponding author. University of California at San Francisco Psoriasis and Skin Treatment Center, 515 Spruce Street, San Francisco, CA 94118.
E-mail address: john.koo@ucsfmedctr.org (J. Koo).

ence exacerbation of their skin conditions from stress, and stress nonresponders are those for whom their emotional states seem to have nothing to do with the natural course of their skin diseases.

Primary psychiatric disorders refer to cases in which patients have no real skin disease but present instead with serious psychopathology. All of the skin manifestations are self-induced. This category includes conditions such as delusions of parasitosis, neurotic excoriations, factitial dermatitis, and trichotillomania. These conditions often are seen by dermatologists as the prototypes of psychodermatologic disorders because they are more blatantly psychogenic even though there are fewer of these patients than psychophysiologic patients.

Secondary psychiatric disorders are those in which the patients develop emotional problems, such as depression, as a result of having a skin disorder, usually as a consequence of disfigurement from the skin disorder. For certain conditions, such as vitiligo or alopecia areata, the psychosocial impact of the skin disease is the primary difficulty experienced by the patient, because these conditions generally are not life threatening or symptomatic.

Cutaneous sensory disorders refers to conditions in which patients have unpleasant sensations on the skin, such as itching, burning, stinging, crawling, or biting, with no apparent organic etiology; a psychiatric diagnosis may or may not be present.

The last category of psychodermatologic conditions involves clinical situations where psychotropic medications are more efficacious in treating certain bona fide skin conditions than traditional therapeutic agents used in dermatology. For example, the antidepressant, doxepin, is a more powerful antipruritic agent than most of the traditional antihistamines, such as diphenhydramine (Benadryl) or hydroxyzine (Atarax).

The second way to classify psychodermatologic cases is by the nature of the underlying psychopathology. This helps guide the selection of an appropriate psychotropic agent for each psychodermatologic case. Most psychodermatologic cases fall into four psychiatric diagnoses: depression, obsessive-compulsive disorder, anxiety, and delusional disorder. For example, if the underlying psychopathology involves depression, the treatment is an antidepressant. It does not matter if patients present with a primary psychiatric disorder, such as neurotic excoriations resulting from depression; a psychophysiologic disorder, such as psoriasis exacerbated by depression; or secondary depression resulting from disfigurement; as long as the underlying psychopathology is depression, an antidepressant is the most appropriate choice of treatment.

The determination of the category of psychodermatologic disorders and the decision about the underlying psychiatric diagnosis are made independent of each other. Any one of the four psychopathologies—depression, obsessive-compulsive disorder, anxiety, and delusional disorder—can be found in any one of the different categories of psychodermatologic disorders.

**Treatment of depression**

Depression frequently is encountered in dermatology practices. Patients report depressed mood or anhedonia (ie, inability to feel pleasure). Feelings of worthlessness, hopelessness, and excessive guilt are common. Patients also may report somatic symptoms, such as loss of appetite, weight loss, sleep disturbance, decreased energy, and difficulty concentrating. Preoccupation with physical health may occur. The symptoms may cause significant social or occupational dysfunction, significant subjective distress, or impairment in functioning.

Selective serotonin reuptake inhibitors (SSRIs) are the first-line treatment for depression. Probably the only tricyclic antidepressant (TCA) worth considering as a possible first-line antidepressant in dermatology is doxepin because of its combined antipruritic, antihistaminic, and antidepressant effects. There also are two antidepressants with different mechanisms of action other than SSRIs that are worth keeping in mind when treating psychodermatologic patients who have depression: venlafaxine (Effexor) and bupropion (Wellbutrin). Nefazodone (Serzone) recently was removed from the market because of cases of hepatic toxicity.

*Selective serotonin reuptake inhibitors*

SSRIs are the most widely prescribed class of antidepressants. They also are the first-line treatment for obsessive-compulsive disorder. The SSRIs include paroxetine (Paxil), sertraline (Zoloft), citalopram (Celexa), escitalopram (Lexapro), and fluoxetine (Prozac). Fluvoxamine (Luvox) is also an SSRI. It is not commonly used, however, to treat depression, because it is associated with many drug interactions with cytochrome P-450 metabolized medications, and the other SSRIs are just as effective.

The side-effect profiles of SSRIs are more alike than different given their similar mechanisms of action. Gastrointestinal effects, such as nausea and diarrhea, are the most common side effects. Giving the medication with food often alleviates the nausea. Nausea usually improves after several days. Insomnia may occur with any of the SSRIs, but fluoxetine tends to be more activating and is more likely to produce anxiety and insomnia than the other SSRIs. SSRIs should be given in the morning if insomnia occurs. Sedation is more likely to occur with paroxetine. If sedation occurs, the medication should be given at bedtime. SSRIs can be associated with sexual dysfunction. Most SSRI studies reveal an incidence of approximately 40% for sexual difficulties, most commonly involving difficulties with orgasm [4]. When sexual side effects occur, switching to another class of antidepressant that causes less sexual dysfunction, such as bupropion, is recommended.

The dosing guidelines of SSRIs are listed in Table 1. Like other antidepressant treatments, full clinical response to SSRIs is gradual. The onset of response to SSRIs usually begins approximately 2 to 3 weeks after the optimal therapeutic dosage is reached, and 4 to 6 weeks are required before the full therapeutic effect is apparent. There is no linear relationship between SSRI dose and response. For partial responders, however, the dosage may be increased to maximize therapeutic effect. The lack of response to one SSRI or inability to tolerate one SSRI is not predictive of the same reaction to another SSRI. Patients showing no improvement after 6 weeks of SSRI treatment at the usual effective dosage should switch to another SSRI or to another class of antidepressant, such as venlafaxine or bupropion.

On discontinuation, some patients may experience dizziness, lethargy, nausea, irritability, and headaches. These symptoms can be prevented by tapering the medication slowly over several weeks when discontinuing the drug.

Table 1
Dosing guidelines for selective serotonin reuptake inhibitor

| Generic name | Trade name | Standard dosage range |
|---|---|---|
| Paroxetine | Paxil | Start 20 mg every AM, max 50 mg/d |
| Sertraline | Zoloft | 50 mg every day, max 200 mg/d |
| Citalopram | Celexa | Start 20 mg every day, max 40 mg/d |
| Escitalopram | Lexapro | Start 10 mg every day, max 20 mg/d |
| Fluoxetine | Prozac | Start 20 mg every AM, max 80 mg/d |

*Other noteworthy antidepressants*

Although SSRIs currently are the most frequently prescribed antidepressants, they are effective in only 60%–70% of patients. Furthermore, some patients may be unable to tolerate the side effects of SSRIs. Two antidepressants provide important alternatives to SSRIs in the pharmacologic therapy of depression: venlafaxine and bupropion. Although these antidepressants share with SSRIs a similar level of efficacy and time to onset of action, they have different mechanisms of action and side-effect profiles.

*Venlafaxine*

Venlafaxine is a novel antidepressant that is believed to act by selectively inhibiting serotonin and norepinephrine reuptake with little effect on other neurotransmitter systems [5]. Several clinical studies provide evidence that venlafaxine may offer advantages over conventional therapy in terms of an increased number of responders and improved long-term efficacy [6,7]. In addition, venlafaxine has an anxiolytic effect and may be useful particularly in patients who have mixed symptoms of depression and anxiety [8–11]. A prospective, 12-week, randomized, double blind, placebo-controlled study finds that once-daily venlafaxine extended-release (XR) preparation is more effective than fluoxetine in patients who have major depression and concomitant anxiety [8]. Venlafaxine XR also is shown to be effective for the treatment of anxiety alone [12–14].

Venlafaxine comes in two formulations: immediate release and XR. Immediate release treatment begins with 75 mg per day in two divided doses with food. The dosage can be increased by 75 mg per day after several weeks of treatment for partial responders. The usual effective dosage is 75–225 mg per day on a twice-daily schedule. XR treatment begins with 37.5–75 mg per day with food. The maximum recommended dose is 225 mg per day.

Venlafaxine has a relatively benign side-effect profile. The most common side effects are insomnia and nervousness. Nausea, sedation, fatigue, sweating, dizziness, headache, loss of appetite, constipation, and dry mouth also are common. Like SSRIs, venlafaxine may cause sexual dysfunctions in approximately 10% of patients after several weeks of treatment. Venlafaxine is reported to cause hypertension in approximately 3% of patients and seems to be dose related. Blood pressure should be monitored during venlafaxine therapy. Although venlafaxine-induced hypertension may be managed with standard antihypertensives, the authors recommend switching to another class of antidepressants if hypertension develops.

Venlafaxine can produce dizziness, insomnia, dry mouth, nausea, nervousness, and sweating with abrupt discontinuation. Consequently, it should be tapered slowly over several weeks.

*Bupropion*

Bupropion differs from all other types of antidepressants in its chemical structure and in its proposed mechanism of action. Bupropion is a relatively weak inhibitor of dopamine reuptake with modest effects on norepinephrine reuptake and no effect on serotonin reuptake [15]. Bupropion is shown as effective as SSRIs in the treatment of depression but causes few sexual side effects [16,17]. In addition, bupropion may be considered for depressed patients who have sleep difficulties, because bupropion promotes normal sleep pattern [18,19].

Bupropion comes in two formulations: immediate and sustained release. For immediate release, treatment begins at 200 mg per day, given as 100 mg twice daily. After 4–7 days, the dosage may be increased to 300 mg per day, given as 100 mg three times per day. The usual effective dosage is 200 to 300 mg per day, divided in two to three equal daily doses. For sustained release, treatment begins with 150 mg per day, given as a single daily dose in the morning. After 4–7 days, the dosage may be increased to 300 mg per day, given as 150 mg twice daily if the 150 mg initial dose is adequately tolerated. The usual adult target dosage is 300 mg per day given as 150 mg twice daily.

In general, bupropion is a well-tolerated medication. The most common side effects are insomnia, agitation, headache, constipation, dry mouth, nausea, and tremor. A rare but serious adverse effect of bupropion is seizure induction. The incidence of seizures in patients receiving buprorion increases above the therapeutic dosages of 300 mg per day [20]. Bupropion should not be used in patients who have a history of seizure or who have conditions, such as bulimia, that potentially may lower the seizure threshold. This medication should be avoided in drug or alcohol abusers.

*Doxepin*

The TCA doxepin (Sinequan) probably is the ideal agent for the treatment of depressed patients who have neurotic excoriations. In addition to its antidepressant effect, doxepin has strong antipruritic effect because it is a powerful $H_1$ antihistamine. To stop the excoriating behavior, it is important to treat patients' depression and put an end to the itch/scratch cycle. Moreover, the majority of depressed patients who present with excoriations seem to be suffering from an agitated depression in which the patients paradoxically become more restless, angry, and argumentative when depressed. For these patients, the most common side effect of doxepin, sedation, can be therapeutic.

The usual starting dosage of doxepin for depression is 25 mg per day at bedtime. The dosage can be titrated with 10–25 mg increments every 5–7 days, as tolerated, up to the usual therapeutic range for depression, which is anywhere from 75 to 300 mg per day. In general, it takes at least 2 weeks after the therapeutic dosage is reached before the antidepressant effect is observed. Some patients may require 6–8 weeks of treatment before responding. The other therapeutic effects of doxepin, however, such as the antipruritic effect, effects in calming patients down, and improving insomnia, generally occur immediately. If patients show no response, despite taking a large dose of doxepin for several weeks, it may be helpful to check a serum doxepin level to see if it is within the therapeutic range for depression.

The most common side effect of doxepin is sedation. The sedative side effect usually can be avoided by taking it at bedtime. More persistent sedation may require lowering the dosage or changing the time of administration of doxepin. For example, if patients complain of difficulty waking up in the morning, this usually can be overcome by taking doxepin earlier than bedtime or by dividing the dose so that patients take some of the dose when they get home and the rest at least 1–2 hours before bedtime. This way, patients are less likely to experience excessively high peak serum level and the resultant sedation the next morning. The other side effects of doxepin are similar to those of other older TCAs, including cardiac conduction disturbances, weight gain, orthostatic hypotension, and anticholinergic side effects, such as dry mouth, blurry vision, constipation, and urinary retention. TCAs may slow cardiac conduction, resulting in intraventricular conduction delay, prolongation of the QT interval, and atrioventricular block. Therefore, TCAs are contraindicated in patients who have preexisting conduction defects, arrhythmias, or recent myocardial infarction. A pretreatment EKG is recommended to rule out the presence of prolonged QT in older patients or any patients who have a history of cardiac conduction disturbance. In addition, an EKG should be repeated to rule out dysrhythmia if doxepin is used in dosages of 100 mg per day or higher. Doxepin also should be used with caution in patients who have a history of seizure disorder or manic-depressive disorder because it can lower the seizure threshold and precipitate a manic episode.

Abrupt discontinuation of TCAs may lead to transient dizziness, nausea, headache, diaphoresis, malaise, insomnia, and REM rebound, with uncomfortably vivid dreams. Consequently, they should be tapered gradually over several weeks after prolonged treatment with TCAs. Slow taper also decreases the likelihood of relapse of depressive symptoms.

**Treatment of obsessive-compulsive tendency**

An obsession is a repugnant thought that intrudes repetitively into the thought process of a patient. Compulsion refers to repetitious, stereotyped behavior that is difficult for patients to suppress. The diagnosis of obsessive-compulsive tendency may be justified if either the obsession or the compulsion is of sufficient intensity to interfere with a patient's lifestyle or cause significant subjective distress. Some patients may present only with obsession, whereas others present only with compulsive behaviors. For example, some patients may obsess about the "unsightly greasiness" of their face without engaging in any special activity to try to correct the greasy complexion, whereas other patients may present with an irresistible compulsion to pick their acne without having any special thought process associated with their compulsion.

An obsession can be mistaken for a delusion, because in both cases patients present with a mental preoccupation involving an overvalued idea. The key distinction between obsession and delusion is the presence or absence of insight on the part of the patient. Most adult patients who have obsessive-compulsive tendencies usually recognize and acknowledge the excessive, unreasonable, and destructive nature of their obsessions and compulsions, but are unable to stop obsessive thoughts or their compulsive behaviors. In contrast, delusional patients truly believe in the validity of their delusional thoughts. Frequently, patients who have obsessive-compulsive tendencies are apologetic for their thoughts or behaviors. For example, a patient who has acne excoriée may say, "I know I am not supposed to be doing this, and I know that if I keep picking on my acne I might really scar myself, but I can't stop picking because when I try to stop, I feel this tremendous urge to pick my acne." The presence of such a compulsive urge that intensifies until patients finally give in and engage in the compulsive activity—despite the presence of good insight—helps differentiate obsessive-compulsive tendency from delusional disorder. Unfortunately, not all patients are so typical in their clinical presentation, and, in some cases, obsessive-compulsive tendency and delusion can be difficult to differentiate.

There are many manifestations of obsessive-compulsive tendencies in dermatology. Skin findings in obsessive-compulsive tendencies include eczematous eruptions related to excessive washing, hair loss related to trichotillomania or compulsive hair pulling, and excoriations related to neurodermatitis or compulsive skin picking. Obsessive-compulsive tendencies usually have a chronic course, and few patients achieve true remission [21]. Although symptoms may wax and wane over time, the disorder rarely resolves spontaneously without appropriate treatment [22,23].

SSRIs are the first-line treatment for obsessive-compulsive disorder (see previous discussion of depression.) Obsessive-compulsive symptoms often require higher doses of an SSRI and take longer to respond then when treating depression. In obsessive-compulsive disorder, initial response to a SSRI can take 4–8 weeks, and maximal response may take as long as 20 weeks. Complete remission is unusual. A 10- to 12-week trial with a SSRI at therapeutic dosage is the minimum necessary to confirm true failure to respond. A failure to respond to one SSRI does not predict failure to respond to another [24]. For nonresponders, a 10-week trial of a SSRI followed by a switch to another SSRI is the recommended practice by the authors if a psychiatric referral is not feasible. Therapy should be continued for at least 6 months to 1 year once a therapeutic response is achieved [22]. Medications should be tapered slowly during discontinuation and should be restarted if symptoms reappear.

No matter which medication is used, patients must be told that these medications are not magic bullets. They can be helpful in overcoming obsessive thoughts or compulsive behaviors, but they are no substitute for the patients' own motivation to stop destructive behaviors. Therefore, patients should be encouraged to keep up their own efforts and vigilance in controlling their compulsive behaviors while they undergo treatment with anti–obsessive-compulsive medications.

**Treatment of anxiety**

Patients who have anxiety disorder report excessive anxiety and stress, which may revolve around valid concerns about money, jobs, marriage, health, and so forth. Patients also may report restlessness or feeling on edge, difficulty concentrating or mind going blank, and irritability. In addition to subjective feelings, patients who have excessive anxiety and stress may experience physiologic manifestations of anxiety that may include palpitations, lightheadedness, dizziness, sweaty palms, difficulty breathing, trembling, muscle aches and soreness, and sleep disturbance. The subjective anxiety or the associated physical symptoms can cause significant distress and impairment in functioning.

Psychodermatologic cases involving anxiety often can be divided into two groups: acute and chronic anxiety. The acute and time-limited episode of anxiety usually involves a specific situational stress, such as increasing demand at work, interpersonal difficulty, or a financial crisis. The situational stress can exacerbate a stress-responder's skin disorder. The use of an anxiolytic agent may be indicated for a few weeks to avert a flare of the skin condition and improve mental stability until patients recover from the crisis, especially if nonpharmacologic approaches are either not feasible or not adequate to control the anxiety. The decision as to the treatment of choice for psychodermatologic cases involving anxiety should take into account if the anxiety is acute (short term) or chronic.

## Benzodiazepines

Benzodiazepines are useful especially in the management of acute situational anxiety. Unlike patients who have chronic anxiety, many of these patients who have acute situational anxiety have adequate coping skills and usually recover from the crisis after a few weeks. This period of stress can be long enough, however, to exacerbate their skin disorder. Benzodiazepines take effect immediately and almost always can relieve anxiety if given in adequate doses.

For acute anxiety in dermatology patients who have not tried benzodiazepines before, treatment can begin with alprazolam (Xanax), half a 0.25-mg tablet up to four times per day, on an as-needed basis.

Benzodiazepines generally are well tolerated. For short-term use ($\leq$6 weeks), the main side effect is sedation, but usually this subsides after several days of treatment or can be controlled by dosage adjustment. It is helpful for patients to take an initial dose at home in the evening to see how it affects them when treatment is initiated, especially with regard to the possible sedative effect. Patients should be cautioned against driving after taking benzodiazepines.

Because of the potential risk of addiction with long-term use, physicians should try to limit the duration of treatment with benzodiazepines to no more than 3 to 4 weeks. In many cases, the situational stress resolves during the treatment period.

## Buspirone

Buspirone (Buspar) is preferred for the treatment of chronic anxiety because it is an antianxiety medication that is nonsedating and does not cause dependency. Its main disadvantage, however, is its delayed onset of action and, therefore, buspirone cannot be used on an as-needed basis. Buspirone must be administered for at least 2 weeks before a significant therapeutic effect occurs. Because of the slow onset of action, this agent is not appropriate for the treatment of acute situational stress, because the therapeutic effect may not become evident until after the stressful event has resolved.

The starting dosage is 15 mg per day given as 7.5 mg twice daily and increased to 15 mg twice daily after 1 week. The maximum dosage is 60 mg per day. Most patients respond to dosages between 15 and 30 mg per day. The 15- and 30-mg tablets are scored to be bisected or trisected easily.

Buspirone generally is well tolerated. Most patients experience no adverse effects. The most common side effects are nausea, headache, dizziness, and fatigue. Patients treated previously with benzodiazepines or who have a history of substance abuse seem to have a decreased response to buspirone, because it lacks the euphoria, sedation, and immediate action these patients may have come to expect with anxiety relief.

## Antidepressants

Antidepressants, such as paroxetine (20–50 mg per day), low-dose doxepin ($\leq$50 mg per day), and venlafaxine XR (75 and 150 mg per day), also are shown to be useful for the treatment of chronic anxiety (see earlier discussion) [12–14,25,26].

# Treatment of delusional disorder

The delusional disorders encountered most often by a dermatologist are monosymptomatic hypochondriacal psychosis (MHP). Patients who have MHP are characterized by the presence of an "encapsulated" delusional ideation that revolves around one particular hypochondriacal concern. This can be associated with hallucinatory experiences that are compatible with the delusion. For example, the most common MHP seen by dermatologists is delusions of parasitosis. Many patients who have delusions of parasitosis experience cutaneous sensations of crawling, biting, and stinging along with their delusions. MHP is different from schizophrenia in that individuals who have schizophrenia have other psychologic disturbances in addition to delusions.

*Pimozide*

The most commonly used pharmacologic treatment for delusions of parasitosis is the antipsychotic medication pimozide. Careful titration of pimozide dosage is the key to safe use of this medication. Because of the possibility of extrapyramidal adverse effects, such as stiffness and restlessness, patients should begin treatment at a low initial dosage of 1 mg daily, which can be increased by 1 mg increments every 4–7 days until either optimal clinical response is reached or patients are taking 4–6 mg per day. Even though dosages as high as 10 mg per day are used in dermatologic settings, the authors generally do not recommend going beyond 4–6 mg per day because the risk of side effects increases.

Once the delusions of parasitosis no longer interfere significantly with patients' capacity to work or enjoy life, this clinically effective dosage is maintained for at least 1 month. The dosage of pimozide can be decreased gradually by 1 mg as quickly as every 1–2 weeks until either the minimum effective dosage is determined or patients successfully are tapered off pimozide altogether. Although some patients who have delusions of parasitosis can be tapered off pimozide successfully after 2–4 months, 5–6 months of treatment is a more reasonable expectation. If delusions of parasitosis recur after pimozide is discontinued, patients can be restarted on pimozide in a time-limited fashion. Long-term use of pimozide is best avoided to minimize the risk of tardive dyskinesia developing in these patients. This side effect is characterized by abnormal involuntary rhythmic movements of the face, mouth, tongue, or jaw, which sometimes may be accompanied by involuntary movements of the trunk and extremities. Tardive dyskinesia is the most worrisome adverse effect of pimozide, because it may be irreversible. No cases of pimozide use for MHP causing tardive dyskinesia are reported except for one questionable case. Lindskov reports a patient who had delusions of parasitosis and a "slight twitching of her lips" which "has been present since treatment" [27]. Although the original investigators never labeled this explicitly as tardive dyskinesia, another investigator later interpreted this case as "tardive dyskinesia" [28].

The most common side effects of pimozide are the acute forms of extrapyramidal side effects manifested by stiffness and a feeling of inner restlessness called akathisia. Akathisia is manifested outwardly by difficulty remaining still and fidgeting or pacing. Even though only a minority of patients treated with pimozide experience extrapyramidal side effects, it is advisable for clinicians to explain the possibility of developing such adverse effects before starting pimozide and to give a prescription for either benztropine 1–2 mg up to four times per day or diphenhydramine 25 mg up to four times per day in case patients begin to have symptoms of extrapyramidal side effects. The advantage of benztropine over diphenhydramine is that the former agent is not sedating. Because some patients may have considerable ambivalence about taking pimozide, if they develop extrapyramidal side effects and do not have the means to control them right away, they may decide never to take pimozide. Such a decision can be tragic, because without proper treatment, delusions of parasitosis can last for decades with virtual incapacitation of many of these patients. As long as the extrapyramidal side effects can be controlled with one of the two medications described above, patients can continue with treatment with pimozide and even increase the dose until the optimal dosage is reached.

There are reports of sudden death, presumably cardiac related, in patients who had chronic schizophrenia and who were treated with high-dose pimozide above 10 mg per day [29]. Pimozide theoretically can cause arrhythmias by prolonging the QT interval. To date, the authors have not seen any EKG change from low-dose pimozide used to treat MHP. For those who have a history of cardiac conduction abnormalities or arrhythmia, a pre- and posttreatment EKG should be checked. For those who are young and healthy and have no history of cardiac arrhythmias, it is controversial whether or not an EKG is warranted if the dosage is less than 10 mg per day [29].

*Atypical antipsychotics*

Three atypical antipsychotics—risperidone (Risperdal), olanzapine (Zyprexa), and quetiapine (Seroquel)—are the most frequently prescribed medications for the treatment of psychosis. These newer antipsychotic agents are dopamine and serotonin receptor antagonists. Atypical antipsychotics have greatly reduced the incidence of extrapyramidal side effects and tardive dyskinesia because they are more selective in binding to the receptors that are believed related to antipsychotic effects but not to the other receptors that are related to side effects [30–33]. These atypical antipsychotics, with a much safer side-effect profile, may prove useful for the treatment of MHP. The optimal dosage range for MHP is not established for any of these agents. Studies comparing pimozide with the atypical antipsychotics in the treatment of delusions of parasitosis have not yet been done.

Atypical antipsychotics should be used with caution in patients who have a history of seizures or with conditions, such as Alzheimer's disease, that potentially lower the seizure threshold. During premarketing testing, seizures occurred in 22 (0.9%) of 2500 olanzapine-treated patients, 18 (0.8%) of 2387 quetiapine-treated patients, and 9 (0.3%) of 2607 risperidone-treated patients [34].

*Risperidone*

Risperidone treatment for nondermatologic psychoses begins with 1 mg twice daily, and the dosage may be increased slowly every 5–7 days to the usual effective dosage of 4–6 mg per day on a twice-daily schedule. After titration, patients may take the entire dose at bedtime. Because the optimal dosage for MHP is not established, the authors generally recommend an even more cautious 1-mg once-daily starting dosage. The most common side effects are anxiety, dizziness, and rhinitis. Dose-related side effects include sedation, fatigue, and accommodation disturbance. Risperidone is known to prolong the QT interval and should be used with caution in patients who have abnormal baseline QT intervals or those taking other medications that can prolong the QT interval (eg, antiarrhythmics, such as quinidine or procainamide) [30–32,35]. As the only available atypical antipsychotic with minimal anticholinergic effects (eg, dry mouth, blurry vision, urinary retention, and constipation), risperidone may be considered the agent of choice for the elderly [36,37]. Risperidone is reported effective in the treatment of delusions of parasitosis [38].

*Olanzapine*

Olanzapine treatment for nondermatologic psychoses begins with 5–10 mg per day. The usual effective dosage is 10–15 mg per day. Once again, because the optimal dosage for MHP is not established, the authors recommend a lower starting dosage for dermatologic use. The most common side effects are sedation, anticholinergic effects, and weight gain.

*Quetiapine*

Quetiapine treatment for nondermatologic psychoses starts with 25 mg two times per day. The usual effective dosage is 150–750 mg per day. Again, because the optimal dosage for MHP is not established, the authors recommend a lower starting dosage for dermatologic use. The most common side effects are mild somnolence and mild anticholinergic effects. Quetiapine is associated more often with orthostatic hypotension than the other atypical antipsychotics but usually is manageable with careful dose adjustment, and patients frequently become partially or fully tolerant to it [39].

## Use of psychotropic medications for treating purely dermatologic conditions

Certain psychotropic medications are known to be useful in treating purely dermatologic conditions. The class of medications with the most well-documented analgesic effect is the older tertiary TCAs, such as doxepin and amitriptyline [40–45]. If pruritus is the primary problem, doxepin is the preferred agent. Alternatively, if various manifestations of pain, such as burning, stinging, biting, or chafing, are the primary sensations, amitriptyline is the preferred starting agent.

*Doxepin for pruritus and other dermatologic conditions*

Doxepin frequently is used to treat pruritus when more conventional antipruritic agents, such as diphenhydramine or hydroxyzine, are inadequate. There are several advantages of using doxepin for the control of pruritus compared with the conventional antipruritic agents. First, doxepin has a higher affinity for the histamine receptors than the traditional antihistamines and, therefore, exert a more powerful antipruritic effect. For example, the affinity of doxepin for $H_1$ receptor in vitro is approximately 56 times that of hydroxyzine and 775 times that of diphenhydramine [46]. Second, the therapeutic effect of doxepin is much longer than either of these $H_1$-antihistamine medications. Because of its long half-life, doxepin taken once daily, usually at bedtime, is adequate to provide therapeutic benefit up to 24 hours. Therefore, patients who have severely pruritic conditions, such as atopic dermatitis, who complain of waking up in the middle of the night even though they are taking hydroxyzine or diphenhydramine before bedtime, usually find that when they switch to doxepin, they can sleep throughout the night. Third, doxepin normalizes sleep curves. When patients spend more time in a deeper state of sleep, the amount of nighttime excoriation often diminishes dramatically. Doxepin also can be helpful in treating patients who have chronic urticaria or other disorders mediated by histamines who have failed treatment with traditional antihistamines [47,48].

The dosing guideline for doxepin is discussed previously in the treatment of depression section. There are no good data regarding the optimal dosage for the treatment of conditions, such as pruritus or urticaria. A wide range in dosing is possible depending on individual patients. For example, the dosage of doxepin adequate for control of pruritus may range from as little as less than 10 mg at bedtime (often using doxepin liquid preparation, which is 10 mg/mL) to as much as the maximum dosage for the treatment of depression 300 mg at bedtime.

*Amitriptyline*

For various manifestations of pain sensations, such as burning, stinging, biting, or chafing, amitriptyline is the preferred agent over doxepin because of better documentation of its efficacy as an analgesic. When TCAs are used as analgesics, the dosage required tends to be less than the dosage required for its antidepressant effect. Patients can be started at 25 mg at bedtime and titrated to the maximally effective dosage. For use as an analgesic, a dosage of 50 mg per day or less usually suffices. Side effects of amitriptyline are the same as for doxepin and include sedative, cardiac, anticholinergic, and α-adrenergic side effects, including orthostatic hypotension, which can be problematic particularly in elderly patients. If patients cannot tolerate these agents, other TCAs, such as imipramine or desipramine may be used [49]. The dosage range for these medications is the similar to that for amitriptyline.

## Summary

The majority of mental illnesses, including psychodermatologic conditions, generally are considered chronic. Psychiatric referral and consultation should be attempted whenever feasible. Yet, for a significant proportion of patients who refuse psychiatric referral, the judicious use of psychotropic medications by dermatologists may provide much-needed assistance in the recovery of these patients from psychodermatologic disorders when no other avenue of assistance exists. Though detailed explanations regarding the use of selected old and new psychopharmacologic agents were discussed in this article, the reader is advised to consult standard textbooks on psychopharmacology and the *Physician's Desk Reference* for a more complete description regarding the indications for the use of these medications.

## References

[1] Fried R. Nonpharmacological treatments in psychodermatology. In: Koo J, Lee CS, editors. Psychocutaneous medicine. New York: Marcel Dekker; 2003. p. 411–26.

[2] Koo J. Psychodermatology: a practical manual for clinicians. Curr Probl Dermatol 1995;7:199–234.

[3] Koo J, Pham CT. Psychodermatology: practical guidelines on pharmacotherapy. Arch Dermatol 1992;128: 381–8.

[4] Settle Jr EC. Antidepressant drugs: disturbing and potentially dangerous adverse effects. J Clin Psychiatry 1998;59(Suppl 16):25–30.

[5] Montgomery SA. Venlafaxine: a new dimension in antidepressant pharmacotherapy. J Clin Psychiatry 1993;54:119–26.

[6] Clerc GE, Ruimy P, Verdeau-Pailles J. A double-blind comparison of venlafaxine and fluoxetine in patients hospitalized for major depression and melancholia. Int Clin Psychopharmacol 1994;9:139–43.

[7] Lecrubier Y, Bourin M, Moon CA, et al. Efficacy of venlafaxine in depressive illness in general practice. Acta Psychiatr Scand 1997;95:485–93.

[8] Silverstone PH, Ravindran A for the Venlafaxine XR 360 Canadian Study Group. Once-daily venlafaxine extended release (XR) compared with fluoxetine in outpatients with depression and anxiety. J Clin Psychiatry 1999;60:22–8.

[9] Rickels K, Pollack MH, Sheehan DV, et al. Efficacy of extended-release Venlafaxine in nondepressed outpatients with generalize anxiety disorder. Am J Psychiatry 2000;157:968–74.

[10] Davidson JR, DuPont RL, Hedges D, et al. Efficacy, safety, and tolerability of venlafaxine extended release and buspirone in outpatients with generalized anxiety disorder. J Clin Psychiatry 1999;60:528–35.

[11] Gelenberg AJ, Lydiard RB, Rudolph RL, et al. Efficacy of venlafaxine extended-release capsules in nondepressed outpatients with generalized anxiety disorder: a 6-month randomized controlled trial. JAMA 2000;238:3052–88.

[12] Haskins JT, Aguiar L, Pallay A, et al for the Venlafaxine XR 210 Study Group. Double-blind, placebo-controlled study of once daily venlafaxine XR in outpatients with generalized anxiety disorder [abstract]. Presented at the 11th Congress of the European College of Neuropsychopharmacology. Paris France, Oct. 31–Nov. 4, 1998.

[13] Haskins JT, Rudolph R, Aguiar L, et al for the Venlafaxine XR 214 Study Group. Double-blind,

[13] placebo-/comparator-controlled study of once daily venlafaxine XR and buspirone in outpatients with generalized anxiety disorder [abstract]. Presented at the 11th Congress of the European College of Neuropsychopharmacology. Paris, France, Oct. 31–Nov. 4, 1998.

[14] Haskins JT, Rudolph R, Aguiar L, et al for the Venlafaxine XR 218 Study Group. Venlafaxine XR is an efficacious short- and long-term treatment for generalized anxiety disorder [abstract]. Presented at the 11th Congress of the European College of Neuropsychopharmacology. Paris, France, Oct. 31–Nov. 4, 1998.

[15] Richelson E. Biological basis of depression and therapeutic relevance. J Clin Psychiatry 1991;52(Suppl): 4–10.

[16] Modell JG, Katholi CR, Modell JD, et al. Comparative sexual side effects of bupropion, fluoxetine, paroxetine, and sertraline. Clin Pharmacol Ther 1997;61: 476–87.

[17] Kavoussi RJ, Segraves RT, Hughes AR, et al. Double-blind comparison of bupropion sustained release and sertraline in depressed outpatients. J Clin Psychiatry 1997;58:532–7.

[18] Ware JC, McBrayer R, Rose V. REM sleep enhancement by nefazodone, trazodone, and buspirone. Sleep Res 1993;22:51.

[19] Nofzinger EA, Reynolds III CF, Thase ME, et al. REM sleep enhancement by bupropion in depressed men. Am J Psychiatry 1995;152:274–6.

[20] Davidson J. Seizures and bupropion: a review. J Clin Psychiatry 1989;50:256–61.

[21] Leonard HL, Swedo SE, Lenane MC, et al. A 2- to 7-year follow-up study of 54 obsessive-compulsive children and adolescents. Arch Gen Psychiatry 1993; 50:429–39.

[22] Rasmussen SA, Eisen JL. Treatment strategies for chronic and refractory obsessive-compulsive disorder. J Clin Psychiatry 1997;58(Suppl 13):9–13.

[23] Swedo SE, Rapoport JL, Leonard H, et al. Obsessive-compulsive disorder in children and adolescents: clinical phenomenology of 70 consecutive cases. Arch Gen Psychiatry 1989;46:335–41.

[24] Leonard HL. New developments in the treatment of obsessive-compulsive disorder. J Clin Psychiatry 1997;58(Suppl 14):39–45.

[25] Pollack MH, Zaninelli R, Goddard A, et al. Paroxetine in the treatment of generalized anxiety disorder: results of a placebo-controlled, flexible-dosage trial. J Clin Psychiatry 2001;62:350–7.

[26] Haskell DS, Gambill JD, Gardos G, et al. Doxepin or diazepam for anxious and anxious-depressed outpatients? J Clin Psychiatry 1978;39:135–9.

[27] Linskov R. Delusions of infestations treated with pimozide. Acta Derm Venereol 1985;65:267–70.

[28] Driscoll MS, Rothe MJ, Grant-Kels JM, et al. Delusional parasitosis: a dermatologic psychiatric and pharmacologic approach. JAAD 1993;29:1023–33.

[29] Schatzberg AF, Cole JO, DeBattista C. Manual of clinical psychopharmacology. 3rd edition. Washington, DC: APA Press; 1997. p. 154–5.

[30] Meltzer HY. New drugs for the treatment of schizophrenia. Psychiatr Clin North Am 1993;16:365–85.

[31] Deutch AY, Moghaddam B, Innis RB, et al. Mechanisms of action of atypical antipsychotic drugs: implications for novel therapeutic strategies for schizophrenia. Schizophr Res 1991;4:121–56.

[32] Gerlach J. New antipsychotics: classifications, efficacy and adverse effects. Schizophr Bull 1991;17:289–309.

[33] Davis KL, Kahn RS, Ko G, et al. Dopamine in schizophrenia: a review and reconceptualization. Am J Psychiatry 1991;148:1474–86.

[34] Physicians' desk reference. Montvale (NJ): Medical Economics; 1998.

[35] Lieberman JA. Prediction of outcome in first-episode schizophrenia. J Clin Psychiatry 1993;54(Suppl):13–7.

[36] Casey DE. Side effect profiles of new antipsychotic agents. J Clin Psychiatry 1996;57(Suppl 11):40S–5S.

[37] Prescribing information. Risperdal (risperidone). Titusville (NJ): Janssen Pharmaceutica; 1996.

[38] De Leon OA, Furmaga KM, Canterbury AL, et al. Risperidone in the treatment of delusions of infestation. Int J Psychiatry Med 1997;27:403–9.

[39] Hansen TE, Casey DE, Hoffman WF. Neuroleptic intolerance. Schizophr Bull 1997;23:567–82.

[40] Watson CP, Evans RJ, Reed K, et al. Amitriptyline versus placebo in postherpetic neuralgia. Neurology 1982;32:671–3.

[41] Max MB, Schafer SC, Culnane M, et al. Amitriptyline, but not lorazepam, relieves postherpetic neuralgia. Neurology 1988;38:1427–32.

[42] Watson CPN, Chipman M, Reed K, et al. Amitriptyline versus maprotiline in postherpetic neuralgia : a randomized, double-blind crossover trial. Pain 1992;48: 29–36.

[43] Freinmann C, Harris M, Cawley R. Psychogenic facial pain: presentation and treatment. BMJ 1984; 288:436–8.

[44] Urban BJ, France FD, Steinberger EK, et al. Long-term use of narcotic/antidepressant medication in the management of phantom limb pain. Pain 1986;24: 191–6.

[45] Eberhard G, von Knorring L, Nilsson HL, et al. A double-blind randomized study of clomipramine versus maprotiline in patients with idiopathic pain syndromes. Neuropsychobiology 1988;19:25–34.

[46] Bernstein JE, Whitney DH, Soltani K. Inhibition of histamine-induced pruritus by topical tricyclic antidepressants. J Am Acad Dermatol 1981;5:582–5.

[47] Figueiredo A, Ribeiro CA, Goncalo M, et al. Mechanism of action of doxepin in the treatment of chronic urticaria. Fund Clin Pharmacol 1990;4:147–58.

[48] Lawlor F, Greaves MW. The development of recent strategies in the treatment of urticaria as a result of clinically oriented research. Z Hautkr 1990;65:17–27.

[49] Kishore-Kumar R, Max MB, Schafer SC, et al. Desipramine relieves postherpetic neuralgia. Clin Pharmacol Ther 1990;47:305–12.

# Current Therapy

# Laser Treatment of Vascular Lesions

### Chrys Delling Schmults, MD

*Department of Dermatology, University of Pennsylvania Medical Center, 2 Rhoads Pavilion, 3400 Spruce Street, Philadelphia, PA 19104, USA*

Lasers and other light sources have been developed that remove or improve many vascular lesions that were previously untreatable. Port-wine stains are the most notable example. Many port-wine stains are unresectable, but now can be removed in their entirety noninvasively via laser therapy. Vascular lasers and light sources represent a major advance in dermatology for cosmetic and noncosmetic applications. This article reviews the common vascular conditions amenable to laser therapy and the approaches and devices used.

## Guiding principles in laser therapy

The theory of selective photothermolysis was developed by Anderson and Parish [1]. In simple terms, it postulates that a laser can work by heating to the point of destruction a specific targeted structure within the skin. The targeted structure is destroyed without destroying surrounding tissue because the wavelength of laser light used is absorbed preferentially by the targeted structure and not by surrounding tissue. In the case of vascular lesions, the targeted structure is hemoglobin within blood vessels. The hemoglobin is heated, which also heats and destroys the endothelial cells of the blood vessel walls. In an ideal treatment, the vessel is damaged to the point that blood no longer can course through it. Hemoglobin has three wavelengths of light at which it absorbs a maximal amount of energy: 418 nm, 542 nm, and 577 nm. Vascular lasers have been developed to use these absorption peaks to heat and destroy blood vessels selectively.

A second important principle in laser therapy is that of thermal relaxation time. Simply stated, thermal relaxation time is a measurement of the amount of time it takes for a structure to be heated to the point that heat escapes from it to adjacent structures. The larger the structure, the longer the thermal relaxation time because it takes longer to heat a larger object. In laser therapy, the goal is to heat the target structure maximally, but to stop energy input before the heat begins to escape and damage adjacent structures.

The next important concept is that of pulse duration and the need to match pulse duration to the thermal relaxation time of the target. The pulse duration is the amount of time over which a given dose of light is administered to the skin. For example, q-switched lasers have short pulse durations in the nanosecond range. If 5 Joules of light energy is administered with a q-switched laser, that 5-J dose is given very rapidly over nanoseconds. In contrast, vascular lasers have much longer pulse durations in the millisecond range. With a vascular laser, the same 5-J dose of light may be administered over 1 ms, 40 ms, or 1000 ms; much more slowly than with a q-switched laser.

For a given structure in the skin, the amount of energy absorbed and the subsequent heating and destruction that occur vary greatly between the two previous scenarios. In the first example, when the light dose is given quickly (nanoseconds), only very small structures (with subsequently short thermal relaxation times) are heated significantly. The larger structures did not have a chance to heat up because the energy was given so rapidly. Q-switched nanosecond lasers are used to heat and destroy small structures within the skin, such as particles of tattoo pigment or melanin. Conversely, lasers with longer pulse durations administer a given dose of light relatively slowly.

*E-mail address:* chrysalyne.schmults@uphs.upenn.edu

They heat and destroy larger structures with longer thermal relaxation times. Blood vessels, which are much larger than particles of tattoo pigment, are heated and destroyed by lasers with pulse durations in the millisecond range (termed "long-pulsed lasers"). It follows that larger vessels require longer pulse durations than small vessels for maximal destruction and clinical improvement; this is generally borne out in clinical practice, although multiple other factors come into play as discussed below.

Mismatch of pulse duration and thermal relaxation time can result in adverse effects. Using a pulse duration that is too short (brief) for the targeted structure leads to underheating of that structure and poor efficacy. It also may lead to destruction of smaller unintended targets with shorter thermal relaxation times. Use of pulse durations that are too long can lead to overheating of the target structure. Heat may escape into adjacent structures causing damage.

Finally, another important principle is that longer wavelengths of light penetrate more deeply into the skin. Deeper lesions require a longer wavelength for efficacy. Conversely, more superficial lesions respond to shorter wavelengths.

Two other important terms in laser therapy are "fluence" and "spot size." The fluence is the energy delivered to a given area of skin. It is measured in units of $J/cm^2$. An increase in fluence is an increase in energy emitted by the laser. Increasing the fluence can increase efficacy, but also can increase the risk of scarring if safe parameters are not observed. Spot size is the size of the laser beam administered to the skin surface. In most cases, it is circular, although rectangular spot sizes also are available. Use of a 5-mm spot size means that a circular beam of light measuring 5 mm in diameter is administered to the skin. In general, moving to a larger spot size requires a decrease in energy (a lower fluence) and vice versa. Larger spot sizes also tend to have more scatter (and slightly less efficacy) at the periphery. This difference is usually not noticeable clinically, especially with spot sizes 10 mm and smaller.

In practice, the interaction between laser light and tissue is complicated. Perfectly selective photothermolysis is not yet possible. Multiple structures within the skin absorb laser light to various degrees. If too much energy is absorbed by nontarget structures, blistering, scarring, and dyspigmentation can result. Absorption by epidermal melanin is particularly problematic, especially in patients with Fitzpatrick skin types IV through VI. In these patients, pigmentary alterations (hyperpigmentation and hypopigmentation) resulting from damage to melanocytes are common. Epidermal melanin absorption also can lead to blistering and to injury of nearby dermal structures, resulting in scar formation. Absorption of light by melanin decreases with longer wavelengths. In the case of vascular lasers, longer wavelength lasers still have a high incidence of melanin-related adverse effects (see treatment tip #3 later).

In addition to the direct effects of laser energy on the skin, there are secondary effects of laser injury, such as the inflammatory response. Inflammation and the subsequent changes it produces may play a large role in the ultimate clinical improvement seen with laser therapy. This inflammatory response may help to explain why vascular lesions usually do not disappear immediately with laser treatments, but rather fade gradually in the days and weeks after treatment.

**Brief history of vascular laser development**

Port-wine stains were the initial vascular lesions extensively studied in laser therapy. Argon 488-nm and 514-nm and continuous wave dye 577-nm and 585-nm lasers were used initially. They were associated with a relatively high risk of scarring and pigmentary change [2,3]. Ablative lasers, such as the 10,600-nm carbon dioxide and 2940-nm erbium: yttrium aluminum garnet (Er:YAG) lasers, also were used [4]. These did not target the vasculature, but rather obliterated the lesion as the laser energy was absorbed primarily by water ubiquitous in the skin. Because destruction of a portion of the dermis was necessary for lesion removal, some form of scarring was the norm. Copper vapor 510-nm and 578-nm lasers represented an improvement over the previous lasers above [5]. However, the pulsed dye laser (PDL) largely replaced other lasers in the treatment of port-wine stains.

The PDL with wavelengths ranging from 585 to 600 nm was perfected by Anderson and his group in the 1980s [1,6]. It has become the treatment of choice for port-wine stains. Subsequently the KTP 532-nm laser was found to be useful in the treatment of fine telangiectasias, and intense pulsed light (IPL) systems are effective for diffuse facial erythema. The newer long-pulsed 532-nm KTPs, PDLs, 755-nm alexandrite, diode (with wavelengths 800–900 nm), and 1064-nm neodynium:yttrium aluminum garnet (Nd:YAG) lasers may be helpful in the treatment of leg varicosities and other vascular lesions. Currently a wide array of lasers and light sources are available to the clinician for treatment of vascular lesions, and new devices are being developed constantly.

Many different types of vascular lesions have been shown to resolve or substantially improve with laser therapy, including port-wine stains, hemangiomas,

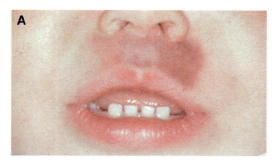 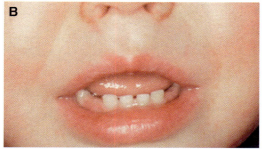

Fig. 1. Port-wine stain in a child before (*A*) and after (*B*) treatment with pulsed dye laser with near-total resolution. (Courtesy of David J. Goldberg, MD, Hackensack, NJ Westwood, NJ, and New York, NY.)

diffuse facial erythema, facial telangiectasia, sclerotherapy-induced matted telangiectasia, spider telangiectasias of the legs, cherry angiomas, spider angiomas, pyogenic granuloma, and vascular malformations arising from CREST syndrome and Osler-Weber-Rendu disease. These lesions are discussed subsequently. Other skin conditions, such as psoriasis, verrucae, and scars, sometimes improve with treatment by vascular lasers. However, because these lesions are not primarily vascular in nature, effects on the vasculature only partially explain the improvements attained. These lesions are not discussed in this article.

## Port wine stains

PDLs remain the mainstay of therapy for port-wine stains. Currently, several devices are commercially available. These lasers have wavelengths ranging from 585 to 600 nm. The early PDLs had fixed pulse durations of 0.45 ms. Newer models have been developed with longer pulse widths. These longer pulse durations better match the 1- to 10-ms thermal relaxation times of port-wine stain vessels. Longer wavelengths of 595 nm and 600 nm penetrate more deeply, enhancing effectiveness. However, these wavelengths are farther from the hemoglobin absorption peak of 577 nm, so higher fluences are required. These higher fluences can cause damage to epidermal melanin. Subsequently, cooling devices have been employed to cool and protect the epidermis while heat is generated in the dermal vessels below. Multiple spot sizes often are available on a single laser via interchangeable hand pieces with 3-, 5-, 7-, and 10-mm round spot sizes commonly seen. Some devices also have rectangular spot sizes that can be used to trace out individual vessels.

The aforementioned modifications have resulted in PDLs with better safety and efficacy in the treatment of port-wine stains. However, complete removal is still not possible in all patients. Overall, approximately 50%–60% of patients have a 75% lightening. A 50% or greater improvement is seen

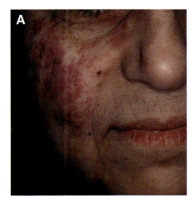 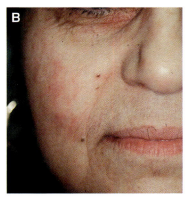

Fig. 2. A thicker port-wine stain in an adult before treatment (*A*) and after (*B*) treatment with improvement, but incomplete clearance after several pulsed dye laser treatment sessions. (Courtesy of David J. Goldberg, MD, Hackensack, NJ Westwood, NJ, and New York, NY.)

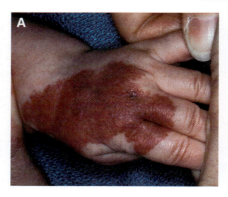 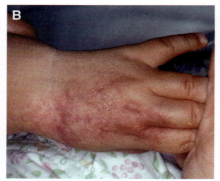

Fig. 3. Port-wine stain on the hand of a child before (*A*) and after (*B*) several treatments with a pulsed dye laser, showing marked improvement, but incomplete resolution. (Courtesy of David J. Goldberg, MD, Hackensack, NJ, Westwood, NJ, and New York, NY.)

in 70%–80% [7]. Thick lesions remain particularly problematic, so treatment should be done in childhood if possible before thickening occurs (Figs. 1 and 2). Large lesions (>20 cm) and lesions of the legs and hands also respond less well (Fig. 3). In most patients, multiple treatments (≥4–10) are required. Optimal treatment parameters are difficult to define from the literature because controlled comparative studies are few, and new lasers are constantly replacing older models. Although often equivalent, the 600-nm wavelength has been shown to improve clearance in some patients (50%) compared with 585-nm wavelength. A higher fluence must be used, however, to compensate for the lower hemoglobin absorption. The higher fluence may result in more dyspigmentation [8].

The main side effect of PDLs is purpura, which generally lasts 5–14 days. Although newer PDLs may generate less purpura, many practitioners believe that treatment is not effective for port-wine stains without purpura. A purpuric response is the chief clinical marker used during treatment. The lowest fluence that produces purpura should be used.

Lasers other than the PDL have been shown to be effective in the treatment of port-wine stains. The long-pulsed 1064-nm Nd:YAG laser has been shown to have efficacy equivalent to the PDL, but with an increased risk of scarring in one study [9]. In a study comparing IPL systems with PDLs, most patients had superior improvement with the PDL, but a subset (6 of 32) had better clearing after IPL therapy [10]. The 532-nm KTP laser has been used to treat port-wine stains refractory to PDL treatment. Adverse effects were increased, however, because higher fluences are needed, and the shorter wavelength results in more epidermal absorption of energy [11]. The long-pulsed 1064-nm Nd:YAG laser also seems to be effective in port-wine stains resistant to PDL. No adverse effects were found in this study [12].

## Hemangiomas (strawberry nevus)

Hemangiomas appear early in infancy, have a growth period of 6–9 months, and usually spontaneously involute during early childhood. Because they resolve on their own, treatment generally is reserved for problematic lesions, such as lesions with a risk of visual or airway obstruction, ocular malformation, bleeding, ulceration, or rapid growth. In these scenarios, a laser may halt growth of the lesion, but cannot remove it. Intralesional or occasionally oral steroids are generally superior to laser therapy in slowing the growth of rapidly proliferating hemangiomas. Laser therapy is useful, however, when steroid therapy is contraindicated or in the case of bleeding or ulcerated hemangioma. One to two PDL treatments generally lead to healing of the ulcerated area, with 5–6 $J/cm^2$ generally being effective [13,14]. Some clinicians also treat early hemangiomas to "nip them in the bud." Studies have not been done to determine if early treatment alters the natural course of hemangiomas. Lasers also can improve the telangiectasia that often remains after a hemangioma has regressed.

## Spider and varicose veins

Sclerotherapy remains the gold standard of noninvasive treatment for spider varicosities of the legs. Progress is rapidly being made in laser technology, however. Laser therapy currently is indicated for matted telangiectasias and other vessels that are too small to accommodate a sclerotherapy needle. It also can be used in patients who cannot tolerate sclerotherapy because of needle phobia or allergy to sclerosing agents.

Compared with port-wine stains, spider veins often require longer wavelengths to enhance penetration to deep vessels. Spider and varicose veins also require longer pulse widths of 20–50 ms or longer because vessels are larger (0.1–5 mm) than vessels comprising port-wine stains. Hyperpigmentation is common even in light-skinned individuals; this usually resolves with time.

Long-pulsed PDLs have been shown to clear vessels with diameters less than 0.5 mm completely. For vessels 0.5–1 mm, improvement, but not clearance, is achieved [15]. Long-pulsed 532-nm KTP and 532-nm Nd:YAG lasers also have been shown to improve, and sometimes clear, lesions [16,17]. The 532-nm Nd:YAG had a high incidence of adverse effects with 10% scarring and 94% hyperpigmentation rates. The long-pulsed 755-nm alexandrite also improved, but did not clear vessels after a single treatment. More than one third of patients had hyperpigmentation [18]. Diode lasers use a small hemoglobin absorption peak at 915 nm in treating vascular lesions. The longer wavelength penetrates more deeply to treat deeper and generally larger vessels. A 940-nm diode laser had no effect on small vessels, but was found to improve larger spider veins of 0.8–1.4 mm in most (88%) patients [19].

In a comparative study, a long-pulsed 1064-nm Nd:YAG laser was found to be superior to long-pulsed 755-nm alexandrite and 810-nm diode lasers for spider veins [20]. Initially the long-pulsed 1064-nm Nd:YAG laser was found to be inferior to sclerotherapy [21]. However, a more recent study has shown them to be equivalent [22]. Diode lasers also are improving, with 6 of 35 patients having complete clearance 6 months after two treatments with a long-pulsed diode laser [23]. Newer devices with longer pulse durations, higher fluences, and combined laser/radiofrequency technology show promise and soon may prove superior to sclerotherapy [24].

A drawback to laser therapy and sclerotherapy is that the usual underlying cause of spider veins, incompetence of a large underlying vein, is not treated. Subsequently, new spider veins continue to form after treatment. Spider and large varicose veins have been shown to respond well to intravenous occlusion of deep incompetent veins with laser or radiofrequency devices [25,26]. This is a minimally invasive technique, however, requiring cannulation of the incompetent vein under ultrasound guidance. It is not discussed in this article.

## Facial telangiectasia and diffuse facial erythema

KTPs, PDLs, and IPL systems are the three devices primarily used in treating facial erythema and telangiectasia. As opposed to lasers, which deliver light of only a single wavelength, IPL systems deliver light comprised of a broad range of wavelengths. Various filters are used to block out portions of the light spectrum and administer wavelengths suitable for a particular lesion. Although KTP, PDL, and IPL all may improve diffuse erythema and discrete telangiectasias, IPL systems generally are best for diffuse erythema, whereas PDL and KTP systems are best for individual telangiectasias. Clearance sometimes may be achieved in a single treatment, but two to three treatments generally are required for telangiectasia, and two to five treatments are required for diffuse erythema. Reformation of lesions is common because photodamage and rosacea often underlie facial erythema and telangiectasia. The more recently developed long-pulsed Nd:YAG lasers also can be used to treat facial telangiectasia (Fig. 4).

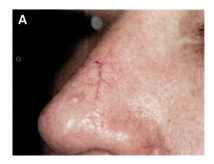
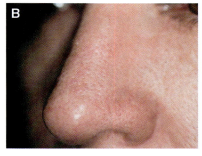

Fig. 4. Telangiectasia of the nasal sidewall before (*A*) and after (*B*) treatment with the millisecond Nd:YAG laser with total resolution. (Courtesy of David J. Goldberg, MD, Hackensack, NJ, Westwood, NJ and New York, NY.)

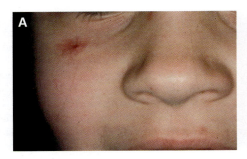 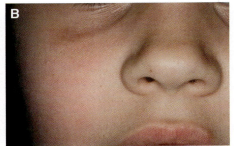

Fig. 5. Spider angioma on the cheek of a child before (*A*) and after (*B*) treatment with the pulsed dye laser with resolution of the lesion and hyperpigmentation, which resolved spontaneously. (Courtesy of David J. Goldberg, MD, Hackensack, NJ, Westwood, NJ, and New York, NY.)

KTP lasers are equipped with small spot sizes of less than 1 mm and are ideally suited for tracing out individual telangiectasias. In a study comparing four different KTP lasers, all were found to have equal efficacy [27]. Although no adverse effects occurred in this study, there is a risk of blistering with KTP lasers if the operator does not keep the laser tip moving during treatment. This risk may be minimized if epidermal cooling is employed [28]. There is no purpura as with PDL treatment.

PDLs can be used to clear individual telangiectasias and diffuse erythema. PDLs have a circular spot size, and treatment areas should not overlap by more than 30%. PDLs generally do not allow for clearance of diffuse erythema in a single treatment. Between treatments, patients may have a meshwork of clear areas separated by areas of erythema. Patients should be made aware of this in advance. Although newer PDLs generate less purpura, it seems that purpura is still required for optimal lesion clearance in many cases [29].

IPL systems are ideal for treating diffuse erythema. IPL systems have large rectangular spot sizes, and overlap of treatment areas is less problematic compared with PDLs. It is easier to clear large areas of diffuse erythema in fewer treatments.

## Miscellaneous lesions

### Pediatric spider angiomas and pyogenic granulomas

Spider angiomas usually occur on the face in children. If they are of cosmetic concern to the child, they usually can be cleared in one to two treatments with either the PDL [30] or the KTP laser (Fig. 5). Pyogenic granuloma is another common childhood lesion amenable to laser treatment. Although they generally resolve spontaneously, these lesions may create cosmetic concern and often bleed profusely, making rapid resolution desirable. Pyogenic granulomas are easily treated in one to two treatments, particularly with the PDL (Fig. 6).

### Syndromes and other conditions with vascular anomalies

Many diseases and syndromes have cutaneous vascular lesions as a feature [31]. Lasers currently have a limited role in the treatment of more severe disorders, such as Klippel-Trénaunay-Weber or Maffucci syndrome, in which malformation of large, dilated, or deep vessels is involved. Disorders with more superficial lesions, such as the lesions seen in

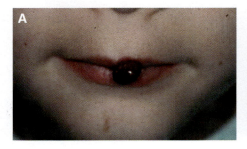 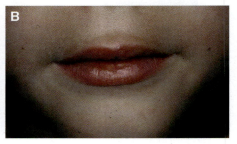

Fig. 6. Pyogenic granuloma on the lip before (*A*) and after (*B*) treatment with the pulsed dye laser with complete resolution. (Courtesy of David J. Goldberg, MD, Hackensack, NJ, Westwood, NJ, and New York, NY.)

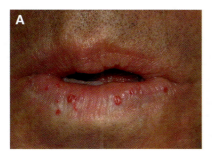
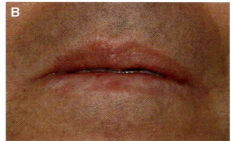

Fig. 7. Vascular malformations of the lip in a patient with Osler-Weber-Rendu disease before (*A*) and after (*B*) treatment with the pulsed dye laser. Total resolution is achieved briefly, but new lesions continue to form. This patient is retreated every 6–8 weeks.

hereditary hemorrhagic telangiectasia (also known as "Osler-Weber-Rendu disease") or CREST syndrome, are amenable to laser therapy. PDL and KTP lasers may be used to treat these lesions, which may be of cosmetic concern or cause difficulty due to bleeding in the case of hereditary hemorrhagic telangiectasia. Complete resolution is not always possible, and patients are likely to continue to develop new lesions. Control rather than cure is achieved (Fig. 7).

Patients with multiple telangiectasias of the mouth, lips, palms, or soles should be asked about a history of nosebleeds (epistaxis) and a family history of similar lesions. If the patient reports such a history, he or she may have hereditary hemorrhagic telangiectasia and should be referred to a pulmonologist, gastroenterologist, and possibly a neurologist to rule out vascular anomalies in other organs. Pulmonic arteriovenous fistulas are particularly life-threatening.

Sturge-Weber syndrome is important to consider in patients with port-wine stains in the V1 (ophthalmic) distribution of the trigeminal nerve. MRI should be done at birth in such patients and repeated within a few years if normal. An electroencephalogram should be obtained if abnormalities are present on MRI, and the patient should be seen by a neurologist. Glaucoma may develop in patients with periocular port-wine stains of either V1 or 2 (maxillary) distributions. These patients should be followed by an ophthalmologist. Port-wine stains associated with these disorders may respond well to PDL treatment. Treatment should be performed as early as possible.

Cobb syndrome should be considered in patients with vascular malformations overlying the spinal cord. MRI should be performed to rule out vascular malformation within the spinal cord. The patient should be followed by a neurologist for early detection of symptoms even if MRI is negative.

Finally, a wide array of systemic medical conditions, including such varied diseases as lupus, sarcoidosis, lymphoma, and tuberculosis, can present with erythematous or telangiectatic cutaneous lesions. It is important to keep the presentations of these diseases in mind when seeing patients with cutaneous vascular lesions. The wide array of diseases with similar presentations underscores the need for dermatologists to be involved in the care of patients seeking cutaneous laser therapy.

**Complications**

Hyperpigmentation is a common adverse effect of vascular laser therapy (Fig. 8). It occurs in approximately 10%–30% of patients and occurs unpredictably. Patients should be warned in advance of this possibility. It is most common in darker skin types and in patients with tans. However, hyperpigmentation can occur in light-skinned patients as well, even

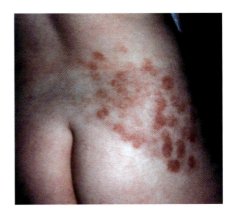

Fig. 8. Hyperpigmentation after pulsed dye laser therapy. This should resolve over months to years. Improvement may be hastened by topical hydroquinone treatment or q-switched Nd:YAG therapy by an experienced practitioner. (Courtesy of David J. Goldberg, MD, Hackensack, NJ, Westwood, NJ, and New York, NY.)

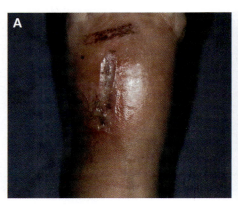 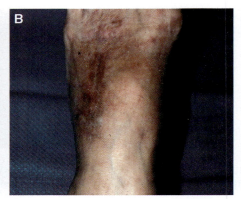

Fig. 9. Severe burn (*A*) leading to scarring (*B*) of the dorsal foot after an intense pulsed light treatment. (Courtesy of David J. Goldberg, MD, Hackensack, NJ, Westwood, NJ, and New York, NY.)

when treatment is performed under correct parameters. It usually resolves with time, but may take months to years to fade completely. Fading may be expedited by use of hydroquinone-containing creams. Sun avoidance is paramount during the resolution phase.

Hypopigmentation also occurs in 2%–3% of patients. It often improves with time, but some cases may be permanent. Atrophic scarring occurs in 1%–5% of patients. If mild, hypopigmentation may improve with time to the point that it is no longer visible. Hypertrophic scarring is rare, occurring in less than 1% of patients when appropriate treatment parameters are used. Dermatitis and ulceration have been reported. Keloid formation has been reported in association with isotretinoin therapy after PDL treatment [32], but not after diode laser therapy [33]. Burns generally occur as a result of overtreatment with an excessive fluence. Care must be taken and lower fluences used on the neck, periocular area, upper lip, and bony prominences, where the risk of burning is increased (Fig. 9).

**Treatment tips**

1. *Take an appropriate history,* noting medications such as nonsteroidal anti-inflammatory drugs and warfarin, which may cause increased purpura, and isotretinoin, which may increase risk of scarring. Many practitioners wait for 1 year after isotretinoin therapy has been completed before performing laser or other elective surgical procedures.
2. *Perform a physical examination* as needed to ensure that the lesion you are treating is benign and does not reflect an underlying medical condition. If there is any question as to the diagnosis, perform a biopsy before any treatment. Examine closely for tan lines and inquire about use of bronzers. Treatment should be delayed until the patient's skin has returned to its natural color.
3. *Note the patient's Fitzpatrick skin type and adjust the treatment accordingly.* Particular care must be taken when treating patients with Fitzpatrick skin types IV and V. In darker skinned individuals, melanin absorbs much of the light output from vascular lasers. This absorption decreases the effectiveness of vascular laser therapy because less light reaches the target vessels in the dermis. A higher fluence is needed to increase the energy to the deeper vessels. However, these higher fluences can cause severe epidermal damage, including blistering, scarring, and dyspigmentation. In a study of Asian patients, cryogen cooling was found to protect the epidermis, allowing for adequate fluences to treat port-wine stains effectively with minimal adverse effect [34]. Safe and effective treatment of vascular lesions patients with type VI skin remains elusive, even in the most experienced hands.
4. *Set realistic patient expectations.* Ensure that patients know approximately how many treatments will be required and whether or not total resolution is likely. Particularly for thicker port-wine stains, spider veins, and hemangiomas, it is important to stress that improvement, rather than clearance, is the goal. If recurrence is likely, as with spider veins, and facial erythema and telangiectasia, this too should be explained. Take standardized

photographs of patients before, during, and after treatment to chronicle the effects of treatment. Discuss common adverse effects, such as dyspigmentation, and rarer ones, such as scarring.
5. *Know thy laser*. Different devices have different settings, so it is paramount to consult the operation manual for the device you are using to establish a safe and appropriate range of laser settings for the lesion you are treating. It also is helpful to obtain advice from colleagues who have experience with the particular laser device you plan to use. Use of too high a fluence can lead to burns and scarring. You also must know how to administer a treatment safely. There are often different distance adapters for different laser hand pieces. These adapters set the focal point for the laser light by determining how far the laser tip is held from the patient during treatment. If they are not used correctly, and the hand piece is not held at the correct distance from the patient, the actual fluence delivered to the skin can be altered, resulting in an ineffective treatment or in burns and scars. Many lasers have adjustable cooling mechanisms or require cooling gels (eg, as with IPL systems) to protect the epidermis and decrease adverse effects. You must be familiar with the proper use of the cooling system for your laser. Finally, almost all lasers require eye protection for the patient and any other personnel in the treatment room (Fig. 10). The type of protection differs depending on the device and the wavelength of light emitted. Failure to use proper eye protection can result in retinal damage. Corneal shields must be used if working over or near the orbit.
6. *Perform test spots* before treating the entire area to establish optimal treatment parameters. These tests should be done in the least obvious location. For each new test spot, increase the fluence at small increments over a safe range. Evaluate in 1 month, then perform treatment to the entire area using the lowest fluence that produced clearing of the lesion. This approach also can be used to determine optimal pulse durations.
7. *Consider anesthetic requirements*. Most adult patients tolerate laser treatment of vascular lesions well without anesthesia if coolants are used appropriately. However, pain may vary by patient and by the lesion being treated. Port-wine stains and spider veins are the most painful lesions to treat. Topical anesthetics, such as EMLA cream, are vasoconstrictors and may make treatment more difficult to administer and potentially less effective. Many children have difficulty tolerating laser treatment. If the treatment area is large, conscious sedation or general anesthesia may be considered. An appropriately trained person other than the laser operator should administer and monitor this anesthesia.
8. *Postoperative care:* After treatment, advise patients to apply cool compresses as necessary for mild discomfort, apply petrolatum or Aquaphor to any areas of crusting, avoid the sun during healing, use sunblock thereafter, and avoid makeup to the area until healed. An exception is PDL-induced purpura, which can be covered by makeup. Green-tinted makeup works best and can be purchased at department stores.
9. *Treatment of erythema and telangiectasia with the PDL:* Begin with the lowest fluence that causes faint purpura. Purpura may be transient, with a brief purpuric flash indicating adequate treatment in some cases. At subsequent treatments, you may increase by 0.5 J/cm$^2$ to maintain efficacy. For most lesions, the maximum fluence is 9–11 J/cm$^2$. Lower fluences are often sufficient for clearance. On delicate areas, such as the neck, eyelids, and upper lip, fluences should be kept lower. A maximum of 6–8 J/cm$^2$ is usually more appropriate in these areas. The maximal energy depends on the laser and lesion in question. Treatment should be stopped when a therapeutic plateau has been reached. Continuing therapy at energy levels higher than those mentioned should be done cautiously and only with experience because the risk of scarring is elevated at higher fluences.
10. *Treatment of port-wine stains with the PDL:* If the lesion was treated in the past with laser or x-ray therapy, examine closely for evidence of scarring and pigmentary change. This may become more obvious as the port-wine stain is removed. Warn patients about purpura and its usual duration of 5–14 days. Use test spots, evaluate at 1 month, and begin with the lowest fluence that resulted in clearance of the lesion. Repeat treatments every 6–8 weeks. Purpura and light crusting can be expected. Blisters or erosions indicate overtreatment, usually with too high a fluence. Most lesion clearance occurs in 4–10 treatments. However, addi-

tional benefits can occur with continued therapy [35].

11. *Using the KTP laser:* There is more room for operator-dependent error with KTP lasers compared with PDLs. The laser tip must be moved constantly during treatment. If the laser is fired repetitively in the same area, overtreatment occurs, as indicated by blistering, erosion, and potentially scarring. When using the KTP, trace the vessels with the laser light moving at a rate that produces transient disappearance of the vessels without epidermal blanching. Using a headlamp and loops may aid in visualizing this therapeutic end point. Erythema is common for the first 24 hours after treatment.

## Tips for entering laser practice

The dermatologist should decide which types of vascular lesions he or she wishes to treat. It is important to consider this initially because no single laser can treat all vascular lesions with equal efficacy. If one's primary interest is diffuse facial erythema, an IPL system might be chosen. If one sees pediatric patients with port-wine stains, pyogenic granulomas, and spider angiomas and adults with facial telangiectasia, the PDL is likely the best choice. As the dermatologist refines his or her expertise in laser therapy, he or she may purchase or rent additional lasers to treat an increasing number of lesions. The temptation to treat all lesions with a single device should be avoided, and it should be recognized that some lesions may be suboptimally treated with the device on hand. Referrals to other physicians should be made as appropriate in these cases.

## Acknowledgments

The author thanks Dr. David J. Goldberg for the kind use of his photographs and Dr. Mussarrat Hussain for his generous assistance with background material.

## References

[1] Anderson RR, Parish JA. Microvasculature can be selectively damaged using dye lasers: a basic theory and experimental evidence in human skin. Lasers Surg Med 1981;1:263–76.
[2] Cosman B. Clinical experience in the laser therapy of port wine stains. Lasers Surg Med 1980;1:133–52.
[3] Lanigan SW, Cartwright P, Cotterill JA. Continuous wave dye laser therapy of port wine stains. Br J Dermatol 1989;121:345–52.
[4] Lanigan SW, Cotterill JA. The treatment of port wine stains with the carbon dioxide laser. Br J Dermatol 1990;123:229–35.
[5] Sheehan-Dare RA, Cotterill JA. Copper vapour laser treatment of port wine stains: clinical evaluation and comparison with conventional argon laser therapy. Br J Dermatol 1993;128:546–9.
[6] Dierickx CC, Casparian JM, Venugopalan V, et al. Thermal relaxation of port-wine stain vessels probed in vivo: the need for 1–10-millisecond laser pulse treatment. J Invest Dermatol 1995;105:709–14.
[7] Kelly KM, Nanda VS, Nelson JS. Treatment of port-wine stain birthmarks using the 1.5-msec pulsed dye laser at high fluences in conjunction with cryogen spray cooling. Dermatol Surg 2002;28:309–13.
[8] Edstrom DW, Ros AM. The treatment of port-wine stains with the pulsed dye laser at 600 nm. Br J Dermatol 1997;136:360–3.
[9] Lorenz S, Scherer K, Wimmershoff MB, et al. Variable pulse frequency-doubled Nd:YAG laser versus flashlamp-pumped pulsed dye laser in the treatment of port wine stains. Acta Derm Venereol 2003;83:210–3.
[10] Strempel H, Klein G. Laser therapy without laser: a controlled clinical trial comparing the flashlamp-pumped dye laser with the Photderm high-energy gas discharge lamp. Lasers Surg Med 1996;11:185–7.
[11] Chowdhury MM, Harris S, Lanigan SW. Potassium titanyl phosphate laser treatment of resistant port-wine stains. Br J Dermatol 2001;144:814–7.
[12] Woo WK, Jasim ZF, Handley JM. Evaluating the efficacy of treatment of resistant port-wine stains with variable-pulse 595-nm pulsed dye and 532-nm Nd:YAG lasers. Dermatol Surg 2004;30(2 Pt 1):158–62.

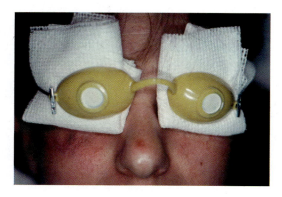

Fig. 10. Eye protection is a must for all persons present in the room during laser therapy. (Courtesy of David J. Goldberg, MD, Hackensack, NJ, Westwood, NJ, and New York, NY.)

[13] Garden JM, Bakus AD, Paller AS. Treatment of cutaneous hemangiomas by the flashlamp-pumped pulsed dye laser: prospective analysis. J Pediatr 1992;120(4 Pt 1): 555–60.

[14] Ashinoff R, Geronemus RG. Capillary hemangiomas and treatment with the flash lamp-pumped pulsed dye laser. Arch Dermatol 1991;127:202–5.

[15] Reichert D. Evaluation of the long-pulse dye laser for the treatment of leg telangiectasias. Dermatol Surg 1998;24:737–40.

[16] Fournier N, Brisot D, Mordon S. Treatment of leg telangiectasias with a 532-nm KTP laser in multipulse mode. Dermatol Surg 2002;28:564–71.

[17] McMeekin TO. Treatment of spider veins of the leg using a long-pulsed Nd:YAG laser (Versapulse) at 532 nm. J Cutan Laser Ther 1999;1:179–80.

[18] Kauvar AN, Lou WW. Pulsed alexandrite laser for the treatment of leg telangiectasia and reticular veins. Arch Dermatol 2000;136:1371–5.

[19] Passeron T, Olivier V, Duteil L, et al. The new 940-nanometer diode laser: an effective treatment for leg venulectasia. J Am Acad Dermatol 2003;48:768–74.

[20] Eremia S, Li C, Umar SH. A side-by-side comparative study of 1064 nm Nd:YAG, 810 nm diode and 755 nm alexandrite lasers for treatment of 0.3–3 mm leg veins. Dermatol Surg 2002;28:224–30.

[21] Lupton JR, Alster TS, Romero P. Clinical comparison of sclerotherapy versus long-pulsed Nd:YAG laser treatment for lower extremity telangiectases. Dermatol Surg 2002;28:694–7.

[22] Levy JL, Elbahr C, Jouve E, et al. Comparison and sequential study of long pulsed Nd:YAG 1,064 nm laser and sclerotherapy in leg telangiectasias treatment. Lasers Surg Med 2004;34:273–6.

[23] Wollina U, Konrad H, Schmidt WD, et al. Response of spider leg veins to pulsed diode laser (810 nm): A clinical, histological and remission spectroscopy study. J Cosmet Laser Ther 2003;5:154–62.

[24] Chess C. Prospective study on combination diode laser and radiofrequency energies (ELOS) for the treatment of leg veins. J Cosmet Laser Ther 2004;6:86–90.

[25] Weiss RA, Weiss MA. Controlled radiofrequency endovenous occlusion using a unique radiofrequency catheter under duplex guidance to eliminate saphenous varicose vein reflux: a 2-year follow-up. Dermatol Surg 2002;28:38–42.

[26] Navarro L, Min RJ, Bone C. Endovenous laser: a new minimally invasive method of treatment for varicose veins—preliminary observations using an 810 nm diode laser. Dermatol Surg 2001;27:117–22.

[27] Goldberg DJ, Meine JG. A comparison of four frequency-doubled Nd:YAG (532 nm) laser systems for treatment of facial telangiectases. Dermatol Surg 1999;25:463–7.

[28] Kauvar AN, Frew KE, Friedman PM, et al. Cooling gel improves pulsed KTP laser treatment of facial telangiectasia. Lasers Surg Med 2002;30:149–53.

[29] Alam M, Dover JS, Arndt KA. Treatment of facial telangiectasia with variable-pulse high-fluence pulsed-dye laser: comparison of efficacy with fluences immediately above and below the purpura threshold. Dermatol Surg 2003;29:681–5.

[30] Geronemus RG. Treatment of spider telangiectases in children using the flashlamp-pumped pulsed dye laser. Pediatr Dermatol 1991;8:61–3.

[31] Paller A, Hirschhorn K, Willner J. Disorders of vascularization. In: Spitz JL, editor. Genodermatoses: a full-color clinical guide to genetic skin disorders. Baltimore: Williams & Wilkins; 1996. p. 88–116.

[32] Bernstein LJ, Geronemus RG. Keloid formation with 585-nm pulsed dye laser during isotretinoin treatment. Arch Dermatol 1997;133:111–2.

[33] Khatri KA. Diode laser hair removal in patients undergoing isotretinoin therapy. Dermatol Surg 2004;30: 1205–7.

[34] Chang CJ, Nelson JS. Cryogen spray cooling and higher fluence pulsed dye laser treatment improve port-wine stain clearance while minimizing epidermal damage. Dermatol Surg 1999;25:767–72.

[35] Kauvar AN, Geronemus RG. Repetitive pulsed dye laser treatments improve persistent port wine stains. Dermatol Surg 1995;21:182–8.

# Cumulative Index 2005

*Note:* Page numbers of article titles are in **boldface** type.

## A

Abdominal contour procedures, **475–493**
  after gastric bypass surgery, 488
  anatomy in, 475–476
  complications of, 488, 492
  in obese patients, 486, 488
  patient consultation and evaluation for, 476–477
  techniques for, 477–482
    full abdominoplasty with or without suction-assisted lipectomy, 481–482
    mini-abdominoplasty, 480
    minimal access abdominoplasty, 482–486
      endoscopically assisted or muscle access abdominoplasty, 485–486
      extended liposuction, 483–484
      open mini-abdominoplasty, 484–485
    modified abdominoplasty, 480–481
    suction-assisted lipectomy, 478–480

Abdominoplasty. *See* Abdominal contour procedures.

Ablative facial resurfacing, **549–559**
  chemical peels in, 370, 550–552
    agents in, 550–551
    postoperative care for, 552
    technique for, 551–552
  combined procedures in, 554
  complications of, 555–559
    erythema, 558
    hyperpigmentation, 557–558
    hypopigmentation, 557
    milia, 557
    scars, 558
  dermabrasion in, 552–553
    instruments for, 552
    technique for, 552–553
  Fitzpatrick skin type and, 549
  indications for, 549
  lasers in, 553–554
  patient preparation for, 549–550
  patient selection for, 549
  results of, 554–555

Ablative lasers, in surgical revisions, 148–149

Abuse, physical and sexual, and posttraumatic stress disorder, 650–651

Acne. *See also* Acne vulgaris.
  depression with. *See* Depression.
  eating disorders and, 597
  emotional impact of, 623
  isotretoin for, suicide due to. *See* Suicide.
  photodynamic therapy for, 204–205
  psychosomatic aspects of, 602, 603–604

Acne vulgaris. *See also* Acne.
  cosmetics for, **575–581**
    cleansers, 576–577
    corneolytics, 577
    definition of, 575
    moisturizers, 577
    retinol, 577
    sulfur, 577
    versus anti-acne drugs, 575–576
    weeks 1 to 4, 577–578
    weeks 4 to 8, 578
    weeks 8 to 12, 578
    weeks 12 to 16, 578
    weeks 16 to 20, 578–579
    weeks 20 to 24, 579

Actinic cheilitis, imiquimod for, 154

Actinic keratoses, imiquimod for, 152, 154, 249–250
  of hands, topical agents for, 516

Acupuncture, in dermatology, 723–724

Acyclovir, indications for, 314–315

Advancement flaps, in auricular reconstruction, 33–38
  in eyebrow reconstruction, 10
  in forehead reconstruction, 4, 7–9
  in lip reconstruction, 46–48, 50–51
  in scalp reconstruction, 19–20

Aging skin, demographics of, 643
  psychosocial aspects of, **643–648**
    body image, 646–647
    Brief Symptom Inventory of, 644
    business interactions, 645
    caregiver reactions, 645
    Eating Disorder Inventory in, 646
    eating disorders, 646–647
    facial expressions, 644–645
    interpersonal interactions, 644–645
    narcissistic personality, 646
    psychologic state, 645–646
    suicidal ideation, 646

Aldara. *See* Imiquimod.

Alefacept. *See* Systemic immune modulators.

Alexithymia, with psoriasis, 685

Allogenic fillers, in facial rejuvenation, 367–368
  in soft tissue augmentation, 353

Alopecia. *See* Hair loss.

Aminolevulinic acid, in photodynamic therapy, 204

Amitriptyline, for dermatologic conditions, 743

Anesthesia, in dermabrasion, 553
  in forehead reconstruction, 2
  in laser therapy, for vascular lesions, 753
  in nasal reconstruction, with dorsal nasal flaps, 78
    with forehead flaps, 89
  in reduction structured rhinoplasty, 533–534
  in rhytidectomy, 418
  topical, in pediatric dermatology, 174
  tumescent, in ambulatory phlebectomy, for varicose veins, 447–448
    in follicular unit transplantation, 401

Angioedema, depression with, 661

Angiomas, spider, in children, laser therapy for, 750

Anthralin, for alopecia areata, 237

Anti-acne drugs, for acne vulgaris, 575–576

Antiandrogen therapy, for female pattern hair loss, 232

Antibiotics, **301–312**
  dalbavancin and oritavancin, 309
  daptomycin, 301–303
    adverse effects of, 302–303
    clinical data on, 301–302
    historical aspects of, 301
    indications for, 301
    interactions with, 302
    mechanism of action of, 301
    pharmacokinetics and dosing of, 302
  gatifloxacin and moxifloxacin, 307–309
    adverse effects of, 308–309
    clinical data on, 308
    historical aspects of, 307
    indications for, 307–308
    interactions with, 308
    mechanism of action of, 307
    pharmacokinetics and dosing of, 308
  in follicular unit transplantation, 400
  in wound healing, 185, 188
  interactions with, 335–336
  linezolid, 303–306
    adverse effects of, 305–306
    clinical data on, 304
    for diabetic foot ulcers, 189
    historical aspects of, 303
    indications for, 303–304
    interactions with, 304–305
    mechanism of action of, 303
    pharmacokinetics and dosing of, 304
    spectrum of activity of, 303
  quinupristin-dalfopristin, 306–307
    adverse effects of, 307
    clinical data on, 306
    historical aspects of, 306
    indications for, 306
    interactions with, 307
    mechanism of action of, 306
    pharmacokinetics and dosing of, 306–307

Antidepressants, for anxiety, 740
  for depression, 737–739
  in dermatology, 731

Antimicrobial dressings, in wound healing, 189–190

Antioxidant therapy, for hypomelanosis, 216

Antipsychotic drugs, for delusional disorders, 741

Antiviral therapy, **313–322**
  acyclovir in, 314–315
  cidofovir in, 316, 318, 319
  experimental vaccines in, 319–320
    for herpesvirus infections, 319
    for human papillomavirus, 319–320
  famciclovir in, 315
  fomivirsen in, 316
  for cytomegalovirus, 314
  for Epstein-Barr virus, 314
  for herpes simplex-1, 313
  for herpes simplex-2, 313–314
  for herpes zoster, 314
  for human papillomavirus, 317–318
  for molluscum contagiosum, 318–319
  foscarnet in, 316–317

ganciclovir/valganciclovir in, 315–316
helicase primase inhibitors in, 317
highly active antiretroviral therapy in, 319
immunomodulators in, 317–318
nucleoside agents in, 314
penciclovir in, 315
valacyclovir in, 315

Anxiety, in dermatology patient, management of, 731, 739–740
with psoriasis, 683–684

Anxiolytics, in dermatology, 731, 739–740

Apligraf, for diabetic foot ulcers, 189

Aptos threads, in suspension procedures, for aging face. *See* Suspension procedures, subdermal suspension threads in.

Aromatherapy, in dermatology, 724

Artecoll, in soft tissue augmentation, 355, 358

Artefill, in soft tissue augmentation, 355, 358

Arterial ulcers, healing of, 188

Ascorbic acid, for hypermelanosis, 217

Atopic dermatitis, cognitive-behavioral therapy for, 726
depression with, 660–661
emotional impact of, 622–623
hypnosis for, 729
in children, massage therapy for.
    *See* Massage therapy.
psychoneuroimmunologic factors in.
    *See* Psychoneuroimmunologic factors.
psychosomatic aspects of, 602

Atypical antipsychotic drugs, for delusional disorders, 741–742

Auricular reconstruction, **23–41**
anatomy in, 23
anterior ear, 26–30
    cartilaginous flaps in, 30
    cartilaginous struts in, 30
    full-thickness perforation in, 27–28
    full-thickness skin grafts in, 26–27
    healing by secondary intention in, 26
    pedicle flaps in, 30
    retroauricular flaps in, 30
    split-thickness skin grafts in, 26–27
free cartilage grafts in, 134–138
    complications of, 138
    contraindications to, 135
    donor site issues in, 135
    future trends in, 138
    graft site preparation in, 137
    harvesting in, 135, 137
    indications for, 135
    placement of, 137
    postoperative care for, 138
inferior helix and earlobe, 38, 41
    advancement flaps in, 38
    full-thickness skin grafts in, 38
midhelix, 36–38
    advancement flaps in, 36–37
    retroauricular flaps in, 37–38
    wedge closure in, 37
postauricular interpolation flaps in, 101, 108–112
posterior ear, 24–26
    healing by secondary intention in, 24
    split-thickness skin grafts in, 24–25
superior helix, 33–35
    advancement flaps in, 33–35
    full-thickness skin grafts in, 33
    split-thickness skin grafts in, 35
    transposition flaps in, 35

Autogenic fillers, in soft tissue augmentation, 351, 353

Autologous fat, in soft tissue augmentation, 353

Autonomic hyperarousal, in posttraumatic stress disorder, 652–653

Avelox. *See* Antibiotics, gatifloxacin and moxifloxacin.

Aversion therapy, for neurodermatitis, 726

Azathioprine. *See* Systemic immune modulators.

Azelaic acid, for hypermelanosis, 217, 219


# B

Baker-Gordon solution peels, in ablative facial resurfacing, 550–551

Bariatric surgery, abdominal contour procedures after, 488

Basal cell carcinoma, imiquimod for, 156–157, 250

Basal cell nevus syndrome, imiquimod for, 157, 160

Benzodiazepines, for anxiety, 740

Betamethasone, for alopecia areata, 234

Biochemotherapy, for melanoma, 325, 328

Biofeedback, in dermatology. *See* Complementary psychocutaneous therapies.

Bleaching products, for hypermelanosis, 219
in hand rejuvenation, 516

Blepharoplasty, **431–442**
  anatomy in, 431–433
    lower eyelid, 432–433
    upper eyelid, 431
    upper eyelid fat pads, 431–432
  complications of, 438–441
    lower eyelid, 439–441
    upper eyelid, 439
  lower eyelid, 435–438
    indications for, 435
    subciliary or transcutaneous approach to, 435–436
      excision of excess skin in, 436
      preoperative marking for, 435–436
      technique for, 436
      wound closure in, 436
    tear trough deformity repair in, 438
    transconjunctival approach to, 436–438
      preoperative marking for, 436
      technique for, 436–438
  upper eyelid, 433–435
    indications for, 433
    preoperative marking for, 434
    surgical planning for, 433–434
    technique for, 434–435
      excision of excess fat, 434–435
      raising myocutaneous flap, 434
      wound closure, 435

Blepharoplasty approach, to midface lift, 510–511

Blindness, blepharoplasty and, 439, 440

Blister grafts, for hypomelanosis, 215

Body dysmorphic disorder, in dermatology patient, case report of, 678–679
  evaluation for, 597

Borderline personality disorder, in dermatology patient, evaluation for, 598

Botulinum toxin, in facial rejuvenation, 369–370
  in neck rejuvenation, 469

Bowen's disease, imiquimod for, 154, 156

Brain-skin axis, in psoriasis, 689

Brainwave spectral feedback, in dermatology, 725

Breast enlargement, after power liposuction, 388

Brief Symptom Inventory, of psychosocial aspects, of aging skin, 644

Bupropion, for depression, 738

Burn wounds, autologous cultured keratinocytes for, 185

Burns, in children, massage therapy for. See Massage therapy.

Buspirone, for anxiety, 740

Butorphanol tartrate, in rhytidectomy, 418

Butyl cyanoacrylate, in skin closure, 193

4-N-Butylresorcinol, for hypermelanosis, 217

Byron ARC unit, in power liposuction, 384

## C

Cadexomer iodine, in wound healing, 190

Calcineurin inhibitors, indications for, 251

Calcipotriol, for hypomelanosis, 213–214

Camouflaging, for melanotic pigmentary disorders, 222

Cancer syndromes, imiquimod for, 157, 160

Carbon dioxide lasers, in hand rejuvenation, 519

Carroll Rating Scale for Depression, of depression associated with acne, 666–667

Cartilaginous flaps, in auricular reconstruction, 30

Cartilaginous struts, in auricular reconstruction, 30

Catastrophic life events, and posttraumatic stress disorder, 651

Cheilitis, actinic, imiquimod for, 154

Chemical peels, for hypermelanosis, 219–221
  in ablative facial resurfacing. See Ablative facial resurfacing.
  in hand rejuvenation, 517–518
  in neck rejuvenation, 471–472

Chemotherapy, for melanoma, 325

Children's Dermatology Life Quality Index, in psoriasis, 708, 712

Chin augmentation, facial implants in, 544

Cidofovir, indications for, 316, 318, 319

Cilostazol, for arterial ulcers, 188

Circumoral rotational-advancement flaps, in lip reconstruction, 51

Cleansers, for acne vulgaris, 576–577

Cobb syndrome, laser therapy for, 751

Cognitive-behavioral therapy, in dermatology. See Complementary psychocutaneous therapies.

Collagens, in facial rejuvenation, 367–368
  in soft tissue augmentation, 347, 350

Complementary psychocutaneous therapies, **723–734**
  acupuncture, 723–724
  aromatherapy, 724
  biofeedback, 724–725
    brainwave spectral feedback, 725
    for hyperhidrosis, 725
    for psychosomatic disorders, 604
    for Raynaud's syndrome, 725
    via electromyography, 725
  cognitive-behavioral therapy, 725–727
    aversion therapy in, 726
    for atopic dermatitis, 726
    for hyperhidrosis, 726
    for lichen simplex chronicus, 726
    for neurodermatitis, 726
    for onychotillomania, 726
    for psoriasis, 688
    for psychoneuroimmunologic factors, in vitiligo, 614
    for psychosomatic disorders, 605
    for urticaria, 726–727
    systematic desensitization in, 726
  herbs and supplements, 731
    antidepressants, 731
    anxiolytics, 731
    interactions with, 336–337
    soporifics, 731
  hypnosis, 727–731
    for alopecia areata, 729
    for atopic dermatitis, 729
    for psoriasis, 729
    for skin picking, 728–729
    for urticaria, 730
    for warts, 730
    to reduce procedure anxiety, 730–731

Composite cartilage grafts, in nasal reconstruction. *See* Nasal reconstruction.

Composite lift, in rhytidectomy, 421

Condylomata acuminata, imiquimod for, 248

Congestive heart failure, infliximab and, 285

Conscious sedation, in pediatric dermatology, 175

Consultation-liaison psychiatry, for psychosomatic disorders, in dermatology patient, 630

Contour threads, in suspension procedures, for aging face, 571

Conversion symptoms, in posttraumatic stress disorder, 596–597

Cook's body peels, in hand rejuvenation, 518

Corneolytics, for acne vulgaris, 577

Cortisol, in psoriasis, 687

Cosmetic units, in surgical revisions, 143

Cosmetics, for acne vulgaris. *See* Acne vulgaris.

Cosmoderm, in facial rejuvenation, 367–368
  in soft tissue augmentation, 353

Cosmoplast, in facial rejuvenation, 367–368
  in soft tissue augmentation, 353

CREST syndrome, laser therapy for, 751

Cross-lip flaps, in lip reconstruction, 52

Croton oil peels, in ablative facial resurfacing, 550–551

Cryotherapy, for hypermelanosis, 221

Cubicin. *See* Antibiotics, daptomycin.

Cultured epidermal cell transplantation, for hypomelanosis, 215

Cyanoacrylates, in skin closure, **193–198**
    and wound hemostasis, 196
    as drug delivery device, 196
    as wound dressings, 195–196
    butyl cyanoacrylate, 193
    indications for, 196
    octyl cyanoacrylate, 193–195
      and infections, 194
      cosmetic outcome of, 194
      cost of, 194–195

Cyclophosphamide. *See* Systemic immune modulators.

Cyclosporine, systemic. *See* Systemic immune modulators.
  topical, indications for, 251

Cyproterone acetate, for female pattern hair loss, 232

Cytokine release syndrome, imiquimod and, 161

Cytokines, in wound healing, 182

Cytomegalovirus infections, antiviral therapy for, 314
  mycophenolate mofetil and, 273

# D

Dalbavancin, indications for, 309

Daptomycin. *See* Antibiotics.

Debulking, in surgical revisions, 147–148

Deep plane lift, in rhytidectomy, 421

Delusional disorders, in dermatology patient, evaluation for, 597–598
　　management of, 740–742

Demyelinating diseases, etanercept and, 281
　　infliximab and, 285

Depigmentation therapy, for hypermelanosis. *See* Hypermelanosis.
　　for hypomelanosis, 215–216

Depression, dysthymia in, diagnostic criteria for, 658
　　in dermatology patient, **657–664**
　　　　depressive equivalents in, 658–659
　　　　developmental considerations in, 659
　　　　diagnosis of, 660
　　　　management of, 661, 736–739
　　　　　　antidepressants in, 737–739
　　　　　　bupropion in, 738
　　　　　　doxepin in, 738–739
　　　　　　selective serotonin reuptake inhibitors in, 736–737
　　　　　　venlafaxine in, 737–738
　　　　premenstrual dysphoric disorder in, 660
　　　　subclinical depression, 659
　　　　suicidal and parasuicidal behavior in, 659
　　　　with acne, 661, **665–674**
　　　　　　and suicide. *See* Suicide.
　　　　　　Carroll Rating Scale for Depression in, 666–667
　　　　　　definition of depression in, 665–666
　　　　　　drug-induced, 667
　　　　　　emotional impact of, 666–667
　　　　　　EuroQol instrument in, 667
　　　　　　Hospital Anxiety and Depression scale in, 666, 667
　　　　　　prevalence of, 666
　　　　　　Short Form 36 in, 667
　　　　with alopecia areata, 661
　　　　with atopic dermatitis, 660–661
　　　　with psoriasis, 660, 683
　　　　with urticaria and angioedema, 661
　　major depressive episode in, diagnostic criteria for, 658

Dermabrasion, for hypermelanosis, 221
　　in ablative facial resurfacing. *See* Ablative facial resurfacing.
　　in surgical revisions, 148

Dermagraft, for diabetic foot ulcers, 189

Dermal fillers, for aging face, 561
　　in hand rejuvenation, 525–526

Dermatitis, atopic. *See* Atopic dermatitis.

Dermatology, evidence-based. *See* Evidence-based dermatology.

Dermatology Quality of Life Index, in psoriasis, 707–708, 712

Dermatology Quality-of-Life Scales, in psoriasis, 708–709, 712

Dermatology Specific Quality of Life scale, in psoriasis, 709, 712

Diabetic foot ulcers, healing of, 188–189

Diffuse unpatterned alopecia, diagnosis of, 396–397

Dimethyl triazino imidazole carboxamide, for melanoma, 325

Diphenylcyclopropenone, for alopecia areata, 236–237

Disabling skin diseases, emotional impact of, **619–627**
　　acne, 623
　　atopic dermatitis, 622–623
　　developmental issues in, 620–621
　　　　age of onset, 620–621
　　　　body image, 620
　　　　self-esteem, 620
　　　　tension regulation, 620
　　hair loss, 623–624
　　on families, 624
　　on society, 624–625
　　psoriasis. *See* Psoriasis.
　　stigma experience in, 682, 684–685
　　　　Indian perspective on, **635–642**
　　　　　　gender in, 639
　　　　　　leprosy, 637–638, 639–640
　　　　　　management strategies in, 640
　　　　　　marital status in, 639
　　　　　　psoriasis, 636
　　　　　　quality of life in, 638
　　　　　　vitiligo, 636–637, 640

Dissociation symptoms, in posttraumatic stress disorder, 596–597

Dorsal nasal flaps, in nasal reconstruction. *See* Nasal reconstruction.

Doxepin, for depression, 738–739
　　for dermatologic conditions, 742–743

Drive for Thinness subscale, of Eating Disorders Inventory, of psychosocial aspects, of aging akin, 646

Drug delivery, cyanoacrylates in, 196

Drug interactions, **335–342**
　　adverse binding interactions between drugs and polyvalent cations, 335–336
　　bisphosphonates, 336

mycophenolate mofetil, 336
quinolone antibiotics, 336
tetracyclines, 335–336
adverse interactions between herbal and
conventional drugs, 336–337
St. John's wort, 336–337
epidermal growth factor receptor inhibitors,
339–340
clinical features of, 339
histopathology of, 340
management of, 340
mechanism of, 340
sulfa allergy, 337–339
definition of, 337
patient advice on, 338–339
versus other antibiotics, 337
with antibiotics. See Antibiotics.
with systemic immune modulators. See Systemic
immune modulators.

Duke boot, for venous ulcers, 188

Dysthymia, diagnostic criteria for, 658

# E

Ear reconstruction. See Auricular reconstruction.

Eating Disorder Inventory, of psychosocial aspects, of aging skin, 646

Eating disorders, in dermatology patient, and acne, 597
and aging skin, 646–647
evaluation for, 597

Ectropion, blepharoplasty and, 440

Ectropion repair, technique for, 149–150

Edema, eyelid, blepharoplasty and, 439, 440
facial, facial implants and, 545
follicular unit transplantation and, 410

Efalizumab. See Systemic immune modulators.

Ego-strengthening therapies, in dermatology, 728

Ego structure, and psychosomatic disorders, in dermatology patient, 603

Electromyography, biofeedback via, 725

Elidel, indications for, 252

Emotional neglect, during early development, and posttraumatic stress disorder, 650

Emotional states, dysregulation of, in posttraumatic stress disorder, 653–654

Endoscopic abdominoplasty, technique for, 485–486

Endoscopic forehead lift, **457–467**
advantages of, 462
aging process and, 457–458
anatomy in, 458–460
fascia, 459
neurovascular structures, 459–460
scalp and forehead musculature, 458–459
forehead and brow facial analysis in, 460
patient selection for, 460–462
brow ptosis and position in, 461
frontal hairline position in, 462
skin quality in, 461
technique for, 462–466
dissection, 463–465
instruments, 462–463
preoperative marking, 462
temporary versus permanent fixation, 465–467

Endotine Midface suspension device, in midface lift, 512–513

Endovenous laser therapy, for varicose veins. See Varicose veins.

Epidermal cell transplantation, for hypomelanosis, 215

Epidermal growth factor receptor inhibitors, interactions with. See Drug interactions.

Epstein-Barr virus, antiviral therapy for, 314

Erbium:YAG lasers, in hand rejuvenation, 519–520
indications for, 202

Erythema, ablative facial resurfacing and, 558
facial, laser therapy for, 749–750, 753

Estlander circumoral cross-lip flaps, in lip reconstruction, 52

Etanercept. See Systemic immune modulators.

Etretinate, for acne, depression due to, 671

EuroQol instrument, of depression associated with acne, 667

Eutectic mixture of local anesthetics, in pediatric dermatology, 174

Evidence-based dermatology, clinical rating scales for, **703–706**
choice of instrument for, 706
construct measurement in, 703
power analysis of, 706
precision in, 704
reliability of, 704–705
standardization of, 706
validity of, 705–706

Excimer laser therapy, for hypomelanosis, 212–213, 214

Expanded polytetrafluoroethylene, in soft tissue augmentation, 359

Extended superficial musculoaponeurotic system flap, in rhytidectomy, 420

Extended supraplatysmal plane skin flap, in rhytidectomy, 421

Extracellular matrix, in wound healing, 183

Extragenital Bowen's disease, imiquimod for, 154, 156

Extramammary Paget's disease, imiquimod for, 161

Extrapyramidal side effects, of antipsychotic drugs, 741

Eyebrow reconstruction. See Forehead reconstruction.

Eyelids, cosmetic surgery on. See Blepharoplasty.

# F

Face-lift. See Rhytidectomy.

Facial expressions, aging skin and, 644–645

Facial implants, for aging face, **541–547**, 561–562
    complications of, 544–546
    patient evaluation for, 542
    results of, 546–547
    technique for, chin augmentation, 544
        malar and submalar augmentation, 542–544

Facial rejuvenation, nonsurgical, **365–371**
    botulinum toxin in, 369–370
    chemical peels in, 370
    temporary augmenting and filling agents in, 367–369. See also Soft tissue fillers.
        collagens, 347, 350, 367–368
        hyaluronic acid, 350–351, 368
        poly-L-lactic acid, 368–369
        Radiance, 369
    topical care, 365–367
        cleansing in, 365–366
        moisturizing, 366
        sun protection, 366–367
        therapeutic creams, 367

Facial resurfacing, ablative. See Ablative facial resurfacing.

Famciclovir, indications for, 315

Fan flaps, in lip reconstruction, 51–52

Fat augmentation, for aging face, 561
    in hand rejuvenation. See Hand rejuvenation.

Fatty acids, unsaturated, for hypermelanosis, 218

Feather Lift, technique for, 423

Female pattern hair loss. See Hair loss.

Fibrin sealants, in short scar face-lift. See Tisseel.

Finasteride, before follicular unit transplantation, 400
    for female pattern hair loss, 232
    for male pattern hair loss, 228–229

Fitzpatrick skin type, and ablative facial resurfacing, 549
    and laser therapy, for vascular lesions, 752

FK-506, indications for, 213–214, 251–252

Flap necrosis, rhytidectomy and, 426–427

Flaps. See specific types, e.g., Advancement flaps.

Flip-flop flaps, in auricular reconstruction, 30, 37–38

Flip-top transplantation, for hypomelanosis, 215

Fluocinolone, for alopecia areata, 235

Flutamide, for female pattern hair loss, 232

Foam sclerotherapy, for varicose veins. See Varicose veins.
    in hand rejuvenation, 522

Follicular unit transplantation, 230–231, 233, **393–414**
    aesthetic issues in, 405–408
        coronal versus sagittal incisions, 408
        frontal hairline and other transition zones, 405–406
        hair direction, 406
        hair distribution, 406–407
        regular versus dense packing, 407–408
    anatomy and physiology of, 393
    complications of, 408–409
        corrective procedures for, 411–412
        facial edema, 410
        folliculitis, 410
        hair loss in donor area, 410–411
        hair loss in recipient area, 411
        improper graft handling and, 409–410
        poor aesthetic judgment and, 409
        poor hair growth and, 409–410
        poor patient selection and, 409
        wide donor scars, 410–411
    individual follicular units in, 394

large sessions for, 394–395
  economizing donor supply in, 394–395
  enhancing unit composition in, 395
  planning for telogen effluvium in, 394
  social issues in, 394
patient preparation for, 400
patient selection for, 395–398
  diffuse unpatterned alopecia in, 396–397
  hair and scalp characteristics in, 397–398
  Norwood classification in, 396
  scalp laxity in, 398
postoperative care for, 404–405
relatively constant distribution of, 395
restoration planning in, 398–399
  photodamage and, 399
  vertex transition point in, 398–399
single strip harvesting in, 395
small recipient sites in, 394
stereomicroscopic dissection in, 395
techniques for, 400–404
  creation of recipient sites, 403–404
  donor harvest, 400
  donor site closure, 402
  follicular unit extraction, 402–403
  graft dissection, 403
  local anesthesia, 401
  operating room setup, 400
  single strip harvesting, 401–402

Folliculitis, follicular unit transplantation and, 410

Fomivirsen, indications for, 316

Foot ulcers, diabetic, healing of, 188–189

Forehead flaps, in nasal reconstruction, 87–93

Forehead lift, endoscopic. See Endoscopic forehead lift.

Forehead reconstruction, **1–11**
advancement flaps in, 4
anatomy in, 1–2
depth of flap development in, 5
for eyebrow defects, 10–11
  advancement flaps in, 10
  H-plasty in, 10
  island pedicle flaps in, 122–123
island pedicle flaps in, 124
lateral, 9–10
  advancement flaps in, 9
  rotation flaps in, 10
  transposition flaps in, 10
local anesthesia in, 2
midline, 5–6
  tissue expansion in, 5–6

paramedian, 6–9
  advancement flaps in, 7–9
  relaxed skin tension lines in, 6–7
  preservation of nerve function in, 2–3
  relaxed skin tension lines in, 3–5
  rotation flaps in, 4–5
  transposition flaps in, 5

Foscarnet, indications for, 316–317

Free cartilage grafts, in auricular reconstruction. See Auricular reconstruction.
in nasal reconstruction. See Nasal reconstruction.

Full-thickness perforation, in auricular reconstruction, 27–28

Full-thickness skin grafts, in auricular reconstruction, 26–27, 33, 38
in ectropion repair, 150
in lip reconstruction, 46
in scalp reconstruction, 16

Furuncles, hypnosis for, 729

Fusiform elliptic excision, in surgical revisions, 143–144

Fusion protein vaccines, for human papillomavirus, 320


# G

Galeotomy, in scalp reconstruction, 15

Ganciclovir/valganciclovir, indications for, 315–316

Gastric bypass surgery, abdominal contour procedures after, 488

Gastrointestinal complications, of azathioprine, 260, 262
of cyclophosphamide, 265
of methotrexate, 267–268
of mycophenolate mofetil, 272

Gatifloxacin. See Antibiotics.

General Health Questionnaire, to assess quality of life, in psoriasis, 707, 708, 711

Geometric broken-line closure, in surgical revisions, 145

German Instrument for the Assessment of Quality of Life in Skin Diseases, in psoriasis, 709, 712

Gillies' flaps, in lip reconstruction, 51–52

Glabridin, for hypermelanosis, 218

Glycolic acid peels, for hypermelanosis, 219–220
in hand rejuvenation, 518

Gore-Tex, in soft tissue augmentation, 359

Gore-Tex suture suspension, in rhytidectomy, 422

Gorlin's syndrome, imiquimod for, 157, 160

Grafts, blister, for hypomelanosis, 215
composite cartilage, in nasal reconstruction.
See Nasal reconstruction.
free cartilage, in auricular reconstruction.
See Auricular reconstruction.
in nasal reconstruction.
See Nasal reconstruction.
punch, for hypomelanosis, 214
skin. See Full-thickness skin grafts; Split-thickness skin grafts.

Growth factors, in wound healing, 182–183

# H

Hair loss, **227–243**
after follicular unit transplantation, 410–411
alopecia areata, 234–240
depression with, 661
diffuse unpatterned, diagnosis of, 396–397
female pattern, 231–235
management of, 232–233
follicular unit transplantation for. See Follicular unit transplantation.
hypnosis for, 729
male pattern, 227–231, 395
management of, 230–231
management of, 239–240
anthralin in, 237
combination therapy in, 239
diphenylcyclopropenone in, 236–237
intralesional steroids in, 235
minoxidil in, 238–239
psoralen plus ultraviolet light therapy in, 237–238
squaric acid dibutylester in, 236–237
systemic steroids in, 235–236
topical steroids in, 234–235
psychosomatic aspects of, 602
telogen effluvium, 233–234
temporal, rhytidectomy and, 427–428
female pattern, management of, antiandrogen therapy in, 232
cyproterone acetate in, 232
finasteride in, 232
flutamide in, 232
hair transplantation in, 233
minoxidil in, 231–232
spironolactone in, 232
male pattern, management of, combination therapy in, 229
finasteride in, 228–229
minoxidil in, 227–228, 229

Hair removal, light therapy in, 202

Hair transplantation. See Follicular unit transplantation.

Hand rejuvenation, **515–527**
chemical peels in, 517–518
dermal fillers in, 525–526
fat augmentation in, 523–525
complications of, 524–525
postoperative care for, 524
results of, 525
technique for, 523–524
intense pulsed light therapy in, 521–522
lasers in, 518–521
noninvasive lasers, 520–521
pigment lasers, 518–519
resurfacing lasers, 519–520
microdermabrasion in, 516–517
radiofrequency devices in, 522
sclerotherapy in, 522–523
topical agents in, 516

Helicase primase inhibitors, indications for, 317

Helix reconstruction. See Auricular reconstruction.

Hemangiomas, laser therapy for, 748

Hematologic complications, of azathioprine, 260
of cyclophosphamide, 265
of methotrexate, 267
of mycophenolate mofetil, 272

Hematomas, facial implants and, 545
retrobulbar, blepharoplasty and, 440–441
rhytidectomy and, 426, 500–501

Hemostasis, in nasal reconstruction, with dorsal nasal flaps, 79
wound, cyanoacrylates and, 196

Herbs and supplements, in dermatology. See Complementary psychocutaneous therapies.

Hereditary hemorrhagic telangiectasias, laser therapy for, 751

Herniated retro-orbital fat, removal of. See Blepharoplasty.

Herpesvirus infections, antiviral therapy for, 313–314
experimental vaccines for, 319

Highly active antiretroviral therapy, indications for, 319

Histoplasmosis, infliximab and, 284

Hospital Anxiety and Depression scale, of depression associated with acne, 666, 667

H-plasty, in eyebrow reconstruction, 10

Human papillomavirus, antiviral therapy for, 317–318
  experimental vaccines for, 319–320
  imiquimod for, 248

Hyaluronic acid, in facial rejuvenation, 368
  in hand rejuvenation, 525–526
  in soft tissue augmentation, 350–351

Hydroquinones, for hypermelanosis, 216–217, 219, 220–221
  in hand rejuvenation, 516

Hylaform, in facial rejuvenation, 368
  in soft tissue augmentation, 350–351

Hyperarousal, autonomic, in posttraumatic stress disorder, 652–653

Hyperbaric oxygen therapy, in nasal reconstruction, with free cartilage grafts, 133

Hyperhidrosis, biofeedback for, 725
  cognitive-behavioral therapy for, 726

Hypermelanosis, management of, 216–222
  chemical peels in, 219–221
  depigmenting agents in, 216–219
    ascorbic acid, 217
    azelaic acid, 217
    bleaching products, 219
    4-N-butylresorcinol, 217
    combination therapies, 218–219
    hydroquinone, 216–217
    kojic acid, 217
    licorice extracts, 218
    monobenzylether of hydroquinone, 217
    monomethyl ether of hydroquinone, 217
    retinoids, 218
    thioctic acid, 218
    unsaturated fatty acids, 218
  dermabrasion in, 221
  future directions in, 223
  lasers in, 221–222
  liquid nitrogen cryotherapy in, 221
  Wood's light examination in, 209–210

Hyperpigmentation, ablative facial resurfacing and, 557–558
  laser therapy and, 751–752

Hypersensitivity reactions, azathioprine and, 262

Hypertension, cyclosporine and, 270

Hypertrophic scars, blepharoplasty and, 439

Hypnoanalysis, in dermatology, 728

Hypnosis, in dermatology. See Complementary psychocutaneous therapies.

Hypomelanosis, management of, 210–216
  camouflaging in, 222
  combination phototherapies in, 213–214
  depigmentation in, 215–216
  future directions in, 223
  immunomodulators in, 213
    steroids in, 213
  melagenin in, 216
  micropigmentation in, 215
  photoprotection in, 222
  phototherapy in, 210–213
    excimer lasers, 212–213
    focused microphototherapy, 212
    psoralens with, 211–212
    ultraviolet A, 211–212
    ultraviolet B, 212
  psychologic support in, 222–223
  surgical, 214–215
    blister grafts, 215
    cultured epidermal cell transplantation, 215
    flip-top transplantation, 215
    melanocyte suspension transplantation, 215
    punch grafts, 214
    split-thickness grafts, 215
  systemic antioxidant therapy in, 216
  tacrolimus in, 213
  psychoneuroimmunologic factors in, 614
    cognitive-behavioral therapy for, 614
  psychosomatic aspects of, 602–603
  stigma experience in, Indian perspective on, 636–637, 640
  Wood's light examination in, 209–210

Hypopigmentation, ablative facial resurfacing and, 557
  imiquimod and, 161
  laser therapy and, 752

Hypothalamic-pituitary-adrenal axis, in atopic dermatitis, 696–697
  in psoriasis, 687–688

# I

Imiquimod, indications for, 246–251, 317–318, 516
  as antineoplastic agent, 249–250
  for human papillomavirus, 248

for nongenital cutaneous warts, 248–249
future directions in, 250–251
hand rejuvenation, 516
skin cancer. *See* Skin cancer.

Immune function, in dermatology patient, psychoneuroimmunologic factors in, 610–611

Immune modulators, for hypomelanosis, 213
in hand rejuvenation, 516
systemic. *See* Systemic immune modulators.

Immunoglobulin E, in atopic dermatitis, 695

Immunotherapy, topical. *See* Topical immunotherapy.

Implants, facial. *See* Facial implants.

Infections, alefacept and, 276
azathioprine and, 262
cyclophosphamide and, 266
efalizumab and, 279
etanercept and, 281
facial implants and, 545–546
infliximab and, 284
methotrexate and, 268
mycophenolate mofetil and, 273
octyl cyanoacrylate and, 194
of free cartilage grafts, 138
rhytidectomy and, 427

Infliximab. *See* Systemic immune modulators.

Infrared light therapy, in neck rejuvenation, 470–471

Intense pulsed light therapy. *See* Light therapy.

Interferons, for melanoma, 323–324

Interleukins, for melanoma, 325, 328

Interpolation flaps, **87–112**
forehead flaps, 87–93
island pedicle flaps, 117
melolabial flaps, 93–101
postauricular pedicle flaps, 101, 108–112
two-staged, in nasal reconstruction, 66–68

Intralesional steroids, in surgical revisions, 143

Intraoral approach, to chin augmentation, 544
to malar and submalar augmentation, 542–544

Island pedicle flaps, **113–127**
advantages of, 115–116
anatomy in, 113
complications of, 116–117
design of, 113–115
disadvantages of, 116–117
in eyebrow reconstruction, 122–123
in forehead and temple reconstruction, 124

in lip reconstruction, 121–122
in medial canthus reconstruction, 124–125
in nasal reconstruction, 123–124
interpolation flaps, 117
myocutaneous flaps, 118–119
transcartilage flaps, 119–121
transposition flaps, 117
tunneling flaps, 117–118
vascular flaps, 118
V-Y advancement flaps, 125

Isotretoin, for acne, and suicide. *See* Suicide.

## J

Jessner solution peels, in ablative facial resurfacing, 550

## K

Karapandzic flaps, in lip reconstruction, 51

Kenalog, for alopecia areata, 235

Keratinocytes, in wound healing, 182–183, 185

Kligman formula, for hypermelanosis, 218

Kojic acid, for hypermelanosis, 217, 219

KTP laser therapy, for vascular lesions, 750, 754

## L

Lagophthalmos, blepharoplasty and, 439

Laser therapy, endovenous, for varicose veins. *See* Varicose veins.
for vascular lesions. *See* Vascular lesions.

Lasers, in ablative facial resurfacing, 553–554, 556
in hand rejuvenation. *See* Hand rejuvenation.
in light therapy. *See* Light therapy.
in neck rejuvenation, 471
in surgical revisions, 143, 148–149

Lentigo maligna, imiquimod for, 160–161

Leprosy, stigma experience in, Indian perspective on, 637–638, 639–640

Leukopenia, cyclophosphamide and, 265
mycophenolate mofetil and, 272

Lichen simplex chronicus, cognitive-behavioral therapy for, 726

Licorice extracts, for hypermelanosis, 218

Lidocaine, in pediatric dermatology, 174–175

Light therapy, **199–207**
    in hand rejuvenation, 521–522
    in neck rejuvenation, 470–471
    lasers and intense pulsed light in, 200–203
        extending therapeutic range of, 201
        for hair removal, 202
        for hypermelanosis, 221–222
        for hypomelanosis, 212–213, 214
        for nonablative dermal remodeling, 202
        for skin resurfacing, 202
        for vascular lesions, 749, 750
        need for trials in, 202–203
    photodynamic therapy in, 204–205
        for acne, 204–205
        for hypomelanosis. *See* Hypomelanosis.
    tissue optics and photobiologic reactions in, 199–200
    ultraviolet light in, 203–204
        for alopecia areata, 237–238
        for hypomelanosis, 211–212
        narrow-band UVB, 203
        novel sources of, 203–204

Linezolid. *See* Antibiotics.

Lingual mucosal flaps, in lip reconstruction, 46

Lip reconstruction, **43–53**
    advancement flaps in, 46–48
        bilateral, 48
        horizontal, 47–48
        perialar crescentic melolabial, 47
    anatomy in, 43–44
    classification of defects in, 45
    for full-thickness defects, 49–52
        advancement flaps in, 50–51
        circumoral rotational-advancement flaps in, 51
        Gillies' flap in, 51–52
        Karapandzic flaps in, 51
        microvascular free flaps in, 52
        pedicle flaps in, 52
        remote tissue flaps in, 52
        staircase-plasty in, 51
        wedge excision and layered repair in, 49–50
    full-thickness skin grafts in, 46
    healing by secondary intention in, 46
    island pedicle flaps in, 121–122
    rotation flaps in, 48–49
    transposition flaps in, 49
    vermilionectomy and vermilion reconstruction in, 46

Lipectomy, suction-assisted, technique for, 478–480
    with full abdominoplasty, technique for, 481–482

α-Lipoic acid, for hypermelanosis, 218

Liposuction, extended, technique for, 483–484
    in neck rejuvenation, 472
    power. *See* Power liposuction.

Liquid nitrogen cryotherapy, for hypermelanosis, 221

Liquiritin, for hypermelanosis, 218

L-M-X anesthetic, in pediatric dermatology, 174

Local flaps, in scalp reconstruction, 17

# M

Major depressive episode, diagnostic criteria for, 658
    in dermatology patient, evaluation for, 594

Malar augmentation, facial implants in, 542–544

Malar fat pad, in rhytidectomy, 416
    mobilization or suspension of, 420–421

Male pattern hair loss. *See* Hair loss.

Massage therapy, for atopic dermatitis, in children, 719–720
        dermatologic assessment in, 720
        participants in, 719
        results of, 720
        standard medical care in, 719
    for burns, in children, 717–719
        attention control group in, 717
        behavior observations in, 718
        participants in, 717
        results of, 718
        standard medical care in, 717

Medial canthal webbing, blepharoplasty and, 439

Medial canthus reconstruction, island pedicle flaps in, 124–125

Medtronic/Xomed PowerSculpt, in power liposuction, 385

Melagenina, for hypomelanosis, 216

Melanin pigmentary disorders. *See* Hypermelanosis; Hypomelanosis.

α-Melanocyte-stimulating hormone, anti-inflammatory effects of, 612–613

Melanocyte suspension transplantation, for hypomelanosis, 215

Melanoma, management of, **323–333**
        advanced disease, 325–328
            biochemotherapy for, 325, 328
            chemotherapy for, 325

combination chemotherapy for, 325
  interleukins for, 325, 328
  radiation therapy in, 330
  stage III, adjuvant therapy for, 323–325
  vaccines in, 328–330
    multipolyvalent, 329
    univalent, 329–330
  metastatic, imiquimod for, 161

Melolabial flaps, in nasal reconstruction. *See* Nasal reconstruction.

Mental status examination, in dermatology patient, *See* Psychiatric evaluation.

Metastatic disease, from malignant melanoma, imiquimod for, 161

Methotrexate. *See* Systemic immune modulators.

8-Methoxypsoralen, for hypomelanosis, 211

Methylprednisolone, for alopecia areata, 235

MicroAire PAL, in power liposuction, 384

Microdermabrasion, in hand rejuvenation, 516–517

Microphototherapy, focused, for hypomelanosis, 212

Micropigmentation, for hypomelanosis, 215

Microvascular free flaps, in lip reconstruction, 52

Midface lift, **505–514**
  anatomy in, 505–508
    facial nerve, 507–508
    fatty layers, 507
    midface volume, 507
    muscles, 506–507
    relationship of infraorbital rim and cornea, 505–506
    sensory nerves, 506
  approaches to, 509–511
    blepharoplasty incision, 510–511
    face-lift incision, 510
    temporal, 510
    transoral, 511
  dissection planes in, 508–509
  suspension in, 511–513
    permanent versus absorbable sutures in, 512
    tissue adhesives in, 512–513

Milia, ablative facial resurfacing and, 557

Mindfulness–meditation-based stress reduction, for psoriasis, 688

Mini-abdominoplasty, technique for, 480, 484–485

Minimal access abdominoplasty. *See* Abdominal contour procedures.

Minoxidil, before follicular unit transplantation, 400
  for alopecia areata, 238–239
  for female pattern hair loss, 231–232
  for male pattern hair loss, 227–228, 229

Moisturizers, for acne vulgaris, 577

Molluscum contagiosum, antiviral therapy for, 319–320

Monfreux method, of foam sclerotherapy, for varicose veins, 444

Monobenzylether of hydroquinone, for hypermelanosis, 217
  for hypomelanosis, 215–216

Monomethyl ether of hydroquinone, for hypermelanosis, 217, 218–219

Monosymptomatic hypochondriacal psychosis, in dermatology patient, management of, 740–742

Moxifloxacin. *See* Antibiotics.

Muscle access abdominoplasty, technique for, 485–486

Mycophenolate mofetil, systemic. *See* Systemic immune modulators.
  topical, indications for, 252, 254

Myelosuppression, azathioprine and, 260
  cyclophosphamide and, 265

Myocutaneous flaps, raising of, in blepharoplasty, 434

Myocutaneous island pedicle flaps, indications for, 118–119

# N

Narcissistic personality disorder, in dermatology patient, and aging skin, 646
  evaluation for, 598

Nasal reconstruction, bilobed transposition flaps in, 59–61
  composite cartilage grafts in, 129–134
    complications of, 134
    contraindications to, 130
    donor site issues in, 131
    graft site preparation in, 132–133
    harvesting in, 131–132
    indications for, 130
    placement of, 132–133
    postoperative care for, 133–134
    preoperative instructions for, 130–131
    suturing in, 133

dorsal nasal flaps in, **73–85**
   anatomy in, 75–76
   historical aspects of, 73–75
   modifications of, 81–83
   pearls and pitfalls of, 83–84
   postoperative care for, 79–81
   preoperative assessment for, 77
   principles of rotation in, 76–77
   technique for, 77–79
     anesthesia and skin preparation, 78
     closure, 79
     drawing, 77–78
     dressing, 79
     hemostasis, 79
     incisions and undermining, 78–79
forehead flaps in, 87–93
free cartilage grafts in, 134–138
   complications of, 138
   contraindications to, 135
   donor site issues in, 135
   future trends in, 138
   graft site preparation in, 137
   harvesting in, 135, 137
   indications for, 135
   placement of, 137
   postoperative care for, 138
island pedicle flaps in, 123–124
melolabial flaps in, **65–71**
   interpolation flaps, 66–68, 93–101
   superiorly based single-stage flaps, 65–66
   turnover flaps, 68, 70

Nasolabial transposition flaps, in lip reconstruction, 49

Natural killer cells, in psoriasis, 688

Nd:YAG laser therapy, indications for, 201

Neck lift, in rhytidectomy, 418–419

Neck rejuvenation, **469–474**
   chemical peels in, 471–472
   injections in, 469
   lasers in, 471
   light therapy in, 470–471
   liposuction in, 472
   neck slings in, 473
   platysmaplasty in, 472–473
   radiofrequency tissue tightening in, 469–470
   rhytidectomy in, 473

Neck slings, in neck rejuvenation, 473

Needle phobia, systematic desensitization for, 726

Nerve function, preservation of, in forehead reconstruction, 2–3

Neurapraxia, rhytidectomy and, 428–429

Neurodermatitis, cognitive-behavioral therapy for, 726

Neuropeptides, anti-inflammatory effects of, 613

Nonablative lasers, in surgical revisions, 143

Nongenital cutaneous warts, imiquimod for, 248–249

Norwood classification, of male pattern hair loss, 396

Nottingham Health Profile, to assess quality of life, in psoriasis, 707, 711–712

Numbing of responsiveness, in posttraumatic stress disorder, 653–654

# O

Obese patients, abdominal contour procedures in, 486, 488

Obsessive-compulsive disorders, in dermatology patient, case reports of, **675–680**
   body dysmorphic disorder, 678–679
   compulsive skin picking, 677–678
   obsessive-compulsive disorder, 675–676
   trichotillomania, 676–677
evaluation for, obsessive-compulsive disorder, 595–596
   obsessive-compulsive personality disorder, 598
management of, 739
with atopic dermatitis, 698–699

Octyl cyanoacrylate, in skin closure. *See* Cyanoacrylates.

Olanzapine, for delusional disorders, 742

Onychotillomania, cognitive-behavioral therapy for, 726

Oritavancin, indications for, 309

Osler-Weber-Rendu disease, laser therapy for, 751

Osteotomy, in reduction structured rhinoplasty, 537

Oxygen tension, in wound healing, 184

# P

Paget's disease, extramammary, imiquimod for, 161

Parasitosis, delusions of, in dermatology patient, management of, 741

Parasuicidal behavior, in dermatology patient, 659

Pediatric dermatology, **171–180**
   adherence to treatment programs in, 175–179
     age factors in, 176
     cognitive factors in, 176
     developmental factors in, 175–176
     family's role in, 177–178
     physician's role in, 178–179
     psychologic factors in, 177
     social and emotional factors in, 176–177
   office visit in, 171–173
     for adolescents, 172–173
     for infants, 171–172
     for school-aged children, 172
     for toddlers and preschool-aged children, 172
   pain and intrusive procedures in, 173–175
     nonpharmacologic approaches to, 173–174
       in adolescents, 174
       in infants, 173
       in school-aged children, 174
       in toddlers and preschool-aged children, 173–174
     pharmacologic approaches to, 174–175
       conscious sedation, 175
       lidocaine, 174–175
       topical anesthetics, 174

Pedicle flaps, in auricular reconstruction, 30, 101, 108–112
   in lip reconstruction, 52

Peels, chemical, for hypermelanosis, 219–221
   in ablative facial resurfacing. *See* Ablative facial resurfacing.
   in hand rejuvenation, 517–518
   in neck rejuvenation, 471–472

Penciclovir, indications for, 315

Penis, Bowen's disease of, imiquimod for, 156

Pentoxifylline, for arterial ulcers, 188

Peptide-based vaccines, for human papillomavirus, 320

Perialar crescentic melolabial advancement flaps, in lip reconstruction, 47

Perioral reconstruction. *See* Lip reconstruction.

Personality disorders, in dermatology patient, evaluation for, 598

Pexiganan, for diabetic foot ulcers, 189

Phenol compounds, for hypermelanosis, 216–217

Phenol peels, in ablative facial resurfacing, 550–551, 556

Phenolic-thioether, for hypermelanosis, 217

Phlebectomy, for varicose veins. *See* Varicose veins.

Photodamage, and follicular unit transplantation, 399

Photodynamic therapy, for hypomelanosis. *See* Hypomelanosis.
   in hand rejuvenation, 516
   in neck rejuvenation, 470
   indications for, 204–205

Photodynamic therapy, for psoriasis, 688

Photomodulation, in neck rejuvenation, 470

Photoprotection, against hypomelanosis, 222

Physical abuse, and posttraumatic stress disorder, 650–651

Pigment lasers, for hypermelanosis, 221–222
   in hand rejuvenation, 518–519

Pigmentary disorders, melanin. *See* Hypermelanosis; Hypomelanosis.

Pimecrolimus, indications for, 252

Pimozide, for delusional disorders, 741

Platysmaplasty, in neck rejuvenation, 472–473

Poly-L-lactic acid, in facial rejuvenation, 368–369
   in hand rejuvenation, 526

Polymethylmethacrylate, in soft tissue augmentation, 355, 358

Port wine stains, laser therapy for, 747–748, 753–754

Postauricular pedicle interpolation flaps, in auricular reconstruction, 101, 108–112

Posttraumatic stress disorder, cutaneous effects of, **649–656**
     catastrophic life events and, 651
     emotional neglect during development and, 650
     physical and sexual abuse and, 650–651
   in dermatology patient, evaluation for, 596–597
   responses to, 652
     autonomic hyperarousal, 652–653
     dysregulation of internal emotional states, 653–654
     intrusive re-experiencing of trauma, 652
     numbing of responsiveness, 653–654

Power liposuction, **383–391**
   advantages of, 385–388
     avoidance of contour irregularities, 388
     better sculpting, 386
     less bruising, 387

less patient discomfort, 387
less surgeon fatigue, 385
more precision, 386
patient safety, 387
breast enlargement after, 388
cannula designs in, 383–384
reciprocating cannulas, 384
ultrasonic cannulas, 384, 390
complications of, 390–391
equipment for, 384–385
Byron ARC unit, 385
Medtronic/Xomed PowerSculpt, 385
MicroAire PAL, 385
Wells-Johnson unit, 384
historical aspects of, 383–384
patient preparation for, 389
technique for, 389–390
standing epidural liposuction, 389–390

Prednisone, for alopecia areata, 235

Procedure anxiety, hypnosis for, 730–731

Psoralens, for alopecia areata, 237–238
for hypomelanosis, 211–212

Psoriasis, **681–694**
efalizumab for, 279–280
emotional impact of, 621–622, 681–686
alexithymia, 685
anxiety, 683–684
depression, 660, 683
disability and quality of life, 682–683
interpersonal interactions, 684–685
on families, 685–686
personality styles, 685
stigma, 682, 684–685
exacerbation of, 686–688
cortisol in, 687
hypothalamic-pituitary adrenal axis in, 687–688
natural killer cells in, 688
stress and, 686–687
management of, 688–689
cognitive-behavioral therapy in, 688
future directions in, 689
hypnosis in, 729
mindfulness–meditation-based stress reduction in, 688
phototherapy in, 688
mycophenolate mofetil for, 273
psychosomatic aspects of, 602
quality of life scales in, **707–716**
Children's Dermatology Life Quality Index, 708, 712
Dermatology Life Quality Index, 707–708, 712
Dermatology Quality-of-Life Scales, 708–709, 712
Dermatology Specific Quality of Life, 709, 712
General Health Questionnaire, 707, 708, 711
German Instrument for the Assessment of Quality of Life in Skin Diseases, 709, 712
Nottingham Health Profile, 707, 711–712
patient's willingness to pay and, 710
Psoriasis Disability Index, 709, 712, 714
Psoriasis Index of Quality of Life, 710, 714
Psoriasis Life Stress Inventory, 709, 714
Quality Adjusted Life Year, 710
Salford Psoriasis Index, 710, 714
Short Form 36, 707, 708, 710–711
Sickness Impact Profile, 707, 708, 711
Skindex, 708, 712
time trade-off and, 710
stigma experience in, Indian perspective on, 636
ultraviolet light therapy for, 203

Psoriasis Disability Index, to assess quality of life, in psoriasis, 709, 712, 714

Psoriasis Index of Quality of Life, in psoriasis, 710, 714

Psoriasis Life Stress Inventory, to assess quality of life, in psoriasis, 709, 714

Psychiatric evaluation, of dermatology patient, **591–599**
mental status examination in, 592–598
for body dysmorphic disorder, 597
for delusional disorder and other psychoses, 597–598
for major depressive disorder, 594
for obsessive-compulsive disorder, 595–596
for personality disorders, 598
for posttraumatic stress disorder, 596–597
for social phobia, 596
for suicide risk, 594–595
patient history in, 591–593

Psychiatry, consultation-liaison, for psychosomatic disorders, in dermatology patient, 630

Psychoanalytic therapy, for psychosomatic disorders, in dermatology patient, 604

Psychocutaneous therapies, complementary. *See* Complementary psychocutaneous therapies.

Psychoneuroimmunologic factors, in dermatology patient, **609–617**
and immune function, 610–611

α-melanocyte-stimulating hormone in, 612–613
neuropeptides in, 613
personality and coping styles in, 611–612
   social relationships in, 611–612
with atopic dermatitis, 613, **695–701**
   false contamination, 698–699
   hygiene hypothesis, 698
   hypothalamic-pituitary-adrenal axis in, 696–697
   immunoglobulin E in, 695
   importance of mental scenario, 699
   infant response to stress, 697
   maternal caring behavior, 697
   obsessive-compulsive disorder, 698–699
   temperament and stress, 697–698
with urticaria, 613–614
with vitiligo, 614
   cognitive-behavioral therapy for, 614

Psychopharmacology, in dermatology, **735–744**
for anxiety, 739–740
for delusional disorders, 740–742
for depression. *See* Depression.
for obsessive-compulsive disorders, 739
for purely dermatologic conditions, 742–743
psychiatric disorder classification in, 735–736

Psychoses, in dermatology patient, evaluation for, 597–598
   management of, 740–742

Psychosomatic disorders, in dermatology patient, **601–608, 629–633**
acne, 602, 603–604
alopecia areata, 602
atopic dermatitis, 602
consultation-liaison psychiatry for, 630
ego structure and, 603
management of, 604–605
   biofeedback in, 604
   cognitive-behavioral therapy in, 605
   psychoanalytic, 604
   supportive counseling in, 604–605
   systematic desensitization in, 605
psoriasis, 602
research on, 630–631
sexuality and, 603–604
specific symptoms of, 631–633
vitiligo, 602–603

Pulley stitch, in scalp reconstruction, 16–17

Pulsed dye laser therapy, for vascular lesions, 746, 747–748, 750, 753–754

Punch grafts, for hypomelanosis, 214

Purpura, blepharoplasty and, 439

Pyogenic granulomas, in children, laser therapy for, 750

## Q

Q-switched laser therapy, for hypermelanosis, 221–222
in hand rejuvenation, 518–519

Quality Adjusted Life Year scale, in psoriasis, 710

Quetiapine, for delusional disorders, 742

Quinolone antibiotics, interactions with, 336

Quinupristin-dalfopristin. *See* Antibiotics.

## R

Radiance, in facial rejuvenation, 369
in soft tissue augmentation, 358

Radiation therapy, for melanoma, 330

Radiofrequency closure, for varicose veins. *See* Varicose veins.

Radiofrequency tissue tightening, in neck rejuvenation, 469–470

Raynaud's syndrome, biofeedback for, 725

Reciprocating cannulas, in power liposuction, 384

Reduction structured rhinoplasty, **529–540**
anesthesia in, 533–534
historical aspects of, 529
postoperative care for, 537–540
preoperative evaluation for, 529–533
   clinical photography in, 532
   patient consultation in, 532–533
   patient history in, 530
   physical examination in, 530–532
   radiography and laboratory tests in, 532
surgical planning for, 533
technique for, 534–537

Relaxed skin tension lines, in forehead reconstruction, 3–7
in surgical revisions, 142–143

Remote tissue flaps, in lip reconstruction, 52

Renal complications, of cyclosporine, 270

Renova, in facial rejuvenation, 367

Reproductive complications, of cyclophosphamide, 265
of methotrexate, 268

Resiquimod, indications for, 318

Responsiveness, numbing of, in posttraumatic stress disorder, 653–654

Restylane, in soft tissue augmentation, 350–351

Resurfacing lasers, in hand rejuvenation, 519–520

Retin-A, in facial rejuvenation, 367

Retinoids, for acne, depression due to, 671
  for hypermelanosis, 218–219
  in facial rejuvenation, 367

Retinol, for acne vulgaris, 577

Retroauricular flaps, in auricular reconstruction, 30, 37–38

Retrobulbar hematomas, blepharoplasty and, 440–441

Retro-orbital fat, herniated, removal of. *See* Blepharoplasty.

Revisions, surgical. *See* Surgical revisions.

Rhinoplasty, reduction structured. *See* Reduction structured rhinoplasty.

Rhytidectomy, **415–430**
  anatomy in, 416–417
    deep compartments, 417
    fat, 416
    platysma, 417
    skin, 416
    superficial compartments, 416
    superficial musculoaponeurotic system, 417, 420
  complications of, 426–429, 500–501
    flap necrosis, 426–427
    hematomas, 426, 500–501
    neurapraxia, 428–429
    temporal hair loss, 427–428
    wound infections, 427
  fibrin sealants in. *See* Tisseel.
  historical aspects of, 415–416
  in neck rejuvenation, 473
  midface. *See* Midface lift.
  postoperative care for, 426
  preoperative consultation and evaluation for, 417–418
    for anesthesia, 418
    medical history in, 418
  techniques for, 418–426
    deep plane or composite lift, 421
    extended superficial musculoaponeurotic system flap, 420
    extended supraplatysmal plane skin flap, 421
    neck lift, 418–419
    short scar lift, 422
    S-lift, 421–422
    standard two-plane lift, 419–420
    subperiosteal lift, 421

  suspension lifts, 422–426
    Feather Lift, 423
    two-plane lift with mobilization or suspension of malar fat pad, 420–421
    Webster lift, 421

Risperidone, for delusional disorders, 742

Rotation flaps, in forehead reconstruction, 4–5, 10
  in lip reconstruction, 48–49
  in scalp reconstruction, 17–19

# S

Salford Psoriasis Index, in psoriasis, 710, 714

Salicylic acid peels, in hand rejuvenation, 518

Scalp laxity, and follicular unit transplantation, 398

Scalp reconstruction, **13–21**
  advancement flaps in, 19–20
  anatomy in, 13–15
  full-thickness skin grafts in, 16
  galeotomy in, 15
  healing by secondary intention in, 16
  local flaps in, 17
  margin control in, 15
  primary closure in, 16–17
  pulley stitch in, 16–17
  rotation flaps in, 17–19
  split-thickness skin grafts in, 16
  tissue expansion in, 17
  towel clamps in, 17
  transposition flaps in, 20–21

Scars, ablative facial resurfacing and, 558
  donor site, follicular unit transplantation and, 410–411
  hypertrophic, blepharoplasty and, 439

Scleral show, blepharoplasty and, 440

Sclerotherapy, for varicose veins. *See* Varicose veins.
  in hand rejuvenation, 522–523

Sculptra, in facial rejuvenation, 368–369

Sedation, conscious, in pediatric dermatology, 175

Selective serotonin reuptake inhibitors, for depression, 736–737
  for obsessive-compulsive tendency, 739

Sexual abuse, and posttraumatic stress disorder, 650–651

Sexuality, and cutaneous disorders, 603–604

Short Form 36 score, of depression associated with acne, 667
  to assess quality of life, in psoriasis, 707, 708, 710–711

Short scar lift, fibrin sealants in. *See* Tisseel.
in rhytidectomy, 422

Sickness Impact Profile, to assess quality of life, in psoriasis, 707, 708, 711

Silicone fillers, in soft tissue augmentation, 358–359

Silver-based antimicrobial dressings, in wound healing, 189

Skin, aging. *See* Aging skin.

Skin cancer, imiquimod for, **151–164**
actinic cheilitis, 154
actinic keratoses, 152, 154
adverse reactions to, 161–162
basal cell carcinoma, 156–157
Bowen's disease, 154, 156
cancer syndromes, 157, 160
cutaneous melanoma metastases, 161
extramammary Paget's disease, 161
invasive squamous cell carcinoma, 156
lentigo maligna, 160–161
mechanism of action of, 151–152
safety of, 161–162

Skin closure, cyanoacrylates in. *See* Cyanoacrylates.

Skin diseases, disabling. *See* Disabling skin diseases.
in children, massage therapy for.
*See* Massage therapy.

Skin equivalents, in wound healing, 185

Skin grafts. *See* Full-thickness skin grafts;
Split-thickness skin grafts.

Skin picking, compulsive, case report of, 677–678
hypnosis for, 728–729

Skin resurfacing, lasers in, 202

Skindex, to assess quality of life, in psoriasis, 708712

S-lift, in rhytidectomy, 421–422

Social anxiety disorder, in dermatology patient, evaluation for, 596

Social phobia, in dermatology patient, evaluation for, 596

Soft tissue fillers, **343–363**. *See also*
Facial rejuvenation.
adverse effects of, 346
allogenic, 353, 367–368
autogenic, 351, 353
autologous fat, 353
collagens, 347, 350, 367–368
expanded polytetrafluoroethylene, 359
historical aspects of, 343

hyaluronic acid, 350–351, 368
manufacturers of, 360–362
minimizing risks of, 344
optimizing outcome of, 346
polymethylmethacrylate, 355, 358
preoperative preparation for, 343–344
Radiance, 358, 369
silicone, 358–359
synthetic, 355
techniques for, 344–346
methods of delivery, 345–346
needle selection, 344
xenogenic, 346–347

Soporifics, in dermatology, 731

Spider angiomas, in children, laser therapy for, 750

Spironolactone, for female pattern hair loss, 232

Split-thickness skin grafts, for hypomelanosis, 215
in auricular reconstruction, 24–25, 26–27, 35
in scalp reconstruction, 16

Squamous cell carcinoma, imiquimod for, 249–250
invasive, imiquimod for, 156

Squaric acid dibutylester, for alopecia areata, 236–237

St. John's wort, versus conventional medications, interactions with, 336–337

Staircase-plasty, in lip reconstruction, 51

Standing epidural liposuction, technique for, 389–390

Stem cells, in wound healing, 184

Sterile chonditis, free cartilage grafts and, 138

Steroids, for alopecia areata. *See* Hair loss.
for hypomelanosis, 213
in immunosuppressive therapy, 251
intralesional, in surgical revisions, 143

Strawberry nevi, laser therapy for, 748

Stress, effects of, on psoriasis, 686–687

Sturge-Weber syndrome, laser therapy for, 751

Subciliary approach, to blepharoplasty.
*See* Blepharoplasty.

Subclinical depression, in dermatology patient, 659

Subdermal threads, in suspension procedures, for aging face. *See* Suspension procedures.

Submalar augmentation, facial implants in, 542–544

Subperiosteal lift, in rhytidectomy, 421

Suction-assisted lipectomy, technique for, 478–480
  with full abdominoplasty, technique for,
    481–482

Suicidal ideation. *See also* Suicide.
  in dermatology patient, 659
    aging skin and, 646
    evaluation for, 594–595

Suicide. *See also* Suicidal ideation.
  in dermatology patient, isotretinoin and,
    667–671
    case reports of, 668
    causal connection in, 667–668
    cohort studies of, 668
    mechanism of action of, 671–672
    population-based studies of, 668, 670–671

Sulfonamides, interactions with. *See*
  Drug interactions.

Sulfur, for acne vulgaris, 577

Superficial musculoaponeurotic system, in rhytidectomy. *See* Rhytidectomy.

Surgical revisions, **141–150**
  ablative lasers in, 148–149
  cosmetic units in, 143
  debulking in, 147–148
  dermabrasion in, 148
  ectropion repair in, 149–150
  flap refinements in, 142–143
  fusiform elliptic excision in, 143–144
  geometric broken-line closure in, 145
  intralesional steroids in, 143
  nonablative lasers in, 143
  relaxed skin tension lines in, 142
  techniques for, 141–143
    suturing, 141
  timing of, 143
  V-Y and Y-V advancement repairs in,
    145–146
  W-plasty in, 144
  Z-plasty in, 146–147

Suspension procedures, for aging face, **561–573**
  contour threads in, 571
  subdermal suspension threads in, 562, 564,
    566–571
    anesthesia in, 566
    complications of, 569–571
    results of, 569
  versus other procedures, 561–562
  in rhytidectomy, 422–426

Symptom substitution, in dermatology, 728

Synercid. *See* Antibiotics, quinupristin-dalfopristin.

Systematic desensitization, for needle phobia, 726
  for psychosomatic disorders, in dermatology
    patient, 605

Systemic immune modulators, **259–300**
  alefacept, 275–278
    adverse effects of, 276
      immune system, 276
      infections, 276
      injection site reactions, 276
      oncogenic potential, 276
    dosage and monitoring of, 278
    efficacy of, 276–277
    indications for, 277
    mechanism of action of, 275–276
    pharmacology of, 275–276
    usage guidelines for, 277–278
  azathioprine, 259–260, 262–263
    adverse effects of, 260, 262
      gastrointestinal, 260, 262
      hematologic, 260
      hypersensitivity reactions, 262
      oncogenic potential, 262
      opportunistic infections, 262
    dosage and monitoring of, 263
    indications for, 262–263
    interactions with, 263
    pharmacology of, 260
    usage guidelines for, 263
  cyclophosphamide, 263, 265–266
    adverse effects of, 265–266
      gastrointestinal, 265
      hematologic, 265
      oncogenic potential, 265
      opportunistic infections, 266
      reproductive toxicity, 265
      urologic, 265
    dosage and monitoring of, 266
    indications for, 266
    interactions with, 266
    pharmacology of, 263, 265
    usage guidelines for, 266
  cyclosporine, 269–272
    adverse effects of, 270
      nephrotoxicity and hypertension, 270
      oncogenic potential, 270
    dosage and monitoring of, 271–272
    indications for, 251, 270–271
    interactions with, 271
    pharmacology of, 269–270
    usage guidelines for, 271
  efalizumab, 278–280
    adverse effects of, 278–279
      immune system, 279
      infections, 279

oncogenic potential, 278–279
    thrombocytopenia, 279
  dosage and monitoring of, 280
  efficacy of, 279
  indications for, 279–280
  interactions with, 280
  mechanism of action of, 278
  pharmacology of, 278
  usage guidelines for, 280
etanercept, 280–283
  adverse effects of, 280–282
    demyelinating disease, 281
    immune system, 281
    infections, 281
    injection site reactions, 281–282
    oncogenic potential, 280–281
  dosage and monitoring of, 283
  efficacy of, 282
  indications for, 282
  interactions with, 283
  mechanism of action of, 280
  pharmacology of, 280
  usage guidelines for, 282–283
infliximab, 283–287
  adverse effects of, 283–285
    congestive heart failure, 285
    demyelinating disease, 285
    immune system, 284–285
    infections, 284
    infusion reactions, 285
    oncogenic potential, 283–284
  dosage and monitoring of, 287
  efficacy of, 285–286
  indications for, 286
  interactions with, 287
  mechanism of action of, 283
  pharmacology of, 283
  usage guidelines for, 286–287
methotrexate, 267–269
  adverse effects of, 267–268
    gastrointestinal, 267–268
    hematologic, 267
    oncogenic potential, 268
    opportunistic infections, 268
    reproductive toxicity, 268
  dosage and monitoring of, 269
  indications for, 268–269
  interactions with, 269
  pharmacology of, 267
  usage guidelines for, 269
mycophenolate mofetil, 272–275
  adverse effects of, 272–273
    gastrointestinal, 272
    hematologic, 272

infections, 273
oncogenic potential, 272–273
  dosage and monitoring of, 274
  indications for, 252, 254, 273–274
  interactions with, 274
  pharmacology of, 272
  usage guidelines for, 274

# T

Tacrolimus, for hypomelanosis, 213, 214
  indications for, 251–252

Tardive dyskinesia, antipsychotic drugs and, 741

Tazarotene, for hypermelanosis, 218

Tear trough deformity, blepharoplasty for, 438

Telangiectasias, facial, laser therapy for, 749–750, 753
  hereditary hemorrhagic, laser therapy for, 751

Telogen effluvium, management of, 233–234

Temple reconstruction, island pedicle flaps in, 124

Temporal approach, to midface lift, 510

Temporal hair loss, rhytidectomy and, 427–428

Tequin. See Antibiotics, gatifloxacin and moxifloxacin.

Tessari method, of foam sclerotherapy, for varicose veins, 444–445

Tetracyclines, interactions with, 335–336

ThermaCool device, in neck rejuvenation, 469–470

Thioctic acid, for hypermelanosis, 218

Thrombocytopenia, efalizumab and, 279

Tisseel, in short scar face-lift, **495–504**
  complications of, 499–501
  mechanism of action of, 496
  results of, 498–499
  technique for, 496–498

Tissue adhesives, in midface lift, 512–513

Tissue-engineered skin products, for diabetic foot ulcers, 189

Tissue expansion, in forehead reconstruction, 5–6
  in scalp reconstruction, 17

Topical immunotherapy, **245–258**
  for alopecia areata, 236–237
  immunosuppressive agents in, 251–252, 254
    calcineurin inhibitors, 251
    cyclosporine, 251
    mycophenolate mofetil, 252, 254

pimecrolimus, 252
steroids, 251
tacrolimus, 213, 214, 251–252
Toll-like receptor agonists in, 246–248
Toll-like receptors in, 245–246

Tourbillion method, of foam sclerotherapy, for varicose veins, 445

Transcartilage island pedicle flaps, indications for, 119–121

Transconjunctival approach, to blepharoplasty. See Blepharoplasty.

Transcutaneous approach, to blepharoplasty. See Blepharoplasty.

Transoral approach, to midface lift, 511

Transposition flaps, bilobed, **55–64**
case reports of, 61–64
complications of, 58–59
historical aspects of, 55
in nasal reconstruction, 59–61
technique for, 56–58
in auricular reconstruction, 35
in forehead reconstruction, 5, 10
in lip reconstruction, 49
in scalp reconstruction, 20–21
island pedicle flaps, 117

Tretinoin, for hypermelanosis, 218–219
in facial rejuvenation, 367

Triamcinolone acetonide, for alopecia areata, 235

Triazolam, in rhytidectomy, 418

Trichloroacetic acid peels, in ablative facial resurfacing, 550
in hand rejuvenation, 518

Trichotillomania, in dermatology patient, case report of, 676–677

Tuberculosis, reactivation of, infliximab and, 284

Tumescent anesthesia, in ambulatory phlebectomy, for varicose veins, 447–448
in follicular unit transplantation, 401

Tunneling island pedicle flaps, indications for, 117–118

Turnover flaps, in nasal reconstruction, 68, 70

Twenty-Item Toronto Alexithymia Scale, in dermatology patient, with psoriasis, 685

Two-plane lift, in rhytidectomy, 419–420
with mobilization or suspension of malar fat pad, 420–421

## U

Ulcers, healing of. See Wound healing.

Ultrasound, in power liposuction, 384, 390

Ultraviolet light therapy. See Light therapy.

Urologic complications, of cyclophosphamide, 265

Urticaria, cognitive-behavioral therapy for, 726–727
depression with, 661
hypnosis for, 730
psychoneuroimmunologic factors in, 613–614

## V

Vaccines, experimental, for herpesviruses, 319
for human papillomavirus, 319–320
for melanoma. See Melanoma.

Valacyclovir, indications for, 315

Varicose veins, **443–455**
ambulatory phlebectomy for, 446–448
clinical studies of, 448
complications of, 447
contraindications to, 447
indications for, 447
technique for, 446–447
technologic advances in, 447–448
tumescent anesthesia in, 447–448
endovenous laser therapy for, 451–453, 748–749
810-nm diode laser in, 452–453
versus radiofrequency closure, 453
940-nm diode laser in, 453
980-nm diode laser in, 453
clinical studies of, 452
indications for, 452
radiofrequency closure for, 448–451
complications of, 449
contraindications to, 449
indications for, 449
technologic advances in, 450
versus endovenous laser therapy, 453
versus stripping plus high ligation, 450
with ambulatory phlebectomy, 450
without high ligation, 450–451
sclerotherapy for, 443–446
foam in, 444–446
advantages of, 444
agents for, 444
clinical studies of, 445–446
preparation of, 444–445
versus surgery, 446

Vascular island pedicle flaps, indications for, 118

Vascular lesions, laser therapy for, **745–755**
    anesthesia in, 753
    choice of laser in, 753
    complications of, 751–752
    facial telangiectasias and diffuse erythema, 749–750, 753
    Fitzpatrick skin type in, 752
    fluence in, 746
    hemangiomas, 748
    historical aspects of, 746–747
    history taking in, 752
    patient expectations in, 752–753
    physical examination for, 752
    port wine stains, 747–748, 753–754
    postoperative care for, 753
    pulse duration in, 745, 746
    pulsed dye lasers in, 746, 747–748, 750, 753–754
    spider and varicose veins. *See* Varicose veins.
    spider angiomas and pyogenic granulomas, in children, 750
    spot size in, 746
    syndromes with vascular anomalies, 750–751
    test spots in, 753
    thermal relaxation time in, 745
    wavelengths in, 746

Venlafaxine, for depression, 737–738

Venous ulcers, healing of, 188

Vermilionectomy, in lip reconstruction, 46

Vertex transition point, in follicular unit transplantation, 398–399

Viruslike particles, for human papillomavirus, 319–320

Vision, loss of, blepharoplasty and, 439, 440

Vitamin A, for acne, depression due to, 671

Vitiligo. *See* Hypomelanosis.

V-Y advancement island pedicle flaps, indications for, 125

V-Y advancement repair, in surgical revisions, 145–146

## W

Warts, hypnosis for, 730

Webster flaps, in lip reconstruction, 47

Webster lift, in rhytidectomy, 421

Wedge closure, in auricular reconstruction, 37

Wedge excision, in lip reconstruction, 49–50

Wells-Johnson unit, in power liposuction, 384

Westerhof formula, for hypermelanosis, 219

Wood's light examination, of melanin pigmentary disorders, 209–210

Wound dressings, cyanoacrylates as, 195–196

Wound healing, **181–192**
    antibiotics in, 185, 188
    antimicrobial dressings in, 189–190
    cytokines in, 182
    extracellular matrix in, 183
    growth factors in, 182, 183
    keratinocytes in, 182–183, 185
    of arterial ulcers, 188
    of diabetic foot ulcers, 188–189
    of venous ulcers, 188
    oxygen tension in, 184
    prohealing elements in skin and, 181–182
    serum versus plasma in, 182–183
    skin equivalents in, 185
    stem cells in, 184

Wound hemostasis, cyanoacrylates and, 196

Wound infections, rhytidectomy and, 427

W-plasty, in surgical revisions, 144

## X

Xeroderma pigmentosum, basal cell carcinoma with, imiquimod for, 160

## Y

Y-V advancement repair, in surgical revisions, 145–146

## Z

Z-plasty, in surgical revisions, 146–147

Zyderm, in facial rejuvenation, 367
    in soft tissue augmentation, 347

Zyplast, in facial rejuvenation, 367
    in soft tissue augmentation, 347

Zyvox. *See* Antibiotics, linezolid.

**United States Postal Service**
**Statement of Ownership, Management, and Circulation**

| 1. Publication Title | 2. Publication Number | 3. Filing Date |
|---|---|---|
| Dermatologic Clinics | 0 7 3 3 - 8 6 3 5 | 9/15/05 |

| 4. Issue Frequency | 5. Number of Issues Published Annually | 6. Annual Subscription Price |
|---|---|---|
| Jan, Apr, Jul, Oct | 4 | $205.00 |

7. Complete Mailing Address of Known Office of Publication (*Not printer*) (*Street, city, county, state, and ZIP+4*)

Elsevier, Inc.
6277 Sea Harbor Drive
Orlando, FL 32887-4800

Contact Person: Gwen C. Campbell
Telephone: 215-239-3685

8. Complete Mailing Address of Headquarters or General Business Office of Publisher (*Not printer*)

Elsevier, Inc., 360 Park Avenue South, New York, NY 10010-1710

9. Full Names and Complete Mailing Addresses of Publisher, Editor, and Managing Editor (*Do not leave blank*)

**Publisher** (*Name and complete mailing address*)
Tim Griswold, Elsevier, Inc., 1600 John F. Kennedy Blvd., Suite 1800, Philadelphia, PA 19103-2899

**Editor** (*Name and complete mailing address*)
Alexandra Gavenda, Elsevier, Inc., 1600 John F. Kennedy Blvd., Suite 1800, Philadelphia, PA 19103-2899

**Managing Editor** (*Name and complete mailing address*)
Heather Cullen, Elsevier, Inc., 1600 John F. Kennedy Blvd., Suite 1800, Philadelphia, PA 19103-2899

10. Owner (*Do not leave blank. If the publication is owned by a corporation, give the name and address of the corporation immediately followed by the names and addresses of all stockholders owning or holding 1 percent or more of the total amount of stock. If not owned by a corporation, give the names and addresses of the individual owners. If owned by a partnership or other unincorporated firm, give its name and address as well as those of each individual owner. If the publication is published by a nonprofit organization, give its name and address.*)

| Full Name | Complete Mailing Address |
|---|---|
| Wholly owned subsidiary of | 4502 East-West Highway |
| Reed/Elsevier, US holdings | Bethesda, MD 20814 |

11. Known Bondholders, Mortgagees, and Other Security Holders Owning or Holding 1 Percent or More of Total Amount of Bonds, Mortgages, or Other Securities. If none, check box. ☐ None

| Full Name | Complete Mailing Address |
|---|---|
| N/A | |

12. Tax Status (*For completion by nonprofit organizations authorized to mail at nonprofit rates*) (*Check one*)
The purpose, function, and nonprofit status of this organization and the exempt status for federal income tax purposes:
☐ Has Not Changed During Preceding 12 Months
☐ Has Changed During Preceding 12 Months (*Publisher must submit explanation of change with this statement*)

PS Form 3526, October 1999 (*See Instructions on Reverse*)

| 13. Publication Title | 14. Issue Date for Circulation Data Below |
|---|---|
| Dermatologic Clinics | July 2005 |

| 15. Extent and Nature of Circulation | | Average No. Copies Each Issue During Preceding 12 Months | No. Copies of Single Issue Published Nearest to Filing Date |
|---|---|---|---|
| a. Total Number of Copies (*Net press run*) | | 2225 | 1900 |
| b. Paid and/or Requested Circulation | (1) Paid/Requested Outside-County Mail Subscriptions Stated on Form 3541. (*Include advertiser's proof and exchange copies*) | 984 | 948 |
| | (2) Paid In-County Subscriptions Stated on Form 3541 (*Include advertiser's proof and exchange copies*) | | |
| | (3) Sales Through Dealers and Carriers, Street Vendors, Counter Sales, and Other Non-USPS Paid Distribution | 292 | 284 |
| | (4) Other Classes Mailed Through the USPS | | |
| c. Total Paid and/or Requested Circulation (*Sum of 15b. (1), (2), (3), and (4)*) | | 1276 | 1232 |
| d. Free Distribution by Mail (*Samples, complimentary, and other free*) | (1) Outside-County as Stated on Form 3541 | 62 | 71 |
| | (2) In-County as Stated on Form 3541 | | |
| | (3) Other Classes Mailed Through the USPS | | |
| e. Free Distribution Outside the Mail (*Carriers or other means*) | | | |
| f. Total Free Distribution (*Sum of 15d. and 15e.*) | | 62 | 71 |
| g. Total Distribution (*Sum of 15c. and 15f.*) | | 1338 | 1303 |
| h. Copies not Distributed | | 887 | 597 |
| i. Total (*Sum of 15g. and h.*) | | 2225 | 1900 |
| j. Percent Paid and/or Requested Circulation (*15c. divided by 15g. times 100*) | | 95% | 95% |

16. Publication of Statement of Ownership
☐ Publication required. Will be printed in the **October 2005** issue of this publication. ☐ Publication not required

17. Signature and Title of Editor, Publisher, Business Manager, or Owner

*Janet Zimmerman* — Manager of Subscription Services    Date: 9/15/05

I certify that all information furnished on this form is true and complete. I understand that anyone who furnishes false or misleading information on this form or who omits material or information requested on the form may be subject to criminal sanctions (including fines and imprisonment) and/or civil sanctions (including civil penalties).

**Instructions to Publishers**

1. Complete and file one copy of this form with your postmaster annually on or before October 1. Keep a copy of the completed form for your records.
2. In cases where the stockholder or security holder is a trustee, include in items 10 and 11 the name of the person or corporation for whom the trustee is acting. Also include the names and addresses of individuals who are stockholders who own or hold 1 percent or more of the total amount of bonds, mortgages, or other securities of the publishing corporation. In item 11, if none, check the box. Use blank sheets if more space is required.
3. Be sure to furnish all circulation information called for in item 15. Free circulation must be shown in items 15d, e, and f.
4. Item 15h., Copies not Distributed, must include (1) newsstand copies originally stated on Form 3541, and returned to the publisher, (2) estimated returns from news agents, and (3), copies for office use, leftovers, spoiled, and all other copies not distributed.
5. If the publication had Periodicals authorization as a general or requester publication, this Statement of Ownership, Management, and Circulation must be published; it must be printed in any issue in October or, if the publication is not published during October, the first issue printed after October.
6. In item 16, indicate the date of the issue in which this Statement of Ownership will be published.
7. Item 17 must be signed.

*Failure to file or publish a statement of ownership may lead to suspension of Periodicals authorization.*

PS Form 3526, October 1999 (*Reverse*)

## *Changing Your Address?*

Make sure your subscription changes too! When you notify us of your new address, you can help make our job easier by including an exact copy of your Clinics label number with your old address (see illustration below.) This number identifies you to our computer system and will speed the processing of your address change. Please be sure this label number accompanies your old address and your corrected address—you can send an old Clinics label with your number on it or just copy it exactly and send it to the address listed below.

We appreciate your help in our attempt to give you continuous coverage. Thank you.

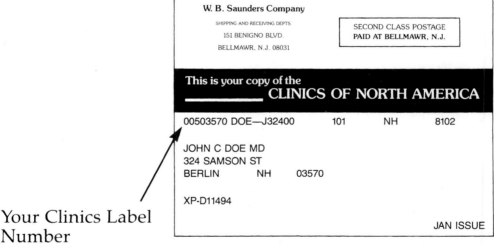

**Your Clinics Label Number**
Copy it exactly or send your label along with your address to:
**W.B. Saunders Company, Customer Service**
Orlando, FL 32887-4800
Call Toll Free 1-800-654-2452

Please allow four to six weeks for delivery of new subscriptions and for processing address changes.